18
9930

Developments in Psychiatric Research

Developments in Psychiatric Research

Essays based on the Sir Geoffrey Vickers Lectures of the Mental Health Foundation (formerly Mental Health Research Fund)

Edited by J. M. Tanner
for the Mental Health Foundation

HODDER AND STOUGHTON
LONDON SYDNEY AUCKLAND TORONTO

ISBN 0 340 20977 1 Boards

Printed in Great Britain for
Hodder and Stoughton Educational,
a division of Hodder and Stoughton Ltd,
Mill Road, Dunton Green, Sevenoaks, Kent,
by J.W. Arrowsmith Ltd, Bristol

Phototypesetting by Print Origination
Bootle, Merseyside L20 6NS

Foreword

When the original Mental Health Research Fund was formed, spectacular advances in other branches of medicine had come about as a result of patient and devoted research backed by reasonably adequate funds, adequate numbers of workers and adequate facilities for the exchange of ideas. Psychiatry was still only growing in recognition as a medical discipline and the problem of mental disorder was scarcely acknowledged, in spite of its magnitude. Thus an organization was formed with the object of providing for this field what other medical charities had so successfully provided in their own particular spheres.

In 1949 a meeting of practising psychiatrists, professional research workers and interested laymen was held at the Royal Society of Medicine, where it was decided that the objects of the organization should be to promote:

(a) Research on the causation, prevention and cure of nervous and mental illness;

(b) Research on fundamental problems related to mental health, such as the physiology of the nervous system;

(c) Research on the forms of social structure most likely to lead to the improvement of the mental quality and stamina of the community, and most likely to reduce the incidence of addiction, delinquency and crime.

At this meeting the Mental Health Research Fund was inaugurated. Its initial momentum was assured by the characteristic action of one of our distinguished founders who, passing a cheque for £100 across the table, said to our newly elected Secretary 'Go and buy some notepaper—nothing will happen if we don't have it'. This proved a decisive stimulant because it soon became apparent that if we were to ask the public for money, we must know how best to use it. In the meetings which later led to the formation of the Research Committee, doctors and scientists first of all chose a remarkable layman as their Chairman—Sir Geoffrey Vickers, V.C. (after whom the lectures published in this book were named). Secondly, they decided that they must try to get a clear view of the field with the help of those engaged in it. In March 1952, just twenty-five years ago, at Magdalen College, Oxford, for two days there sat round the conference table neuroanatomists, pharmacologists, psychiatrists, biochemists, professors of sociology, practitioners of psychoanalysis, and experts in animal behaviour, the physiology of the nervous system and the endocrinology of the mentally sick. The terms of reference were broad: 'What are the ignorances which today principally hamper our understanding of the nature, prevention and cure of mental illness? What advances in research are most likely to remove these and so help reduce the population of mental hospitals and institutions for delinquents?' Sir Geoffrey Vickers chaired this conference and summed it up. The papers were edited by J.M. Tanner, M.D., who edits the present book, and published under the title of *Prospects in Psychiatric Research* (Blackwell, 1953).

Not only was this conference useful in itself, but for the first time it gave specialists in widely differing fields the opportunity of meeting others who previously were only names to them and of hearing about their work. It also achieved its object in providing an indication of the main lines research was taking. It was in effect the Research Committee's first project.

As a result of the Oxford Conference, it was decided that as money became available we would act as a funding body and that we would not undertake research directly ourselves. It has all along been our reason for creating an independent charitable foundation that, with State medicine (including State research), there must be an alternative source of funds to which a research worker can apply. This inevitably meant that we did not propose to support research projects for which Government money was likely to be available, a principle which has been maintained throughout our existence. Neither have we at any time sought Government assistance or grants for our activities, although we have always maintained close liaison with the Medical Research Council.

In the early Fifties it was often stated that there was plenty of money for research into mental disorder, but a lack of available talent to whom support could be given. It soon became apparent that, with just one Chair of Psychiatry in the universities and no career structure, such potential research workers as there were could not be expected to remain in the field if they could see no senior posts which would allow them to pursue their research interests. This was a vicious circle which happily today has been broken: there are now twenty-two established chairs and an adequate career structure.

Our contribution towards solving the problem at that time was to initiate our grant-giving programme by establishing Fellowship awards, the first of which was made in October 1954. The idea behind them was to stimulate application for research in mental disorder in the belief that each successful holder of a Fellowship (which was usually for two or three years) would be encouraged to make a research career in this field. We have since awarded fifty-seven Fellowships, and in spite of the creation of a more adequate research career structure by the State we are continuing with our Fellowship scheme. The success of the policy has been borne out by the number of Fellowship holders who have continued their research careers with outstanding success.

Fellowships were only a part of our programme. Our Research Committee were rightly concerned with the quality of the research for which grant applications were received and furthermore laid down that applicants must be working in a recognized research establishment. We have never been a wealthy organization and over the years the number and quality of applications have often been dependant on whether it was generally known that there were sufficient funds to make it worthwhile applying. On the other hand, looking back over the awards made in the last twenty years, it is clear that the competition for our limited funds has helped produce a body of high-quality work which has contributed to the significant advances that have occurred in the treatment of the mentally disordered. We have also made a number of small grants where a quick answer and help could assist a project which would otherwise have remained uncompleted. The encouragement of students and nurses by means of prize essays and grants to student electives, the encouragement of travel to overseas research institutions or conferences, have also all played a part in our supporting the research structure.

The Research Committee itself has become a unique institution. We know of no other similar multi-disciplinary body independent of Government support. It consists of some twenty members from widely different disciplines and serving in an entirely voluntary capacity. It has held 175 meetings since 1954, and 84 members have served on it on a rotational system—no one serving more than six years in one spell. From the first informal meeting twenty-five years ago it has remained the wish of the Committee that it should be chaired by a layman. Sir Geoffrey Vickers chaired the Committee through the first fifteen years. He made a unique contribution to its development, and the series of annual lectures which provide the substance of this book was appropriately named after him. He was succeeded by Mr Duncan Dewdney. Mr Dewdney and Professor Tanner, who served as Honorary Secretary from the beginnings of the Research Committee until the end of 1976, ensured the continued smooth working of this scientific body.

Well over £1,000,000 has been spent on research since 1954 and although at first sight this looks a substantial sum in relation to the number of mentally disordered, it is not. Research into mental health, in spite of much devoted voluntary work, has never attracted massive public support as so many other disorders of the body have successfully done. Maybe the very term, mental health, when the appeal is in fact for the mentally ill, fails to convey to the public that it includes such widespread disorders as schizophrenia, suicide and depression, as well as mental retardation. Public attitudes towards such disorders have undoubtedly improved enormously, but a sense of shame still prevents many who might have a direct interest in helping promote research from doing so. Perhaps if everyone concerned appreciated the enormous advances in treatment that have occurred during the last twenty-five years, there would be a concerted public and voluntary effort to accelerate our efforts.

This is not the place to catalogue the improved outlook for the mentally disordered. Although no cure for schizophrenia has yet been found, its treatment by the use of drugs has improved the prospects of the patients out of all recognition and radically altered a situation where previously the disease usually resulted in the patient spending the rest of his or her life in hospital. The suicide rate in Britain has fallen since 1963 from 12 to 8 per 100,000. There have been many developments of drugs for the treatment and prevention of depression, together with a substantial advance in methodology and measuring techniques which can be brought to bear upon important problems of basic and applied research. Add this and many advances in other related fields to the improvement brought about by the Mental Health Act of 1959 to the transformation of the mental hospitals and the establishment of outpatient treatment in general hospitals, and we have a picture which has vastly changed since we started our work.

In 1972 the Mental Health Research Fund amalgamated with the Mental

Health Trust, which had been established to encourage projects for helping the mentally disordered in the community. As the Mental Health Foundation we continue to have the Research Committee as originally constituted, together with a Projects Committee supporting pioneer ideas for communities to help themselves deal with the mentally disordered in their midst. Inflation has already sadly eroded our resources in real terms, but if circumstances permit us to continue our work, we believe that voluntary endeavour has still a worthy contribution to make.

The Vickers Lectures were started in 1963. Not only do they provide a record of scientific thought at the time they were given, but their updating for this book shows the advance or lack of advance made in their subjects since the research was originally carried out. We are most grateful to the lecturers for reviewing and rewriting their material, and for allowing it to be represented in this book.

I.T. Henderson
Vice-Chairman
Mental Health Foundation
March 1977

Contents

The Contributors

Mary D. Salter Ainsworth
Professor of Psychology and Psychiatry, University of Virginia. USA

David H. Clark
Consultant Psychiatrist, Fulbourn Hospital, Cambridge, England

Trevor C.N. Gibbens
Professor of Forensic Psychiatry, Institute of Psychiatry, University of London, England

David A. Hamburg
President, Institute of Medicine, National Academy of Sciences, USA; formerly Professor of Psychiatry, Stanford University School of Medicine, USA

Sir Denis Hill
Professor of Psychiatry, Institute of Psychiatry, University of London, England

Seymour S. Kety
Professor of Psychiatry, Harvard Medical School; Director, Psychiatric Research Laboratories, Massachusetts General Hospital, USA

Paul E. Polani
Professor of Paediatric Research, Guy's Hospital Medical School, University of London, England

Heinz F.R. Prechtl
Professor of Developmental Neurology, University of Groningen, Holland

Michael Rutter
Professor of Child Psychiatry, Institute of Psychiatry, University of London, England

Michael Shepherd
Professor of Epidemiological Psychiatry, Institute of Psychiatry, University of London, England

Eliot Slater
Formerly Director of the Medical Research Council Psychiatric Genetics Unit, Institute of Psychiatry, University of London, England

Peter Townsend
Professor of Sociology, University of Essex, England

Sir Geoffrey Vickers, V.C.
Formerly Chairman of the Research Committee, Mental Health Research Fund (now the Mental Health Foundation)

Lyman C. Wynne
Professor and Chairman, Department of Psychiatry, University of Rochester, USA

The Editor

J.M. Tanner
Honorary Secretary, Research Committee, Mental Health Research Fund and Mental Health Foundation, 1951-1976; Professor of Child Health and Growth, Institute of Child Health, University of London, England.

1. Social development in the first year of life: maternal influences on infant-mother attachment

Mary D. Salter Ainsworth

For twenty years my major research endeavour has been an investigation of the social development of infants in the first year of life. No small part of my interest in this research stems from my belief, which is shared by many others, that how a child develops socially is highly relevant to his later mental health. Since a large proportion of a baby's social behaviour occurs in interaction with his mother figure, I have devoted myself chiefly to observing mother-infant interaction in many of the situations that constitute an infant's waking day. I have been particularly interested in investigating the development of the attachment of a baby to his mother. I have sought to identify the infant behaviours that mediate the growth of that relationship and the situations in which they are most likely to be activated. I have also been concerned with individual differences in the nature of the attachment relationship, and with learning something about the influences that shape these individual differences. It is clear that the nature of the interaction a baby has experienced with his mother throughout the first year is among the most important influences on the kind of attachment relationship he eventually forms with her. It is with this aspect of mother-infant interaction that this paper deals.

In any interaction between two members of a dyad it must be assumed that each makes a contribution to the interaction. Each influences the behaviour of the other. Together with my research colleagues, I have been attempting to disentangle these contributions, to ascertain in what ways the mother seems to have the greater influence on the baby's behaviour and in what ways the baby seems to have the greater influence on the mother. We have not been concerned primarily with sorting out these influences within any single interaction, however, or within any limited time period. Rather, we have taken a developmental perspective. We have examined changes of behaviour over time in our endeavour to discover whether it seems to be infant or mother who has the more potent long-term influence on the other, and in what aspects of behaviour such influence is manifested. This report focuses on developmental changes in attachment behaviours and on situations in which attachment behaviours seem especially likely to be activated or intensified.

I have found it productive to work within the ethological-evolutionary theory of attachment developed by Bowlby (1, 2, 3), to which I myself have made contributions (4, 5, 6). I believe, however, that the findings reported here are independent of their theoretical context.

I have investigated two samples of mother-infant pairs, one in Uganda (4) and another that I studied more recently and more intensively in the United

The Sir Geoffrey Vickers Lecture of 19 February 1975.

States. It is upon the behaviour of the American sample that this report is based.

Method

Sample

The sample consists of twenty-six white, middle-class mother-infant pairs, living in the Baltimore area. The families were originally contacted through paediatricians in private practice, usually before the baby's birth. Sixteen of the babies are boys; ten are girls. Only six were first-born—all of them boys. All infants were reported to be normal at birth. Only four were breast fed. Three of the mothers had part-time work at some time during the baby's first year, but only one worked full-time.

Observations and records

Our observations of the sample were both intensive and comprehensive. They were carried out in the course of visits to the home, once every three weeks, from 3 to 54 weeks after the baby's birth. Each visit lasted approximately four hours, so that we have about 72 hours of observation of each mother-infant pair. There were four visitor-observers in all, each of whom followed his assigned cases throughout the baby's first year. As a reliability check, however, I myself took care to visit each home several times, with or without the regular visitor.

One can never wholly ignore the possibility that an observer may affect the interaction that is being observed. To hold this effect to a minimum, we counted on the very frequent, very long visits to encourage the families to act unselfconsciously and naturally. Furthermore we were participant observers, responsive to the overtures of both mother and baby, in the belief that this was less threatening than maintaining a purely spectator role. We assiduously avoided interfering, giving advice, or implying any criticism or judgement. We were truly interested in the characteristics and development of each individual baby, and perhaps this helped the mother to ignore the fact that she also was being observed. In appreciation of the cooperation we received, we paid all of the baby's routine paediatric bills for the first year.

The observer noted as much as possible of what happened during the visit— everything the baby did, especially everything that occurred when he was interacting with another person, and as much as possible of what the mother and other members of the household did and said. After the visit, the observer dictated from notes a narrative record of what had transpired during the visit. It is these narrative records that constitute the raw data.

Data analysis

Although narrative records such as these are rich in detail and preserve sequences of interaction, they are notoriously difficult to analyse. We finished our home visits in August 1967. Ever since then we have been busy analysing data, but the analysis is not yet complete. A fundamental task has been to identify the most useful dimensions in terms of which behaviour may be assessed, and then to devise methods of measuring them. Since the resulting measures of maternal and infant behaviour are numerous, it is more convenient to describe them in conjunction with the presentation of findings.

A 'strange situation' in the laboratory

A standardized laboratory situation was devised to supplement home observations (7, 8, 9). This was labelled 'the strange situation' because the environment was unfamiliar to the baby, and hence might activate 'fear of the strange' (10). Each baby, accompanied by his mother, was introduced to this situation when he was approximately 51 weeks old. We were interested to see how he would explore this unfamiliar environment both when his mother was present and when she was absent, how he would react to a stranger when away from home, and how he would respond to two brief separations from his mother in this unfamiliar environment and to reunion with her afterwards. There were striking individual differences in these various responses. We have concluded that these—especially the responses to reunion—reflect important qualitative differences in the nature of the infant's attachment to his mother. Indeed, for research purposes, we now use this procedure as a situational test for the assessment of attachment.

We could distinguish three main groups of infants on the basis of their behaviour in this standardized situation at twelve months of age. The largest group we have come to identify as secure in their attachments to their mothers. They responded to reunion by seeking to be close to their mothers. Most of them wanted to be picked up, and resisted any early attempt by the mother to put them down. All of this heightened seeking of proximity and contact was, however, relatively unambivalent. Another group responded similarly except that their seeking of contact and interaction was mingled with conspicuously angry resistance. We refer to this as the ambivalent group. Finally, another group avoided the mother upon reunion. They either ignored her altogether, or mingled proximity seeking with looking away, turning away, or moving away from her. This we call the avoidant group. There is reason to believe that both the ambivalent and avoidant infants are anxious in their attachment relationships.

We have now tested 106 one-year-olds in this situation and have ascertained that classification of infants can be replicated with a high degree of reliability by trained persons working 'blind' (11). Furthermore, the codings, from which we derived the measures of behaviour of infant and mother at home, were done by many student assistants who had no knowledge of either the strange-situation classifications or any other assessments.

Results

Infant crying

The first set of findings I shall report pertains to infant crying and maternal responsiveness to it (12). Every instance of an infant's crying that occurred in the course of the 72 hours of observation spread over the first year was coded—noting the circumstances in which the cry took place, how long it lasted, whether or not the mother intervened, how promptly she did so, what she did, and finally what terminated the cry. Infant crying was measured in two ways—the frequency of the episodes of crying per waking hour and the duration of crying in minutes per waking hour. Mother's responsiveness to crying—or rather her unresponsiveness—was measured in two ways: the number of crying episodes she altogether ignored, and the duration of her unresponsiveness, which was the number of minutes her baby cried without or before her intervention.

In this, and in other analyses, we found it convenient to divide the first year into quarters, with approximately sixteen observation hours for each, and to use as our measure the mean score for each quarter. Measures derived from this broad a data base tend to minimize day-to-day variations and hence to be relatively stable.

As might be expected, the duration of crying decreased over the first year, although the mean frequency of episodes did not. There were great individual differences in both, however. For example, the duration ranged in the first quarter from twenty-one minutes per hour to almost no crying at all.

The first and most obvious question to be asked is whether the differences in amount of crying could be attributed to constitutional differences in infant irritability, which ought to be reflected in the first-quarter measures of crying. For each of the two measures, each quarter was correlated with every other quarter. Although all the coefficients in each correlation matrix were positive, only one in each was large enough to be statistically significant (at the 5% level), the correlation between third- and fourth-quarter crying. Thus it seemed not to be until the second half of the first year that crying became a stable infant characteristic. Amount of early crying was not significantly related to amount of later crying. Thus initial constitutional differences did not seem to have a lasting effect on how much babies cried.

Mothers also differed initially in their responsiveness to crying, but, unlike the infants, were fairly consistent throughout the baby's first year. The cross-quarter correlations were all positive and nearly all high enough to be statistically significant. Mothers who ignored crying early on tended to continue to ignore it. Those who responded promptly at first tended to continue to respond promptly. This is the first step in our argument that maternal behaviour affects the amount of infant crying more than amount of infant crying affects maternal behaviour. Babies change over time more than their mothers do.

Next we undertook cross-quarter correlations between infant behaviour and maternal behaviour. Table 1 shows the intercorrelations between fre-

TABLE 1   Correlations between episodes of crying ignored by the mother and frequency of infant crying (extracted from ref. 12)

Episodes of crying ignored by the mother	Frequency of infant crying			
	First quarter	Second quarter	Third quarter	Fourth quarter
First quarter	—	0.56**	0.21	0.20
Second quarter	0.34	—	0.39*	0.36
Third quarter	0.48*	0.32	—	0.52**
Fourth quarter	0.21	0.29	0.40*	—

*$p < 0.05$ **$p < 0.01$

quency of infant crying episodes and number of episodes ignored by the mother. The within-quarter correlation coefficients have been omitted from the table, because they throw no light upon influences of one partner on the other over time. The upper right-hand figures show the correlations between maternal behaviour in one quarter and infant behaviour in subsequent quarters. It may be seen that in each case the more episodes the mother ignored in one quarter, the more frequently the baby cried in the next quarter, and, conversely, the less ignoring in one quarter the less crying in the next.

The figures in the lower left-hand portion of the matrix show the correlations between infant behaviour in one quarter and maternal behaviour in subsequent quarters. It may be seen that first-quarter frequency of infant crying is not significantly related to second-quarter maternal ignoring of crying, nor is second-quarter infant behaviour related significantly to third-quarter maternal behaviour. Third-quarter frequency of infant crying is just as significantly related to fourth-quarter maternal ignoring as is third-quarter maternal ignoring to fourth-quarter frequency of infant crying.

Our interpretation of these intercorrelations is that through the first half of the first year maternal behaviour tends to influence infant behaviour more strongly than infant behaviour influences maternal behaviour. Mothers who ignore crying in the first and second quarters tend to have babies who cry relatively frequently later on, whereas mothers who respond to early infant crying influence their babies to cry less frequently subsequently. By the second half of the first year, however, the influences appear to be reciprocal.

Table 2 shows the intercorrelations between the duration of infant crying and the duration of maternal unresponsiveness. Here again maternal unresponsiveness in the first quarter is significantly related to relatively long crying in the second quarter, whereas the amount of infant crying in the first quarter is not significantly related to duration of maternal unresponsiveness in either the second or third quarters. By the second half of the first year, however, it is clear that there is reciprocal influence to a strong degree.

From all of these findings we have concluded that, within the first part of the first year, maternal responsiveness to infant crying tends over time to reduce the amount the infant cries to a significantly greater extent than does unresponsiveness, whereas the amount the baby cried initially—his constitutional irritability—is not related significantly either to the amount he cries later on, or to how responsive or unresponsive his mother subsequently becomes. In the second half of the first year, however, a vicious spiral seems to

TABLE 2 Correlations between duration of mother's unresponsiveness to infant crying and duration of infant crying (extracted from ref. 12)

Duration of maternal un-responsiveness	Duration of infant crying			
	First quarter	Second quarter	Third quarter	Fourth quarter
First quarter	—	0.45*	0.40*	0.32
Second quarter	0.37	—	0.42*	0.65**
Third quarter	0-12	0.51**	—	0.51**
Fourth quarter	0.41*	0.69**	0.52**	—

*p<0.05   **p<0.01

have become established in some mother-infant pairs. The more unresponsive the mother, the more the baby cries, and his crying seems to make her more reluctant than ever to respond.

We acknowledge that the significant correlations that have led us to these conclusions are not very high, and that we can give only a slight edge to the mother as influencing the baby more strongly, at least in the early months, than he influences her. It is noteworthy, however, that the results do not go strongly in the opposite direction, as extrapolations from learning theory have commonly predicted, and, indeed, as advice commonly given to mothers would have it.

Over many decades mothers have been advised not to respond to the baby when he cries, and especially not to pick him up lest he become 'spoiled' and picking up is exactly what our mothers most frequently did when they responded to crying. If, then, a baby does not learn to cry to get what he wants because his mother responds to him promptly, what does he learn? We suspected that one of the things he learned was to communicate by means other than crying. A measure of infant communication was devised for the fourth quarter, based on facial expression, gesture, and non-crying vocalization, taking into account how varied, how clear, and yet how subtle such communication appeared to be. Table 3 shows the correlations of this measure with the measures of infant crying and of maternal responsiveness to crying. It may be seen that the less the infant cries, the more varied, clear, yet subtle his other modes of communication are. Furthermore, the more unresponsive his mother is to his crying the less expressive are his non-crying communications.

Maternal responsiveness to infant crying tells only part of the story, however. The mother who responds promptly to crying signals tends also to be responsive to infant signals of all kinds. Indeed, if a mother is highly sensitive to infant signals, his entire behavioural repertoire has signal value for her.

Mother-infant interaction relevant to feeding

One of the situations in which maternal sensitivity to infant signals can be well observed is during feeding. A detailed examination was made of interaction relevant to feeding in the babies' first three months (13). Throughout this analysis we were interested in the extent to which the mother's interventions were in response to the baby's signals, so that he was allowed to be an active partner in feeding, in contrast to the extent to which she dominated their

TABLE 3   Correlations between infant communication, crying, and maternal responsiveness to crying (fourth quarter) (extracted from ref. 12)

	Infant communication
Duration of crying	—0.71**
Frequency of crying	—0.65**
Duration of mother's unresponsiveness	—0.63**
Episodes of crying ignored by mother	—0.54**

$**p < 0.01$

transactions. We identified four main dimensions of feeding interaction in which maternal sensitivity to infant signals played a part.

The first related to when the baby was fed. Was this when his behaviour began to signal that he was hungry, or was the mother more concerned with getting him on to a schedule—or even on to three meals a day even in these early months? Or was the mother totally arbitrary, as five of our mothers were, feeding at irregular intervals apparently according to their own complex inner promptings rather than to schedule or to infant signals?

The second dimension referred to the termination of feeding. Was this when the baby signalled that he had had enough, or did the mother either coax or force him to take more? Or, impatient to get on with other activities, did she prematurely put the baby down while he was still hungry? A third dimension was the mother's regard for infant preferences when presenting new foods.

A fourth and perhaps the most important dimension was the extent to which the baby was allowed to pace the rate of his own food intake, whether he was suckled or spoon fed. Did the mother tolerate pauses, or did she constantly tease the baby to keep sucking? Were the holes in the nipple of the bottle so large that the baby got milk so fast that he choked and spluttered? In spoon feeding did the mother shovel the food in or was she sensitive in her pacing? Spoon feeding by a sensitive mother was a joy to behold. The interaction was rhythmical, rather slow in tempo, with the mother constantly taking her cue from the baby's behaviour.

In the original report of this analysis (13) we classified mother-infant pairs in terms of differences in these four dimensions, and found that infants of some classificatory groups were secure in their later attachment relationship with the mother, according to the strange-situation assessments, whereas those of other classificatory groups were anxious. Later, nine-point scales were devised to measure each of the four dimensions of the feeding interaction described above. Since the resulting four sets of scores were found to be highly correlated, they were combined to yield a mean score for each dyad. The point-biserial correlation coefficient between these combined scores and the secure-anxious dichotomy was 0.84.* This suggests a strong positive and highly significant relationship between maternal sensitivity to infant signals relevant to first-quarter feeding and the quality of the later infant-mother attachment relationship.

Incidentally, the 'sensitive' ends of our nine-point scales together provide an excellent definition of what 'demand' feeding can be—something that neither our mothers nor their paediatricians seemed clear about. Indeed we came to disregard totally what the mother told us about whether she fed on demand or according to schedule. Some of the most sensitively responsive mothers insisted that they were feeding by schedule—quite ignoring the 'snacks' they gave between scheduled feedings—whereas some of the most insensitive mothers insisted they were feeding 'on demand'.

We do not suggest that how a baby is fed early on is the crucial variable in determining the later infant-mother relationship. Rather, it seems likely that how a mother fed her baby provided a good sample of how she interacted with

*This finding was obtained in the course of a further analysis of feeding interaction carried out by Dr Russel Tracy.

him generally in the first quarter, and that patterns of interaction established early in the first year tend to persist throughout the intervening months, even though the specific details of the interaction may change substantially, as they certainly do in regard to infant feeding.

Mother-infant interaction in face-to-face situations

Let us next consider interaction in another situation that occurs frequently in the early months—interaction when mother and baby are face-to-face, either when she bends over him in his cot or infant seat, or when she holds him out so that they are *en face*. The part of the study to be reported here is the analysis of how babies who differed in quality of attachment at the end of the first year (i.e. in terms of our strange-situation assessments) interacted with their mothers in the early weeks. For this analysis we used data from home visits between the ages of six and fifteen weeks (i.e. overlapping but not co-extensive with the first quarter), after the baby had clearly become capable of eye-to-eye contact and social smiling (14).

The measures employed were frequency measures—the percentage of face-to-face episodes in which a given behaviour occurred, whether an infant behaviour, a maternal behaviour, or a dyadic behaviour in which mother and infant played reciprocal roles. Table 4 refers to two groups who differed in the quality of their later attachment relationship: a 'secure' group and an 'anxious' group.* It may be seen that infants who later formed secure attachments, more than those who later were anxiously attached, smiled in their early face-to-face interactions with their mothers, and bounced or jiggled about in apparent happy excitement. They fussed or cried less frequently than the anxious group, less frequently responded by merely looking at the mother, and less frequently took the initiative in terminating the interaction. It is worth noting that they did not differ significantly from the anxious group in

TABLE 4   Means of infant measures of early face-to-face interaction for two groups varying in quality of later infant-mother attachment

Infant behavioural measures	Means of groups		p^a
	Secure $N = 9$	Anxious $N = 10$	
Bouncing	21.3%	5.4%	<0.01
Smiling	45.0%	29.5%	<0.025
Vocalizing	29.4%	18.2%	n.s.
Merely looking	9.2%	30.3%	<0.01
Fussing or crying	2.8%	9.6%	<0.025
Terminates episode	11.8%	29.9%	<0.005
Contented state prior to face-to-face episode	85.9%	79.1%	n.s.

a *t*-test used

*In the original classification (9) there were three groups, A, B, and C, to which we now refer as anxious avoidant, secure, and anxious ambivalent, respectively. In this sample Group B had three sub-groups. For the purposes of the analysis reported here, Blehar, Lieberman, and Ainsworth (14) separated Group B into two groups, B_3 which they label 'secure', and a group consisting of B_1 and B_2 which they label 'intermediate'. The 'intermediate' group is omitted in the present report of their analysis.

their state before the interaction began, which suggests that these differences cannot be attributed to the fact that the anxious group was more upset than the secure group to begin with.

TABLE 5   Means of maternal and dyadic measures of early face-to-face interaction for two groups varying in quality of later infant-mother attachment

Maternal and dyadic behavioural measures	Means of groups		p^a
	Secure $N = 9$	Anxious $N = 10$	
Contingent pacing	58.9%	17.3%	<0.001
Encouraging further interaction	25.2%	3.4%	<0.001
Ensuing interaction (dyadic)	47.3%	21.1%	<0.005
Playfulness	18.6%	8.5%	<0.10
Abruptness	0.6%	12.0%	<0.001
Brief interaction (dyadic)	35.6%	62.5%	<0.005
Routine care	6.8%	26.2%	<0.005
Silent, unsmiling initiation of interaction	9.9%	19.7%	<0.05
No response to baby's initiations of interaction	4.6%	15.3%	<0.05
Termination of interaction	40.0%	41.0%	n.s.

[a] *t*-test used

Mothers initiated far more episodes of interaction than did their babies in these early weeks. Indeed the mothers generally may be described as setting the tone of the face-to-face interaction. Table 5 shows the differences in early interaction of the mothers of the babies who were later identified as secure or anxious. It may be seen that there were two behaviours that were much more frequent among the mothers of the secure group than among those of the anxious group—behaviours labelled as 'contingent pacing' and 'encouragement of further interaction'. A mother was identified as showing contingent pacing when she leaned toward the baby, smiling or talking, gently, and in slow tempo, allowing the baby plenty of time to mobilize a response before she gave another gentle burst of stimulation. She was identified as encouraging further interaction if, after little or no initial response from the baby, she did not abandon her effort to get interaction going, but instead gently persisted in her stimulation, increasing her vivacity as he became more responsive. It is not surprising, therefore, that these mothers were more often successful than were the mothers of the babies who later became anxiously attached in getting chains of reciprocal responses going, which tended to prolong the duration of the face-to-face episode. In contrast, the mothers of the babies later identified as anxious, more frequently than mothers of later secure babies, confined face-to-face interaction to routine-care situations, and attempted to initiate interaction silently and with an impassive facial expression. They were more frequently abrupt in their pacing, and hence, not surprisingly, their episodes of face-to-face interaction tended to be of brief duration (i.e. judged to have lasted less than thirty seconds).

Even more interesting were the differences between the secure and anxious groups in regard to differential behaviour to the mother in comparison with

TABLE 6   Means of infant measures of early face-to-face interaction with the mother versus the visitor for two groups varying in the quality of later infant-mother attachment

Infant behavioural measure				Attachment groups		
		Secure			Anxious	
	M[a]	V[a]	p[b]	M	V	p
Bouncing	21.8%	6.0%	< 0.05	5.4%	5.0%	n.s.
Vocalizing	29.4%	13.8%	< 0.05	18.2%	19.9%	n.s.
Merely looking	9.2%	32.1%	< 0.05	30.3%	32.1%	n.s.
Smiling	46.0%	28.5%	< 0.11	29.5%	28.5%	n.s.
Crying or fussing	2.8%	2.2%	n.s.	9.6%	2.1%	< 0.025
Terminates episode	11.8%	31.7%	< 0.01	26.9%	22.5%	n.s
Contented state prior to face-to-face episode	85.9%	89.3%	n.s.	79.1%	83.1%	n.s.

[a] M refers to mother; V to visitor
[b] t-test used

the relatively unfamiliar visitor-observer. It may be seen from Table 6 that the secure group showed the more positive differential behaviour in early face-to-face interaction, vocalizing and bouncing more frequently in interaction with the mother than with the visitor, whereas the anxious group did not display these behaviours differentially. The secure group more frequently merely looked at the visitor when *en face* with her than when *en face* with the mother, and more frequently took the initiative in terminating interaction with the visitor. The anxious group were just as likely merely to look at the mother as at the visitor, and just as likely to terminate interaction with one figure as with the other. The babies who later became anxious differentiated between mother and visitor only in that they more frequently cried or fussed when *en face* with the mother. It seems clear that the group who later became securely attached had learned to discriminate their mothers from relatively unfamiliar persons, and that this occurred at an age before sixteen weeks, which is strikingly early for discrimination via the distance receptors. It is not clear that the group who later became anxiously attached were discriminating between the two classes of figures when they fussed more in interaction with the mother. The visitors were careful to pace their interventions 'contingently' and to 'encourage further interaction'—behaviours in which the mothers of the 'anxious' group were unskilful. It may have been that the apparent discrimination was attributable to markedly different behaviour of the two figures, whereas I do not believe that there was such a behavioural difference in the case of the other group.

Striking though these findings are, neither the face-to-face nor the feeding interaction findings disentangle the relative influences of infant and maternal behaviour upon each other as well as did the analysis of crying. It could always be argued that it was the baby's behaviour in feeding or in face-to-face interaction that made the mother act as she did rather than vice versa. Let us turn to another aspect of our data in which we have been able to sort out direction of effects.

Mother-infant interaction in relation to close bodily contact

Every instance was coded in which a baby was picked up by his mother, under what circumstances the pick-up took place, how he responded to it, what both he and his mother did while she held him, and what he did when he was subsequently put down. We derived several measures of infant behaviour from this coding, and a substantially larger number of maternal measures (15). Here I shall refer to only two infant measures and three maternal measures. We scored as 'positive responses to being held' all instances in which a baby smiled, or moulded his body to that of his mother, or, later in the first year, all instances in which he showed active behaviours such as embracing her, scrambling over her body, exploring her face or body with his hands, and the like. The measure was the percentage of pick-up episodes in which such positive responses were shown. (It is worth noting here that all of the infants in the sample were initially capable of a positive response to being held. If in doubt, we picked the baby up ourselves to see whether he could adjust his posture to the body of the person who held him.) We identified some responses to being held as 'negative'— those in which the baby began to cry, or continued crying without being soothed by the pick-up, or in which he stiffened or squirmed, or, later in the first year, pushed away from or hit at his mother. There was, of course, a proportion of pick-up episodes in which neither positive nor negative responses could be identified.

How were these responses to close bodily contact related to the way in which the mother behaved when she held her baby? Within each quarter we found strong and significant relationships between maternal behaviour and the way in which babies responded to being held and to being put down, but the most salient findings come from an examination of cross-quarter correlations. The three which will be reported here involve qualitative aspects of maternal behaviour that have no direct relationship to how often the mother picked her baby up or how long she held him.

The first of these variables we have labelled 'tender, careful, holding'— rather shamefacedly because TLC has become a cliché. This kind of holding behaviour is characterized both by a gentle slowing down of the mother's usual speed and vigour of movement, and by a pacing of the tempo of her physical handling of the infant to his tempo of response. An estimate was made of how much of a mother's total holding time was characterized by this kind of behaviour, and this was compared with the percentage of pick-up episodes in which the infant responded positively to being held.

The first comparison was of the consistency over time of infants' and mothers' behaviour considered separately. Mothers, although differing widely in amount of tender, careful holding, showed substantial individual consistency in relative amount from the first to the second quarter, and from the second to the third, but this behaviour in any of the first three quarters was essentially unrelated to fourth-quarter behaviour. This, we suggest, was probably because such gentle handling was no longer appropriate for the older, stronger, more competent infant. Infants, on the other hand, showed no consistency in frequency of positive response to being held from the first quarter to any subsequent quarters. Differences in response to being held seemed to take some time to become established as stable, individual differences. Once established, however, they were highly consistent in the second, third, and fourth quarters.

Table 7 shows the cross-quarter correlations between maternal tender,

TABLE 7   Correlations between maternal tender, careful holding infants' positive response to being held

Maternal tender, careful holding	Infant positive response to being held			
	First quarter	Second quarter	Third quarter	Fourth quarter
First quarter	—	0.51**	0.53**	0.46*
Second quarter	0.28	—	0.69**	0.67**
Third quarter	0.38	0.41*	—	0.44*
Fourth quarter	0.26	0.25	0.25	—

*p <0.05   **p <0.01

careful holding and infant positive response to being held. In the upper right-hand portion of the matrix appear the correlations between maternal behaviour in one quarter and infant behaviour in subsequent quarters. It may be seen that all of these are substantial correlations and statistically significant. Babies who have been held tenderly and carefully earlier tend later to respond positively to close bodily contact. In the lower left-hand portion of the matrix appear the correlations between infant behaviour in one quarter and maternal behaviour in subsequent quarters. Although these are all positive correlations, they are smaller than the other set, and only one is large enough to be significant. It seems certain that a positive infant response is not a significant factor in leading the mother to behave more tenderly as time goes on, whereas there is a strong case for inferring that the mother's early tender behaviour has a long-term facilitating effect on infant response to contact, extending even into the fourth quarter.

An opposite trend was found for mother's display of affection when holding her baby. For each mother we determined the percentage of pick-up episodes in each quarter in which she displayed affection, i.e. kissed, hugged, or caressed her baby. Cross-quarter correlations showed that individual differences in this behaviour were highly consistent throughout the first year. Table 8 shows the cross-quarter correlations with infant positive response to being held. It may be seen that only one of the correlations in the upper right-hand portion of the matrix is large enough to be significant. Thus, although affectionate maternal behaviour in the third quarter is significantly related to infant positive response to holding in the fourth, her behaviour in the first

TABLE 8   Correlations between maternal affectionate behaviour and infants' positive response to being held

Maternal affectionate behaviour	Infant positive response to being held			
	First quarter	Second quarter	Third quarter	Fourth quarter
First quarter	—	0.13	0.19	0.22
Second quarter	0.32	—	0.33	0.36
Third quarter	0.36	0.49*	—	0.44*
Fourth quarter	0.28	0.41*	0.51**	—

*p <0.05   **p < 0.01

and second quarters is not significantly related to later infant behaviour. In particular, affectionate display in the first quarter seems essentially unrelated to later positive response by the infants. In the lower left-hand portion of the matrix it may be noted that infant positive response in the first quarter is not significantly related to maternal affectionate behaviour in any of the later quarters. The correlation coefficients are higher in this portion of the table however, and infant positive response in the second and third quarters is related significantly to maternal affectionate display later on. Thus it seems that from the second quarter onward an infant's positive response to being held tends to make his mother relatively more likely to display affection.

Here is an example of a virtuous spiral. Mothers who are tender and careful in their physical handling of the baby in the early months seem to engender in him a tendency to respond positively to close bodily contact. This in turn tends to evoke an affectionate response in the mother, which may contribute all the more to the baby's enjoyment of contact. Without tender, careful behaviour, however, a mother's displays of affection in the early months do not seem to give the baby a positive experience while being held.

A third maternal behaviour has been labelled 'inept holding'. The measure of inept holding was the percentage of total holding time in which the mother handled the baby roughly, or very clumsily or inappropriately, such as when one mother held her baby upside down in her arms without seeming to notice that the toes were where the head should have been. Inept holding was relatively rare, but the amount shown by each mother was a fairly consistent characteristic, especially throughout the first three quarters. Inept maternal holding was compared with infants' negative response to being held. Individual differences in the latter were fairly consistent from the second quarter onward, but initial differences in frequency of negative responses were essentially unrelated to later differences. Thus, maternal behaviour was again more consistent throughout the first year than was infant behaviour.

Table 9 shows the cross-quarter correlations between inept maternal behaviour and negative infant response to being held. The correlations in the upper right-hand portion of the matrix tend to be substantial and significant, suggesting that mothers who handle their babies ineptly in earlier quarters tend to have babies who respond negatively to being held in later quarters. It may be noted in the lower left-hand portion of the matrix that an infant's negative responsiveness in the first quarter is not significantly related to how

TABLE 9   Correlations between inept maternal holding behaviour and infants' negative response to being held

| Maternal inept behaviour | Infant negative response to being held | | | |
	First quarter	Second quarter	Third quarter	Fourth quarter
First quarter	—	0.42*	0.56**	0.24
Second quarter	0.11	—	0.73**	0.35
Third quarter	0.22	0.80**	—	0.47*
Fourth quarter	0.24	0.48*	0.53**	—

*$p < 0.05$ **$p < 0.01$

inept his mother is in later quarters. Negative responses in the second and third quarters, however, are strongly associated with later maternal ineptness in holding. It appears that by the second quarter a vicious spiral has built up, so that maternal ineptness and negative infant response are reciprocally related from then on. Nevertheless there is some reason to believe that the mother began the vicious spiral by her inept handling in the infant's earliest months.

Some might argue that tender, careful, and affectionate maternal behaviour would spoil a baby, addicting him to physical contact, making him eager to cling to his mother and reluctant to leave her to explore the world. Our findings do not support such an argument. Even in the first quarter we found an inverse correlation between positive response to being held and protesting at being put down, and this inverse relationship continues into the latter half of the first year, when infants who have enjoyed being held not only cheerfully accept being put down, but then, as often as not, move off into independent exploratory play. It is the babies who respond negatively to being held who tend to cry when put down, and, in the last quarter, even though they may have resisted being held, they seek to be picked up again after having been put down rather than turning toward exploratory activity.

Infant responses to everyday separation and reunion

Stayton and Ainsworth (16) examined infant responses to the everyday separations that occur at home when the mother leaves the room, and to her subsequent return. The four infant measures used were crying and following in leave-room episodes, and positive greeting or crying in enter-room episodes. It is of interest to examine the relationships of these to the other infant behaviours we have been considering. A table of intercorrelations includes many significant coefficients, some positive and some inverse. Since such tables are difficult to comprehend at a glance, we are including here the results of a factor analysis of fourth-quarter behaviours (see Table 10). This analysis suggested that there were two main factors or dimensions that

TABLE 10   Factor analysis of some fourth-quarter infant behaviours (from ref. 16)

Infant behaviour	Factor I	Factor II
Crying when mother leaves room	0.88	—0.17
Following when mother leaves room	—0.23	—0.16
Positive greeting when mother enters	—0.59	—0.25
Crying and mixed greeting when mother enters	0.66	0.00
Frequency of crying	0.73	0.28
Duration of crying	0.72	0.43
Positive response to being held	—0.34	—0.54
Negative response to being held	0.28	0.63
Stops crying when picked up	—0.06	—0.64
Positive response to being put down	—0.53	—0.49
Negative response to being put down	0.38	0.18
Initiation of pick-up	0.02	—0.60
Initiation of put-down	0.18	0.61

Note: Factor I accounted for 33.24% of the variance and Factor II for 24.63%.

accounted for a substantial amount (58%) of the variance in infant behaviour. Factor I is a bipolar factor, with one pole defined by the frequency of infant crying when mother leaves the room—the frequency of separation anxiety. Other behaviours with high positive loadings—and thus by implication associated with frequency of separation anxiety—are frequency and duration of crying, crying when greeting the mother, and also to a lesser extent a negative response when put down after having been held. The behaviour with the highest loading toward the opposite pole of the dimension, is greeting the mother positively when she enters the room. Other behaviours with high loadings in the same direction are responding positively to being put down, and to a lesser extent responding positively to being held.

It is suggested that Factor I may be interpreted as representing an anxiety versus security dimension of behaviour manifested by the infant at home. Factor II, on the other hand, appears to refer to response to close bodily contact, but this will not be discussed here.

We have seen how infant crying and responses to close bodily contact are related to certain maternal behaviours. Table 11 shows correlations of

TABLE 11 Correlations of separation-related infant behaviours with some maternal behavioural measures (fourth quarter) (extracted from ref. 16)

Maternal behavioural measures	Infant behaviours		
	Crying when mother leaves	Following when mother leaves	Positive greeting
Acknowledgement of baby upon entering room	−0.10	0.08	0.21
Frequency of leaving room	0.14	0.05	−0.31
Duration of unresponsiveness to crying	0.46*	−0.10	−0.40*
Ignoring crying episodes	0.45*	−0.03	−0.42*
Sensitivity-insensitivity	−0.40*	0.40*	0.46*

*$p < 0.05$

separation and greeting behaviours with several measures of maternal behaviour. Crying and mixed greeting have been omitted from this table; they occur too infrequently to yield significant correlations with any of the maternal measures. Only two of the maternal measures refer to maternal behaviour directly relevant to leaving or entering the room: acknowledgement of the baby upon entering, and frequency of leaving the room. Neither of these is significantly related to any of the infant behaviours. The two measures of maternal unresponsiveness to crying are, however, significantly related to separation distress and to positive greeting. Mothers who ignore crying or who are slow to respond to it have babies who more frequently cry in little everyday separations, and who are less likely to give her a happy greeting when she returns. The fifth measure refers to a nine-point rating scale* to assess maternal sensitivity to infant signals and communications in the fourth quarter. It may be seen that following the mother when she leaves and

*This scale and instructions for using it may be found in Ainsworth, Bell and Stayton (19).

greeting her positively when she returns are both significantly related to maternal sensitivity to signals, whereas frequency of crying when the mother leaves the room is significantly related to maternal insensitivity.

Our interpretation of these findings is as follows. Babies who show relatively much separation anxiety in little everyday separations at home may be described as generally anxious in their relations with their mothers. Their mothers tend to have been relatively insensitive and unresponsive to their signals (including crying signals) not merely in the fourth quarter but generally throughout the first year. These unresponsive mothers have not facilitated the growth of trust. On the contrary, their babies seem to lack confidence that their mothers will be accessible and responsive to them when needed. On the other hand, babies who rarely cry when their mothers leave the room may be described as securely attached. Their mothers tend to have been sensitively responsive to their signals, and this consistent responsiveness has engendered in these infants expectations that the mother will be accessible and responsive to him when needed, so that even when she leaves the room he has confidence that she is still available to him. It is as though he knows where she is, could follow her if he chose, and could signal her if he wished, in the confident expectation that she would respond.

Infant behaviour in the strange situation

Involuntary separation in an unfamiliar situation is a different story (9, 11). Even infants who seem very secure at home, and who cry little in minor, everyday separation situations, tend to be distressed when their mothers leave them with a stranger or alone in the laboratory 'strange situation'. They slow down in their playing with toys that had previously absorbed their attention, or stop playing altogether. Sooner or later they begin to search for the mother, and sooner or later almost all of them begin to cry, if not during the first separation at least during the second. Paradoxically, the babies who do not cry

TABLE 12   Measures of behaviour displayed at home by infants in the three strange-situation classificatory groups (mean scores for the fourth quarter)

Measures of home behaviour in the fourth quarter	Strange situation assessments of attachment		
	Anxious avoidant $N = 6$	Secure $N = 13$	Anxious ambivalent $N = 4$
Duration of crying	5.6**	3.0	8.1**
Positive response to holding	10.7**	36.4	16.5*
Negative response to holding	21.2**	6.2	23.0*
Positive response to put-down	59.8	68.7	50.3**
Negative response to put-down	39.2**	27.3	30.8**
Initiation of pick-up	16.2	22.1	9.5*
Crying when mother leaves	20.3**	14.1	29.0**
Following when mother leaves	56.3	55.6	21.3**
Positive greeting	28.2*	39.1	23.0*
Crying and mixed greeting	12.3	9.5	17.3*
Obedience to mother's verbal commands	54.0*	81.2	44.0**

Note: p values pertain to the t-test of differences between each of the anxious groups and the secure group. *$p < 0.05$ **$p < 0.01$.

when separated from their mothers in the strange situation—and these are chiefly infants in the anxious-avoidant group—tend to be among those who are most anxious at home.

Table 12 shows how the three main classificatory groups, distinguished in terms of their strange-situation behaviour, may be distinguished also in terms of their behaviour at home during the fourth quarter. This Table includes only those measures in terms of which differences between groups were statistically significant. The two anxious groups, avoidant and ambivalent, were each compared with the secure group.*

It may be seen that in comparison with the secure group the anxious, avoidant group cried more frequently when the mother left the room, and less frequently greeted her cheerfully when she returned. They cried for longer periods, responded to holding more negatively and less positively, and responded more negatively to being put down. Furthermore, they tended to be less frequently obedient to their mothers' verbal commands (17). It was because they were so clearly anxious in their everyday interactions with their mothers that we were inclined to believe that the avoidant behaviour that they showed in the reunion episodes of the strange situation, as well as their apparent lack of separation anxiety in the laboratory, were defensive.

In comparison with the secure group the anxious, ambivalent group were more likely to cry at home when the mother left the room, and less likely to follow her. They less frequently greeted the mother cheerfully when she returned, and more frequently with a cry. They cried more in general, and responded to holding less positively and more negatively. They also responded to being put down less positively and more negatively. They were less likely to initiate being picked up. Finally, they were less obedient to their mothers' commands.

In general, there is a remarkable degree of congruence between behaviours that characterize the infant-mother relationship at home and those that characterize it in the strange situation. The main discrepancy occurs with the avoidant group, and even this is only an apparent discrepancy if one views those who are avoidant in the strange situation as essentially anxious.

Maternal sensitivity to infant signals

The mothers of the three groups—secure, avoidant, and ambivalent—may also be distinguished in terms of their behaviour at home in the fourth quarter, but these seem relatively unimportant when compared with the evidence that has been assembled in this paper for the influence of behaviour in earlier months of the first year. Throughout all of the aspects of mother-infant interaction that have been discussed here, one attribute of maternal behaviour kept reappearing in various guises as significantly related to positive infant responses at the time and to eventual security of the infant-mother attachment relationship, namely, maternal sensitivity to infant signals. This attribute was reflected not only by the rating scale of that title but also in the following: responsiveness to infant crying, each of the four dimensions of early feeding interaction, contingent pacing and encourage-

*Here the 'secure' group is comprised of all the sub-groups of Group B, two of which had been treated as an 'intermediate' group in a previous analysis.

ment of interaction in face-to-face situations, and tender, careful handling while in close bodily contact.

Infant avoidance and maternal behaviour

The dimension of sensitivity-insensitivity to infant signals does not account for all qualitative differences in the infant-mother attachment relationship, however. It does not account for the fact that some insensitive mothers have babies who develop avoidant behaviour whereas others do not. We have made some progress in understanding how this comes about (18), but here I can do no more than state a few of the conclusions we have reached from our analysis so far. Our first clue was that the mothers of anxious, avoidant babies emerged (in terms of a nine-point rating scale of maternal acceptance-rejection) as rejecting, whereas mothers of anxious non-avoidant babies did not (19). This scale dealt with the frequency with which a mother's loving concern for her baby became overridden by irritation either at his behaviour, or at the extent to which he interfered with her other valued activities. But how do mothers convey such rejection? In addition to obvious overt manifestations of angry irritability, they seem to express it through behaviour relevant to close bodily contact. All of the mothers of the avoidant group were aberrant in such behaviour. Some found close contact with the baby distasteful and some were indifferent to it; in either case they tended relatively often to rebuff the baby when he sought contact. Others made close contact often disturbing or painful to the baby through the physical force they exerted in attempts to control his behaviour. Consequently, it seemed, their babies came to view the prospect of close bodily contact with their mothers as potentially punitive or at least rebuffing. This, we suggest, resulted in conflict.

When circumstances prompt such a baby to seek contact with his mother—as when he is alarmed, uncomfortable, or anxious—his tendency to approach her is incompatible with his tendency to avoid her because of the unpleasant or disappointing experiences he has had relevant to contact with her. He seeks contact, as all babies do, but at the same time he avoids it. In the strange situation this conflict is demonstrated by the fact that when his mother leaves he tends to try to follow her, but when she returns, he tends to avoid her, either by ignoring her or, showing his conflict even more overtly, by beginning to approach her and then turning away. At home, the conflict is shown less dramatically, presumably because attachment behaviour is less strongly activated than it was in the strange situation. Avoidant babies do approach their mothers at home, but they often do so tentatively, by making partial approaches followed by moving off, or by going the whole way and then merely touching her instead of clambering up, and touching her most peripheral parts such as her feet.

Summary

In summary, it seems as though different patterns of maternal behaviour have a potent effect on infant behaviour and on the character of the eventual infant-mother attachment relationship, and that this impact begins to make itself felt in the earliest weeks or months of the baby's life. Nevertheless, I feel I must set some limits to the apparently sweeping claims I may seem to have made in presenting our findings.

1. I do not propose that experience in the first few months, or even in the first year, sets the tone of social relations for all time. Later interaction with the mother figure, interaction with other figures, and a variety of later experiences undoubtedly have an effect, for better or for worse. Nevertheless I believe that early patterns of interpersonal interaction, once established, tend to have their own momentum. Based both upon habitual modes of responding and upon expectations of others, they may not be readily or perhaps entirely reversed by later experience.

2. Our findings cannot safely be projected beyond the end of the first year, although some of my colleagues and students have found evidence to support such projection into the second year or even beyond (e.g. 20, 21). It is tempting to suggest that we have in this investigation some hypotheses about the aetiology of disturbances which appear later in childhood or even in adulthood. The only grounds for entertaining such suggestions, however, is that our findings fit very well with aetiological hypotheses emerging from the clinical literature. A study confined to the first year of life would have doubtful predictive value if a clinical perspective could not be brought to bear on it.

3. It is acknowledged that it is risky to generalize from a small sample of white, middle-class, American infant-mother pairs. Nevertheless I am emboldened to do so by the fact that the findings for this sample are highly congruent with the findings of twenty-eight infant-mother pairs that I observed in country villages in Uganda (4).

4. Nevertheless, a small sample yields a greatly oversimplified picture. Only conspicuous and even obvious trends can be emphasized. However valid they might subsequently prove to be in a larger sample, more complex patterns, or patterns that pertain only to a small minority of cases, must of necessity be passed over.

5. Although our data support the notion that the effect of maternal behaviour on the infant is greater (in making for individual differences) than the effect of infant behaviour on the mother, it might be otherwise in a sample that included infants 'at risk'. With such a sample more evidence might be found for the proposition that constitutional differences in infants have a profound differential effect on maternal behaviour. Furthermore, it should be emphasized that the dimensions of maternal behaviour in our study that seemed to affect the infant significantly were not assessed in absolute terms but rather in terms of how maternal behaviour was geared to infant cues.

Finally, attention should be drawn to the fact that we have been unsuccessful so far in distinguishing significant patterns among the infants whose relations with their mothers were judged to be of clearly secure quality. Similarly we have found that the maternal behaviours associated with secure attachment are all highly correlated. At the outset of the study I had thought that there might be a number of different ways in which a mother might foster the growth of secure attachment, but our findings suggest that the mothers of secure babies resemble each other closely. On the other hand, there seems to be a variety of patterns of anxious infant-mother attachments, only two of which have been identified here, and a variety of patterns of maternal behaviour associated with them. Therefore I believe that Tolstoi was close to the truth when he said: 'Happy families are all alike; every unhappy family is unhappy in its own way.'

Acknowledgements

The research upon which this paper is based has been supported by Grants 62-244 of the Foundations' Fund for Research in Psychiatry and RO1 HD 01712 of the United States Public Health Service, by the Office of Child Development, by the Grant Foundation and by the Spencer Foundation; this support is gratefully acknowledged. I also wish to thank Barbara A. Wittig, George D. Allyn, and Robert S. Marvin II, who carried out many of the observations, and those many others who helped with the 'strange situation' and with the analysis of the data upon which this report is based.

References

(1)   Bowlby, J. (1958) The nature of the child's tie to his mother. *Int. J. Psycho-Anal., 39*, 350-73.
(2)   Bowlby, J. (1969) *Attachment and Loss, Vol. 1, Attachment.* London, Hogarth.
(3)   Bowlby, J. (1973) *Attachment and Loss, Vol. 2, Separation: Anxiety and Anger.* London, Hogarth.
(4)   Ainsworth, M.D.S. (1967) *Infancy in Uganda: Infant Care and the Growth of Love.* Baltimore, The Johns Hopkins University Press.
(5)   Ainsworth, M.D.S. (1969) Object relations, dependency, and attachment: A theoretical review of the infant-mother relationship. *Child Dev., 40*, 969-1025.
(6)   Ainsworth, M.D.S. (1972) Attachment and dependency: A comparison. In *Attachment and Dependency*, Ed. J.L. Gewirtz, pp. 97-137. Washington, D.C., V.H. Winston.
(7)   Ainsworth, M.D.S. and Wittig, B.A. (1969) Attachment and exploratory behaviour of one-year-olds in a strange situation. In *Determinants of Infant Behaviour IV*, Ed. B.M. Foss, pp. 111-360. London, Methuen.
(8)   Ainsworth, M.D.S. and Bell, S.M. (1970) Attachment, exploration, and separation: illustrated by the behavior of one-year-olds in a strange situation. *Child Dev., 41*, 49-67.
(9)   Ainsworth, M.D.S., Bell, S.M. and Stayton, D.J. (1971) Individual differences in strange situation behavior of one-year-olds. In *The Origins of Human Social Relations*, Ed. H.R. Schaffer, pp. 17-58. London, Academic Press.
(10) Hebb, D.O. (1946) On the nature of fear. *Psychol. Rev., 53*, 250-75.
(11) Ainsworth, M.D.S., Blehar, M.C., Waters, E. and Wall, S. (1977) The strange situation: observing patterns of attachment. Hillsdale, N.J., Lawrence Erlbaum Associates. In press.
(12) Bell, S.M. and Ainsworth, M.D.S. (1972) Infant crying and maternal responsiveness. *Child Dev., 43*, 1171-90.
(13) Ainsworth, M.D.S. and Bell, S.M. (1969) Some contemporary patterns of mother-infant interaction in the feeding situation. In *Stimulation in Early Infancy*, Ed. A. Ambrose, pp. 133-70. London, Academic Press.
(14) Blehar, M.C., Lieberman, A. and Ainsworth, M.D.S. (1977) Early face-to-face interaction and its relation to later infant-mother attachment. *Child Dev., 48*, in press.
(15) Blehar, M.C., Ainsworth, M.D.S. and Bell, S.M. (1977) Mother-infant interaction relevant to close bodily contact: A longitudinal study. In preparation.
(16) Stayton, D.J. and Ainsworth, M.D.S. (1973) Individual differences in infant responses to brief, everyday separations as related to other infant and maternal behaviors. *Dev. Psychol., 9*, 226-35.
(17) Stayton, D.J., Hogan, R. and Ainsworth, M.D.S. (1971) Infant obedience and maternal behavior: the origins of socialization reconsidered. *Child Dev., 43*, 1057-69.
(18) Main, M. and Ainsworth, M.D.S. (1975) Behavior relevant to physical contact as a predictor of differences in infant-mother attachment. In preparation.
(19) Ainsworth, M.D.S., Bell, S.M. and Stayton, D.J. (1974) Infant-mother attachment and social development: 'socialisation' as a product of reciprocal responsiveness to signals In *The Integration of a Child into a Social World*, Ed. M.P.M. Richards, pp. 99-135. London, Cambridge University Press.
(20) Main, M. (1973) Exploration, play, and cognitive functioning as related to child-mother attachment. Unpublished Ph.D. dissertation, Johns Hopkins University.
(21) Blehar, M.C. (1974) Anxious attachment and defensive reactions associated with day care. *Child Dev., 45*, 683-92.

2. The therapeutic community: concept, practice and future

David H. Clark

The last twenty years have seen the rise and dominance in institutional psychiatry of a remarkable notion—'the therapeutic community'. It is both an attitude and a method, a system of treatement and a battle cry, a charm and a password. I have been fortunate to take some part in applying this notion to one part of the field of inpatient psychiatric treatment and have attempted, while doing so, to study the effects of what we did.

The idea that life in a residential institution could in itself be therapeutic is an old one and treatment by a way of life has been a claim of specialized institutions down the ages. The Greek Aesculapian temples, many of the monasteries, and the Victorian Public Schools all claimed that their way of living made people better. The early asylums were founded on this notion, and Pinel and Tuke spoke of the value of the 'regimen of the house' and the necessity of 'moral treatment'. During the nineteenth century this vision was largely lost in psychiatric hospitals, and the model of the two-person treatment situation, where one doctor treated one patient, which so successfully dominated medicine, was accepted by psychiatry. The rise of successful individual psychotherapy reinforced this model.

The 1939-45 War tore psychiatrists out of the closed world of their mental hospitals and the cosiness of the psychotherapeutic consulting rooms and plunged them into the turmoil of army training camps, tented hospitals and combatant units and made them forcibly aware of the tremendous power of social factors for affecting men's thinking and feeling. This awakening led to the growth of group psychotherapy, to the development of the War Office Selection Boards and in particular to the growth of social psychiatry and community methods of treatment in Britain, especially at Northfield Hospital (1), in Maxwell Jones's Effort Syndrome Unit at Mill Hill, and later in the Rehabilitation Units for prisoners-of-war returning demoralized and desocialized from captivity (2, 3). In 1945 Karl Menninger and a group of American psychiatrists toured Europe to see new psychiatric developments; they were particularly impressed by this English ferment, and a whole volume of the *Bulletin of the Menninger Clinic* was devoted in 1945 to papers from England. Among these was Main's paper 'The Hospital as a Therapeutic Institution'.

Main (4) began by describing the traditional hospital and what it did to the patient. 'The fine traditional mixture of charity and discipline they receive is a practised technique for removing their initiative as adult beings, and making

The Sir Geoffrey Vickers Lecture of 26 February 1964, with a Comment on Recent Developments written in 1974. An abridged version of the Lecture was published in the *British Journal of Psychiatry*, 1965, *111*, 974-54.

them "patients".' He pointed out how damaging this was to the neurotic whose illness is often precipitated by social factors. He then described Northfield Hospital under the heading 'A Therapeutic Community': 'The Northfield Experiment is an attempt to use a hospital not as an organization run by doctors in the interest of their own greater technical efficiency, but as a community with the immediate aim of full participation of all its members in its daily life and the eventual aim of the resocialization of the neurotic individual for life in ordinary society. Ideally, it has been conceived as a therapeutic setting with a spontaneous and emotionally structured (rather than medically dictated) organization in which all staff and patients engage.' Finally, he discussed what they had learned about the change necessary in the doctor's work, the staff relations needed, the provision for special needs—such as a secluded place to mourn lost comrades.

At the end of the war those who had been interested in social psychiatry dispersed, returning to their hospitals and their private practices, to group therapy or individual psychoanalysis. The seed had, however, been well planted, and gradually took root and grew during the next decade.

The reaons for this were probably the comments of the social scientists on the mental hospitals, the opportunity of radical changes in the mental hospitals offered by physical treatments and tranquillizers, and the continuing work of Maxwell Jones.

Main spoke in his article of the need for the whole hospital to be a 'therapeutic community'. During the last two decades, however, two slightly different uses of the phrase have been developed. The first is the general therapeutic community approach; this is a way of looking at the life of patients in any psychiatric institution and restructuring their lives. The second is the therapeutic community proper, a small face-to-face intensive treatment facility with extensive social restructuring. The therapeutic community approach is particularly associated with T.P. Rees and others who developed it in mental hospitals during the 1950s. The therapeutic community proper is particularly associated with Maxwell Jones, first at the Effort Syndrome Unit at Mill Hill, then at the Prisoner-of-War Rehabilitation Unit at Dartford and from 1947 at the Social Rehabilitation Unit at Belmont.

In the decade after the War a number of social scientists, social psychologists and social anthropologists published critical accounts of psychiatric institutions. These accounts were most welcome tools to those who were beginning to look at the structure of the hospitals critically. The most widely known were the publications of Stanton and Schwartz (5), which took a most searching and perceptive look at the social structure of a private psychoanalytic hospital. Caudill (6), an anthropologist, entered a neurosis unit as a patient and recorded the way in which other patients instructed the newcomer in the proper behaviour of a patient; how good work at occupational therapy gained you weekend passes, while infractions lost you your matches and cigarettes, and what sort of dreams the doctors liked best. Belknap (7) and Dunham and Weinberg (8) in their accounts of State Hospitals delineated the employee culture which drove the long-term patient towards chronicity. Goffman (9), a perceptive sociologist who spent a year in a big Federal Hospital, contributed unforgettable comments on such subjects as 'The underlife of the public institution'. All these taught us a great deal about what life in the hospital can do to a person who stays there for a long time.

The therapeutic community approach was in some degree a revival of the old principles of moral treatment which had been known for a century and a half. One of the reasons why this revival has been effective is the development of effective physical and drug treatment. Widespread electroplexy and judicious leucotomy removed most of the savagery from the old refractory wards, and the extensive use of tranquillizers since 1955 has made contact possible with many patients who were previously unreachable. There are, however, enough hospitals locked, custodial, hostile and dreary, despite the patients being all heavily tranquillized, to show that drug and milieu therapy are both needed and are synergistic.

The World Health Organization published in 1953 the Third Report of their Expert Committee on Mental Health (10). This marks an important point in the spread of the general therapeutic community approach.

They said of the atmosphere of the hospital: 'The most important single factor in the efficacy of the treatment given in a mental hospital appears to the Committee to be an intangible element which can only be described as its atmosphere, and in attempting to describe some of the influences which go to the creation of this atmosphere, it must be said at the outset that the more the psychiatric hospital imitates the general hospital, as it at present exists, the less successful it will be in creating the atmosphere it needs. Too many psychiatric hospitals give the impression of being an uneasy compromise between a general hospital and a prison. Whereas, in fact, the role they have to play is different from either; it is that of a therapeutic community.'

They also spelled out the constituents of this atmosphere and italicized the following:

1. *Preservation of the patient's individuality.*
2. *The assumption that patients are trustworthy.*
3. *That good behaviour must be encouraged.*
4. *That patients must be assumed to retain the capacity for a considerable degree of responsibility and initiative.*
5. *The need for activity and a proper working day for all patients.*

They finally said that 'the creation of the atmosphere of a therapeutic community is in itself one of the most important types of treatment which the psychiatric hospital can provide'.

The 1953 Report mentions little of the part that other patients may play in an individual's recovery or decline. It speaks of self-government, but seems to mean running social clubs and peripheral activities, not direct patient involvement in ward government. There is no mention of community, face-to-face meetings, nor of social analysis of happenings. Although the team approach is later mentioned, the emphasis is still on treatment flowing from the doctor downward, and there is much emphasis on the need for planning, organization and atmosphere creating.

The Committee's concept was one that was not too difficult for doctors to accept. They were still the titular heads and the main determiners of policy. They decided what work was good, and what bad; which doors should be open and when; who should have responsibility over whom.

Other publications followed, notably those of Greenblatt and others (11, 12) and of Cumming (13).

We may remind ourselves of the position now in 1964 in Britain. There has been a striking change in the mental hospital scene; most ward doors in most hospitals are unlocked and the patients are able freely to come and go through them. A number of mental hospitals are fully open-door, though many maintain one or two locked wards. Most patients are occupied, and instead of sullen, surging hordes in the airing courts one now finds workshops and industrial units. The level of work varies, but a fair number of patients are engaged in skilled work for industrial firms, reasonably well paid. Aided by a change in the law, the amount of legal liberty available for patients has changed dramatically. Whereas before the majority of patients were certified, now nearly all are 'informal'. Although a substantial proportion of patients are compulsorily admitted to hospital, the number under compulsory long-term detention is very small, varying between 2% and 10% through the country. Rehabilitation is actively encouraged, many hospitals have patients going out to work, and many long-stay patients have been successfully discharged from hospital. A striking corollary of all this is a fall in the total number of psychiatric patients in British mental hospitals. The peak number was in 1954, when there were 152,000 patients in psychiatric hospitals; the most recent figures, for 1962, showed that there were 131,500 patients in corresponding accommodation. This is the first time for a century and a half that there has been, during peace time, a sustained fall in the total number of people in psychiatric institutions. I think that the development of the therapeutic community approach and the adoption of active rehabilitation and discharge policies in psychiatric hospitals has been a major contributing factor to this decline. There are those who attribute it entirely to the development of the tranquillizing drugs and others who explain it as due to the dying off of cohorts.

The therapeutic community proper, as developed in particular by Maxwell Jones, is a more revolutionary concept and has not been so widely accepted. It has never been rigidly defined, but two statements express its essence. Maxwell Jones (3) has stated: 'A therapeutic community is distinctive among other comparable treatment centres in the way the institution's total resources, both staff and patients are self-consciously pooled in furthering treatment.' Martin (14) has said: 'A therapeutic community is one in which a deliberate effort is made to use to the fullest possible extent in a comprehensive treatment plan the contribution of all staff and patients.'

The therapeutic community proper has certain characteristics:

1. *Size.* It is small, not more than 100 persons. It is small enough for each member to know the others and for community meetings to be held of all those involved.
2. *The community meeting.* Regularly, often daily, all the people in the community—patients, nurses, doctors, social workers, domestics, etc.—meet for a period to consider common problems.
3. *Its underlying philosophy is the psychodynamic hypothesis,* the belief inherent in most psychotherapy and psychological treatment that an individual's difficulties are mostly in relations with other people and that these can be examined in discussions, understood and remedied.

The therapeutic community uses many different methods of dealing with its problems, but certain social methods are outstanding:

4. *Social analysis of events.* Happenings in the unit are discussed in the community group meetings and an attempt made to understand them.
5. *Freeing of communications.* Attention is given to improving the flow of information upward and downward.
6. *Flattening of the authority pyramid.* This happens inevitably, but is regarded as important in itself and is a marked contrast to the traditional ward.
7. *Provision of learning experiences.* There are constant protected situations where patients can try out their ego strength and learn new ways of coping with difficulties.
8. *Role examination.* This applies to all, but especially to the staff. As they examine their work they are able to change to a more effective and helpful way of functioning.

The most famous therapeutic community is Henderson Hospital, Belmont, founded in 1947 as an Industrial Neurosis Unit and operated by Maxwell Jones from then until 1959. In this dilapidated old wing of a former LCC institution, there were no manifest status distinctions; no one wore uniforms and the visitor was often puzzled as to who were all these voluble, active and interesting people milling around and talking so freely. The day opened with community meetings, followed by staff meetings, and in the workshops and therapy groups were further meetings where every happening was discussed and analysed intensively and actively. For a period psychodrama was used, but it was soon found that if these psychopathic individuals just told their tales it was dramatic enough. There were frequent disturbances, drunken episodes, thefts, violence, difficulties with Belmont Hospital (to which the Unit was attached) and with the Management Committee. All these formed excellent fuel for vigorous discussion. The Unit took people whom nobody else could understand or manage; at first it took men who had been unable to find or stay in work, but later it took those formally diagnosed as 'psychopaths' and, by genuinely involving them in the organization and management of the community, for the first time brought them an understanding of the needs and the legitimate demands of society. Those who worked there found it an exciting experience, some of which they convey in the first team book which they wrote about the unit (2).

Rapoport (15), in his analysis of Belmont, described the 'Unit Ideology', which he said was characterized by four themes:

1. *Democratization.* Every person had one vote; everyone's opinion—nurse, doctor or patient—was as good as the next.
2. *Permissiveness.* The members were expected to tolerate disturbed behaviour; discussion was better than discipline.
3. *Communalization.* Equality and sharing were valuable; everyone should express their thoughts and share them with others.
4. *Reality confrontation.* All were expected to face their problems and interpretations were vigorously forced on them.

In his examination he pointed out some of the contradictions inherent in this, the difficulties of certain professional groups, especially doctors and nurses, in fitting in, and suggested that rehabilitation to the outside world sometimes took second place to treatment—i.e. adjustment to the inside world of the Unit.

There have been a number of therapeutic communities directly modelled on this, for example Wilmer (16), Martin (14), Artiss (17) and Moss and Hunter (18).

During the last ten years at Fulbourn Hospital we have been applying the therapeutic approach to the hospital as a whole and also developing therapeutic communities. In 1954 we planned to start a programme of work, freedom and rehabilitation on the long-stay men's side, so R.M. Hoy and I decided to try to measure how things were before the change and how they were after. The measurements were quite simple, such as what work every man was doing and how much freedom he had; whether he was regarded as incontinent or violent; whether he went on weekend leave. We carried out a census of all the long-stay men's wards in October 1954 and repeated it in November 1955 (19). In 1961, E.G. Oram and I carried out another census which we were able to compare with those of 1954 and 1955 (20). From all these surveys there emerged a picture of the sort of change which occurs in a custodial mental hospital when the therapeutic community approach is applied, and the surveys focused attention on one or two problem areas and confounded some of the hypotheses with which we started.

In 1954 there were four long-stay wards with 336 male patients in them, in overcrowded, old hospital buildings. A programme of work for all was introduced, followed by a cautious opening of doors. During the first period there was no increase in the number of staff, but one of the wards was divided. In the first twelve months the percentage of men at work rose from 22% to 52%; the number with parole from 26% to 72%; there was a drop in the amount of incontinence and a marked drop in the amount of sedation with paraldehyde. There had been a rise in the amount of ECT given.

In 1961 many of these changes had gone further. All the ward doors had been opened in 1957; the total population of the long-stay wards had dropped from 336 to 287. The discharge rate of long-stay patients (i.e. patients who had spent over two years continuously in hospital) had risen to double what it had been in the years before 1954 and had remained high. An analysis of the work the men were doing had shown that not only the proportion employed stayed high, but the quality of the work they were doing had risen. Whereas very few in 1954 had been doing work comparable with paid employees, 15% in 1961 were doing such work or were going out to work in Cambridge or were earning a substantial wage in the Industrial Workshop. In 1954, 40% of the men were totally unemployed; in 1961 only 23% were not working at all. In 1955, 26% of the men had parole; in 1955, 72%; and by 1961, 95% of the men had freedom to come and go. The legal status had also changed. In 1954, 72% of the men were certified under the 1890 Acts; in 1961, only 1.4% of the men were under long-term detention under the Mental Health Act (Sections 26, 60, 65 and 72).

E.G. Oram, D.F. Hooper (a research fellow of the Mental Health Research and Trust Fund) and I have published an account of the first therapeutic community proper at Fulbourn Hospital (21). Difficulties had risen in an outlying forty-bed women's ward used for 'convalescence' for short-stay patients. It was run on traditional lines, with a Sister directing the ward work and a Registrar seeing patients individually. An unhappy spirit of disgruntlement had developed, patients were unwilling to go to the ward, and every now and then there were great difficulties over removing entrenched patients to the 'main building'. Oram rearranged the ward life, starting community and other meetings, cutting down on individual interviews and insisting on the patients taking over the housework. There were many fascinating repercussions both within the staff team and throughout the hospital, but after a time the change in the ward was marked. Morale became high; the women were actively discussing the problems they would face when they returned to their husbands, their homes, their jobs and all that appeared to have caused their breakdowns.

We analysed movements of patients through the ward before and after the therapeutic community was established. We compared a group of 91 patients who passed through the ward six months before the therapeutic community, and 120 patients who passed through the ward in a similar six months after the therapeutic community. We showed that there were no significant differences in age, marital status and diagnosis between the two groups, but that under the therapeutic community the length of stay in the ward was significantly shorter (73 compared with 98 days) and that the total length of stay in hospital of the women passing through was shorter (98 compared with 134 days). There was a decline in the transfers to the 'main building'. In the review period before the therapeutic community there were eleven such transfers out of 90 patients and in the second period there were none out of 120. An analysis of the re-admission rate in both periods showed that it was no higher under the therapeutic community than it had been before. This analysis was therefore able to show that the change of the ward to a therapeutic community had speeded the process of rehabilitation from the hospital and decreased the number of people who became chronically resident.

The sociological analysis, however, pointed to certain continuing problems: the ward had become a special culture, different from the rest of the hospital. There was a social gulf between them which staff, particularly nurses, found difficult to span. Some staff, particularly nurses, found it quite difficult to work in this unit.

We have also developed a therapeutic community in what used to be the women's disturbed ward. Ten years ago we had a traditional women's disturbed ward with padded rooms in active use, noisy, turbulent, bare, many women showing violent and degraded habits and requiring strong clothing. In 1957 it became possible to move staff and patients into a clean, attractive, newly decorated, well-equipped ward in another building; at the same time a vigorous Registrar reviewed all the patients, arranged courses of electroplexy, intensive tranquillization, etc. Following these measures the ward became much more presentable and after a time the ward door was opened, for most of the time at least, so that visitors could be taken in there. D.F. Hooper made a social study of this ward the main subject of his Doctoral thesis (22) and of a later paper (23). Apart from questionnaires and studies, the main method he used was participant observation and interaction analysis, recording the number of interactions between staff members and patients in sample periods; these showed that, despite the apparent change, the social structure was still one based on control and minimum interaction. He also showed that long-term members of the ward showed very little change and very few of them were promoted to better wards. There was also evidence that the ward was failing to carry out its primary duty to the hospital of containing those patients so disturbed that they could not be looked after in other wards.

In 1960 we instituted a therapeutic community in this ward with regular community meetings and an emphasis on understanding and an analysis of social events. The initial period of disorganization was more dramatic than in the previous therapeutic community, and for nine months there was a marked rise in violent episodes. Some of these caused great anxiety to both patients and staff, so that the main topic of discussion in ward meetings was the control of violent behaviour. Over the months, however, these incidents were contained and a far more understanding atmosphere developed. The amount of interchange between staff and patients increased immensely, and nurses found the work on the ward, though still perplexing and tiring, far more interesting than it had been before. We have already shown that there has been a marked difference in the fate of the patients who had spent many years in the previous ward; several of them have already left hospital and a substantial number have achieved sufficient independence for promotion to rehabilitation wards with less supervision. Of thirty-six patients who had been in the ward for at least three years before the changeover, ten have subsequently been promoted to better wards or discharged from hospital, and in 1964, four years after the changeover, only four of the original fifty patients are still in the intensive-nursing ward (as we now call it). The development of this therapeutic community has been a most exciting experience and, despite the strain of the work, the morale of the staff has remained high.

We are still working out the full significance of this experiment, but we have seen that a therapeutic community intensive-nursing ward is more capable of absorbing the deeply disturbed patients from the rest of the hospital than the previous control pattern, and I have learned that the most effective way to change the social structure of a ward is to allow the new change to evolve from interaction rather than to impose it by administrative fiat from outside.

What of the future? We have had a revolutionary twenty years in which we have seen the psychiatric hospitals change amazingly and their vast numbers beginning to decline. We have made beginnings with a new form of social therapy—the therapeutic community.

It seems to me that there is one major permanent and general gain. We have become aware of what living in a hospital can do to a person. We have learned that the old medical adage 'primum non nocere' applies as much to medical institutions as to drugs and surgery, and that Florence Nightingale's dry comment that 'it may seem a strange principle to enumerate as the very first requirement in a hospital that it should do the sick no harm' applies not only to the physical dangers, fevers and contagions, but also the mind and feelings of the patient, and that a stay in hospital which preserves or even restores physical health may cripple the patient's personality by the attitudes and behaviour it enforces or rewards. We shall continue to be far more aware of the need for attention to and planning of the patients' milieu in the psychiatric hospitals, in the new general psychiatric units, and in due course in the general hospital wards, though it may be generations before Main's comment is no longer true in the general hospital: 'the fine traditional mixture of charity and discipline they receive is a practised technique for removing their initiative as adult beings'.

Of the future of the strictly defined therapeutic community it is less possible to be certain. This method of reorganizing a psychiatric unit is exciting and rewarding; many of us believe it to be highly effective—for some patients. I think we shall learn the different kinds of therapeutic communities needed for different disabilities. We shall, I think, find it our most effective instrument for some problems—probably the acting-out character disorders—but not so effective for others—such as guilty and self-reproachful depressed people. In some situations the amount of social reorganization (and personal strain involved) will not be justified by the therapeutic gain. But I am sure that for many years we must go on experimenting with this exciting method, and recording and setting forth our results.

Comment on recent developments

My original lecture was a review of a situation at a particular point in time, namely the position of the Therapeutic Community Concept in February 1964. I therefore thought it best to leave it unaltered and append a note on how things have changed since then.

The 1965 article reviewed the rise, since 1946, of the Concept of the Therapeutic Community, detailed its development during the 1950s, attempted to clarify the concept and finally speculated on the possible future.

In the article I distinguished between the 'Therapeutic Community Approach' and the 'Therapeutic Community Proper'. Now it is probably best to speak of the first as 'The Humane, Liberal Approach', the second as 'The Defined Therapeutic Community' and to consider a third group of activities which can best be entitled (after M. Jones) 'Beyond the Therapeutic Community'.

The humane liberal approach to the life of the institutionalized mentally ill, which I previously called 'The Therapeutic Community Approach', has made great strides in the last decade in Britain and other parts of the world. The restatement of the forgotten principles of Moral Treatment (Rees), that idleness, restraint and brutal coercion towards the confined are not only inhumane but also increase chronicity, has been widely accepted. In 1971, only 6.8% of the 99,760 psychiatric patients in England and Wales were legally detained, and only 7.1% of all psychiatric beds were in locked wards. The total inpatient population has fallen from 150,000 in the peak year of 1954 to 90,000 in 1973. Therapeutic workshops are to be found in 60% of British hospitals and the majority of patients are occupied. Many transitional facilities have been developed (halfway houses, hostels, group homes, sheltered workshops, day centres, night hospitals, day hospitals, etc.). It is now accepted that the life people live may determine their fate and in many hospitals there is a conscious effort to make the life of the patients more challenging and more dignified as well as more comfortable.

In 1964 I spoke of the 'Therapeutic Community Proper' describing the small intensive face-to-face therapeutic unit. A better phrase might have been 'The Defined Therapeutic Community'. This form of treatment, this method of organizing a hospital ward, has gained some acceptance, but more slowly.

In Britain, defined therapeutic communities have been developed in a number of hospitals. Some have flourished, others have closed, but the number has risen slowly. In 1970, informal gatherings of workers in British therapeutic communities began; in 1972, an Association of Therapeutic Communities was formed; it holds some three meetings a year and has 20 institutions and organizations as members as well as 161 individual members. I have visited therapeutic communities in a number of countries, including the USA, Japan, Peru, Poland, Sweden and Norway.

Fulbourn Hospital has continued to be active. The work with Oram mentioned in the lecture produced two articles (20, 24) discussing aspects of the work and rehabilitation programme. Of the 23 wards in 1974 in Fulbourn, four are therapeutic communities. The hospital is much more tolerant of the method; an article discussed some of the problems that arise between the developing therapeutic community and the hospital (25). Two articles described the development of a therapeutic community in the 'disturbed wards' of the hospital (26, 27). In the 1960s Myers carried out control studies which showed clearly the effectiveness of the therapeutic community method in helping disturbed patients, compared with a traditional humane ward in another hospital (28).

Many of the pioneers have moved 'Beyond the Therapeutic Community'. Jones at Dingleton (1963-70) first reorganized the hospital as a therapeutic community, but then moved his therapeutic teams out into the local towns to develop a community psychiatric service. Laing and his co-workers, developing patterns of treatment for young schizophrenics, started from a structure similar to a defined therapeutic community but moved far beyond it. Within Shenley Hospital, he and Cooper developed an experimental unit for young male schizophrenics (29). In 1967 they moved out of the National Health Service to Kingsley Hall (1966-69) and are now experimenting with other communal living situations (30). Synanon, which started with a therapeutic house for drug addicts, has now developed an international movement which offers a life-long commitment similar to a medieval monastic order.

Some of those experiments—notably those of Laing—have been most valuable in indicating alternative ways by which the psychiatric professions can help those who come, or are brought, to them. There is a ferment within psychiatry today, especially in social psychiatry, which is heartening or terrifying, depending on one's attachment to the established order. Some of this is associated with the term 'The Therapeutic Community', although much of it, such as the polemics of Szasz, the poetry of Laing or the revolutionary diatribes of the Radical Therapists, has its roots in other fields.

The Therapeutic Community Concept has, therefore, grown far in the decade since the original lecture. The humane liberal approach has proved most acceptable and has been implemented widely, probably because it does not challenge any traditional professional roles or presuppositions. The defined therapeutic community has won slow and grudging acceptance as a possible way of organizing a psychiatric ward, but is still much challenged and resisted; this resistance arises mainly because the method challenges sharply the traditional roles of the mental health professionals, especially the doctors and nurses. Many of the pioneers have moved into other forms of activity 'beyond the therapeutic community' and have linked with revolutionary ferments gradually changing the practice of psychiatry.

References

(1) Taylor, F.K. (1958) A History of group and administrative therapy in Great Britain. *Br. J. med. Psychol., 31,* 153.

(2) Jones, M. (1952) *Social Psychiatry (The Therapeutic Community).* London, Tavistock.

(3) Jones, M. (1962) *Social Psychiatry in the Community, in Hosptals and in Prisons.* Springfield, C.C. Thomas.

(4) Main, T.F. (1946) The hospital as a therapeutic institution. *Bulletin of the Menninger Clinic, 10,* 66-70.

(5) Stanton, A. and Schwartz, M. (1954) *The Mental Hospital.* London, Tavistock.

(6) Caudill W., *et al.* (1952) Social structure and interaction processes on a psychiatric ward. *Am. J. Orthopsychiat., 22,* 314-24.

(7) Belknap, I. (1956) *Human Problems of a State Mental Hospital.* New York, McGraw-Hill.

(8) Dunham, W. and Weinberg, S.K. (1960 *The Culture of the State Mental Hospital.* Detroit, Wayne State University Press.

(9) Goffman, E. (1961) *Asylums.* New York, Anchor Books.

(10) World Health Organization (1953) *Expert Committee on Mental Health, Third Report.* Geneva.

(11) Greenblatt, M., *et al.* (1957) *The Patient and the Mental Hospital.* Glencoe, Illinois: The Free Press.

(12) Greenblatt, M., York, R.H. and Brown, E.L. (1955) *From Custodial to Therapeutic Patient Care in Mental Hospitals.* New York, Russell Sage Foundation.

(13) Cumming, J. and Cumming, E. (1962) *Ego and Milieu.* New York, Atherton Press.

(14) Martin, D.V. (1962) *Adventure in Psychiatry.* London, Cassirer.

(15) Rapoport, R.N. (1960) *Community as Doctor.* London, Tavistock.

(16) Wilmer, H.A. (1958) *Social Psychiatry in Action.* Springfield, C.C. Thomas.

(17) Artiss, K.L. (1959) *The Symptom as Communication in Schizophrenia.* New York, Grune and Stratton.

(18) Moss, M.C. and Hunter, P. (1963) Community methods of treatment with chronic psychotics. *Br. J. med. Psychol., 36,* 85-91.

(19) Clark, D.H. and Hoy, R.M. (1957) Reform in the mental hospital: a clinical study of a programme. *Int. J. soc. Psychiat., 3,* 211-23.

(20) Clark, D.H. and Oram, E.G. (1966) Reform in the mental hospital: an eight year follow-up. *Int. J. soc. Psychiat., 12,* 98-108.

(21) Clark, D.H., Hooper, D.F. and Oram, E.G. (1962) Creating a therapeutic community in a psychiatric ward. *Hum. Relat., 15,* 123-47.

(22) Hooper, D.F. (1960) Change in a Mental Hospital. Ph.D. Thesis, Cambridge University.

(23) Hooper, D.F. (1962) Changing the milieu in a psychiatric ward. *Hum. Relat., 15,* 111-23.

(24) Oram, E.G. and Clark, D.H. (1966) Working for the hospital. *Br. J. Psychiat., 112,* 997-1005.

(25) Clark, D.H. (1965) The Ward Therapeutic Community and its Effects on the Hospital. In *Psychiatric Hospital Care,* Ed. H. Freeman. London, Bailliere, Tindall and Cassell.

(26) Clark, D.H. and Myers, K. (1970) Themes in a therapeutic community. *Br. J. Psychiat., 117,* 389-95.

(27) Mungovan, R. (1968) Evolution of a therapeutic community. *Nursing Times, 64,* 365-6.

(28) Myers, K. and Clark, D.H. (1972) Results in a therapeutic community. *Br. J. Psychiat., 120,* 51-8.

(29) Laing, R.D., Esterson, A. and Cooper, D. (1967) Results of Family Oriented Therapy with Hospitalized Schizophrenics. In *Psychiatry and Anti-Psychiatry.* London, Tavistock.

(30) Barnes, M. and Berke, J. (1973) *Mary Barnes: Two Accounts of a Journey through Madness.* Harmondsworth, Penguin.

3. Psychiatric research in delinquency behaviour

Trevor C.N. Gibbens

When giving the Fourth Mental Health Trust and Research Fund Lecture in 1966 it seemed best, for the sake of brevity, to give an account of the sort of pre-occupations with research in forensic psychiatry which we had had at the Institute of Psychiatry. Now, some years later, it may be permissible to continue the same rather egocentric plan.

The last decade has seen more fundamental changes in the pre-occupations of criminologists than the previous decade. Until the early sixties the key to the understanding of delinquency was felt to lie with psychiatrists, in their explorations of family tensions and personality development. Not enough was known, it was said, but the approach was right; more and better psychiatric treatment of a conventional kind held the key to the future. Social scientists were willing collaborators. The last ten to fifteen years, however, has seen the emergence of criminal sociology, no longer in collaboration but often in sharp opposition to the psychiatric or psychological theories about the predominant causation of crime and its methods of treatment.

The basic cause of this evolution has been the emergence in the UK of a distinguished group of non-medical criminologists who have carried out the most important social scientific work. The impact of the researches has been in three principal fields.

The first has been the research into the extent and distribution of crime. Many crimes are not even reported to the police, and in many instances only between a third and a half of known crimes are cleared up by arrest. Whether the undetected offender differed from the detected and convicted one was an open question, as was the general extent of criminal behaviour. Much progress has been made recently in coming nearer to the truth by two methods—the 'self-report' method by which a random group of the population (usually juveniles, but in Scandinavia (1) army conscripts aged eighteen) are asked to say how many offences of different kinds they have committed with or without detection. The second and more recent method, 'victim report', consists of asking a normal population sample to describe how many times they have been victims of crimes, whether they reported them and the outcome. This information can be compared with police statistics. The results have shown that crime is much more widespread than many believed. Among a sample of 3% of Stockholm schoolboys 57% admitted at least one serious offence and of these 93% were not caught. Between them, these boys claimed that they had committed 1430 serious offences, but the culprit was

A revised form of the Sir Geoffrey Vickers Lecture of 23 February 1966, an abridged version of which was published in the *British Medical Journal*, 1966, 2, 695-8.

known to the police in only forty-one of them. The proportion of crimes for which an offender was apprehended was thus only 2.9% (2). In Oslo 56% of young men entering the army admitted shoplifting and a similar number admitted smashing street lamps and other public property. Among 1400 London boys aged thirteen to sixteen, Belson (3) found that between a half and a third admitted theft in a variety of situations. As far as victim reports are concerned, the US President's Commission of 1967 made enquiries of 10,000 households, and concluded that about half of major crimes were not reported. Those most frequently unknown were burglaries, rapes, aggravated assaults, and larceny of over fifty dollars. Only a third of burglaries were known and 75% of rapes were not reported. It seems likely that the occurrence of minor offences was often forgotten.

In England considerable progress has been made in assessing the extent of recorded delinquency in relation to self report of delinquency. West (4), has very closely followed 411 boys aged from eight to seventeen in a tough London area, including a study of the family situation on four occasions. 24.8% made a court appearance for misbehaviour between the ages of ten and seventeen, but a number were excluded from a definition of juvenile delinquency because of very trivial offences of truancy or minor motoring offences which do not lead to police recording, leaving a figure of 20.4% delinquents (9% recidivists and 11.4% with only one conviction). This agrees closely with Power's (5) figure of 24% in another working-class area of London. In the national survey of children born in one week in March 1966, Douglas (6) found 10.4% convicted of indictable offences throughout the country, and Wadsworth (7) calculated the figure for London as 13.7%. Calculated in the same way West's group would give a figure of 16.3% and taking account of changes in legal definition, 18.7%. In a current study at the institute of genetic aspects of crime, a group of 300 'non-delinquent controls' aged seventeen to twenty-one working in a provincial factory were shown to include 17% with a juvenile conviction. There is little doubt that in the UK and in many other countries, between 15% and 20% of boys will have a juvenile conviction by the age of seventeen. Self-reported studies at ages fifteen and seventeen were made by West. Misbehaviour ranging from the most trivial (travelling without a ticket 89.5%, breaking windows of empty houses 82.2%) to serious offences (housebreaking 9.3%, planned housebreaking 7.1%, shopbreaking 12.7%) were reported. However, when the 80 most serious self-reporting delinquents (who had committed 21 of the 38 possible sorts of misbehaviour) were compared with the 84 convicted delinquents it was found that half of them were among those already convicted. Moreover, the family background factors which had been found to be of principal importance in distinguishing the delinquents among this general population—namely the five features of low family income, large family size, parental criminality, low intelligence and poor parental behaviour—were also in general present in the most serious undetected delinquents. The general conclusion from this very important study supports what one might hope to be true, namely that there is a very wide spectrum of misbehaviour from the most trivial in which virtually all indulge, through risky and very undesirable behaviour, to the most serious and persistent. Police activity, or the frequency of repeated criminal behaviour, results with reasonable accuracy in picking out for conviction the most serious 10%. Other studies support the view that it is the most serious and persistent of the self-reporting delinquents who tend to get convicted.

One hopes that this is the case because it has been questioned by the results of other studies of self-reported crime, especially in the USA, which have given rise to criticism of the juvenile justice system. It raises the question whether the association between convicted delinquency and working-class slum areas is not a consequence of differential police activity and police discretion. These studies have tended to show for example that self-reported offences are found just as commonly in boys from good backgrounds, of high education, of middle-class environments, who do not reach the courts. It has also given rise to the sociological theory of 'labelling'. Stated crudely this maintains that most if not all young people are delinquent, predominatly because this is the normal response to the inequalities of society, that one of the most powerful factors in creating a recidivist delinquent career is arrest and conviction, and the attachment of a label 'delinquent' which alters the attitudes of teacher and parents as well as the boy's self image which persuades him that he is a black sheep. Treatment has tended to consist of isolating him in 're-educational' institutions which concentrate those with similar outlook, with a secret social system dominated usually by the most anti-social and anti-authority among the inmates. As an adult he will be incarcerated in a prison which destroys his identity, leaves his character naked and without the support of those deceptions and pretensions on which the mental health of all of us depend. This makes him irresponsible and lazy, and cuts him off from sexual and family life, which is the most powerful known force towards social integration after adolescence. Psychiatrists, say the neo-criminologists, must share much of the blame by their insistence upon the importance of biological or psychological anomalies, which, when present, are largely irrelevant to the main social causes and cures. In the adult field, by the discussion of personality disorder and psychopathic personality, and recommendations for indefinite detention for 'treatment' (whether or not a treatment exists), they resemble, in the views of the American psychiatrist Professor Szasz (8), the priests of the Inquisition who were considered to be experts in deviance, and involved in gross interference with human liberty!

It has been a novel experience for forensic psychiatrists, who had hitherto prided themselves on being in the vanguard of penal progress, to find themselves on the defensive, accused by sociologists of being the unwitting tools of outmoded policies, and engrossed in irrelevant research. Although unacceptable in their extreme forms, these views have considerable validity and psychiatric research has responded to it. Aspects of labelling and other sociological theories have clearly exercised a considerable influence upon modern penal policy expressed in the Children's Act of 1969, which aimed at reducing the number of juveniles charged or brought to court, and in recent criminal Justice Acts for adults, which seek to reduce the use of imprisonment and set up additional methods of treatment in the community. Few will deny that these are correct policies, if they can be implemented in practice.

Meanwhile it is interesting to observe that psychiatry, which had its greatest impact when it was based upon psychopathological views, especially psychoanalytic ones which were incapable of proof, has become increasingly scientific in its approach to research, while the views of the neo-criminological schools (which are tending to break up into competing subdivisions, as psychoanalysis did fifty years ago) are expressed only in terms of compatibility with a theory, little or no attempt at validation being made (9).

Attempts to validate labelling theory in fact are very difficult to design. Such attempts as have been made have sometimes supported the theory and sometimes not. It should follow that it is better for a delinquent not to be stigmatized by appearing before a court. In America two groups of boys were followed up, each of which had 'self-reported' four fairly serious offences; the second group had been convicted of the last offence. In line with the theory, the convicted boys were more frequently reconvicted later than those who were undetected. Severity of punishment should also have a bad effect upon serious offenders without much previous delinquency. When boys in this group were followed it was found that Negro working-class boys were less often reconvicted after punishment than if they were warned or placed under light supervision, but the opposite was true of middle-class white boys. There are considerable problems of method and interpretation of results in such studies.

Psychiatric aspects of types of crime

For many years this aspect was the principal form of study by clinical psychiatrists, and can produce useful results in the hands of very experienced psychiatrists. It is inevitable that this should be carried out, particularly in response to public or political pressure in relation to new or disturbing varieties of crime. In this way premature stereotyping or public prejudice can sometimes be prevented. Institute members have thus been encouraged to report upon cruelty to children (10), morbid jealousy in husbands seen in psychiatric practice (11), or those in Broadmoor following murder (12), motor car thieves (13), shoplifters (14). The Wolfenden Committee on Homosexuality and Prostitution was the spur to clinical studies by Scott (15) of the varieties of homosexual offender attending an outpatient clinic, with valuable indications of the sort of treatment required, and a clinical study of juvenile prostitutes in a remand home (16). The extent to which Borstal boys had been subjected to attempts at homosexual seduction was also described; it showed that one third had been subjected to approaches whether or not they had shown any response. This threw doubt upon the popular theory that seduction in early adolescence is a cause of homosexuality (17). In recent times public anxiety has stimulated studies of teenage drug addiction (18, 19, 20), battered babies (21, 22), and battered wives (23), as well as more systematic studies of violent offenders by Nichol and Gunn and their colleagues (24).

There are considerable hazards in such studies. At the simplest they are likely to show in any group passing through the hands of a psychiatrist that some 5% are psychotic, 10% grossly disordered in the psychopathic sense, 10% with well-marked neurotic symptomatology or subnormality, and 75% with moderate or negligible personality disorder, whatever the type of crime. Their value lies in the particular pattern of psychological or social dynamics which can be perceived.

The problem for all these studies is one of sampling. The clinical psychiatrist in his daily practice sees a heavily biased sample of those showing any particular behaviour pattern. In spite of the value of Scott's description of convicted homosexuals, it bears little relation to the distribution of abnormality among homosexuals in general. The systematic study by Schofield (25) of three groups of homosexuals—a group in mental hospitals, a group in prison and a group in the community (contacted by the 'snowball' method, consisting in asking subjects to recommend their friends)—revealed a very different distribution. Those in mental hospitals tended to be in conflict about awareness of their tendency, those in prison tended to be pedophiliacs, middle aged, married, involved in other types of crime and with a deprived and disordered upbringing. As American studies have confirmed by the snowball method, there is a large group of socially well adjusted, competent and successful homosexuals, usually more promiscuous than heterosexuals, and tending to go in for what the courts call 'the full offence', i.e. anal intercourse, rather than the inhibited and partial behaviour of those who are in difficulty, social or psychological. Homosexuals, it is fairly clear, tend to get into difficulty when they are 'in the open' between two havens of refuge—on the one side psychological acceptance of their condition, and on the other integration with a well ordered homosexual subculture. Homosexuals in mental hospitals are less represented than their numbers in the community would suggest. Treatment, one may suppose, consists in helping them in one direction or the other. The limited view of the maladjusted homosexual should not blind one to the overall picture.

The internal relationships between selected groups is, of course, a valuable exercise. Nichol and Gunn's (24) study of aggressive offenders in Borstal and an adult prison investigated a relationship between interview history of aggression (carefully rated by two independent observers), and the relationship between this and the Buss-Durkee questionnaire on aggression (which proved to give a very similar result to other methods of investigation) and a standardized psychiatric interview. They were able to calculate that the 90 men convicted of robbery interviewed in prison represented about half of a national sample convicted as heavily.

Very occasionally one worker can examine what is virtually a national sample. D'Orban (26) calculated that the heroin addicted women seen in Holloway were about half of all such cases known to the Home Office. Even more remarkably, his group of child stealers—another controversial group—represented almost a complete national sample (27). Most were schizophrenics who had lost children for one reason or another, but a minority were hysterical and more normal with mixed motivation.

The importance of sampling was demonstrated in a recent study of arson (28). It has been accepted by psychiatrists and the judiciary that arsonists are frequently mentally disordered people with a persistent and irrational tendency to start fires with a sexually perverse motive. Because of the risk to life and enormous financial loss, the crime attracts long sentences and in recent years life sentences. There is no doubt that such arsonists exist, and a study by Hurley and Monahan (29) of the first fifty arsonists admitted to the psychiatric prison of Grendon confirmed this: 10% had previous convictions for arson, 30% had been previously convicted of sex offences and most showed marked sexual perversions. This, and the study of all French arsonists by Pichaud

(30), referred only to those sentenced to imprisonment. Recently Soothill and Pope (28) followed up the subsequent convictions of all arsonists charged or convicted in 1951, for twenty years. The picture is quite different, only 45% being sent to prison or Borstal, though another 9% were committed to hospital; 43% had no previous convictions of any kind compared with only 6% of the Grendon group. Seven arsonists could not be traced and judging from their age in 1951 had probably died. Of the remaining 67 cases only three were subsequently convicted of arson, one in the same year and the other two after thirteen and fifteen years; two of these had been in mental hospitals. Although some of course may have committed arson without detection, the risk seemed much less than had been supposed.

The reverse process, of studying the criminality of those with well defined mental disorder, has been undertaken by Gunn in a series of well controlled studies. He examined all epileptics sent to all prisons in 1966 together with a control group of non-epileptic prisoners, and a group of non-offending epileptics treated at a psychiatric hospital (31). The incidence of epilepsy in prisoners is higher than in the general community, 7.1 per thousand. Yet there was no difference in offence behaviour (32), very few offences could be related to disturbance of consciousness (33), and there was no special relationship with drinking disorders (34); but the offenders showed rather more anxiety, depression and experienced suicidal thoughts and had made suicidal attempts. The early social background of both groups of prisoners was similarly disordered—large families, poverty, parental loss, etc. Gunn and Bonn (32) concluded that conduct disorders in epileptic children were mainly caused by the disordered home background rather than the epilepsy. With adults, analysis was more complex, but it seemed that both organic and social factors accounted for the excess in prison, and that social factors played a bigger role than the organic. The question was raised whether severe deprivation in childhood might not only cause anti-social behaviour but contribute to causing epilepsy by physical deprivation or trauma (31).

Criminal careers

The forensic psychiatrist's practice differs from that of the general psychiatrist in that he is rarely in complete control of the treatment of offenders. He must collaborate with child care and prison authorities, probation officers, or the courts; adding a treatment component to the work of others and often confined to making an accurate diagnosis and, especially, a prognosis. Some assessment of prognosis is constantly demanded by the courts in cases remanded for a medical report and becomes increasingly important when an assessment of future dangerousness has to be made or the Parole Board has to consider release. The heavily biased lessons of clinical experience need to be constantly improved by systematic follow-up studies and a knowledge of normal expectations in criminal careers. Though it often seems to the outsider that forensic psychiatry deals with hopelessly intractable material, the situation is in reality quite the reverse. While medicine to an increasing extent deals with the progressive decay of later life, forensic psychiatrists know that nearly all offenders moderate or abandon criminal behaviour by the time they are forty—at least to the extent of not getting caught! The question is how to accelerate a process of recovery which is likely to occur in the great majority.

There has been a steady accumulation of data about the chances of conviction in the general juvenile population by West (4), Douglas (6) and Power (5), and of the chances of further reconviction, treated partly by these authors and also by the Home Office study in *Sentence of the Court*, which dealt with reconvictions at different ages of first court appearance (1971). The two hundred Borstal boys studied in 1951-53 have now been followed for ten to twelve years and again later (59). At the ten to twelve year stage 45% had no further convictions at any time or extremely minor ones, but the rest had divided themselves into various patterns—5% were 'petty persistent offenders' with repeated fines or very short sentences for minor assaults, probably becoming alcoholics; 5% had committed sporadic offences with long quiescent periods; 15% were 'late recoveries' who were reconvicted for the first three and a half years and appeared as Borstal failures, but were not reconvicted at least in the next five to seven years; 10% were 'late failures', who did well at first but appeared to start a further criminal career three to six years later; and lastly 20% became serious persistent offenders, attracting heavy sentences for major crimes. After ten to twelve years the 'recovery rate' stands at 63% with the possible addition of 3% of the petty persistent and 4% sporadic offenders who appear to be slowing down in their reconvictions.

One of the problems of assessing criminal careers is that although one can count up reconvictions, there is usually no way of assessing the gravity of the offence except by the punishment it received, which is very unreliable. Sellin and Wolfgang (60) attempted to overcome this difficulty by applying a points system for severity, the number of points attached to a particular type of crime being awarded after ratings made by a sample of the general public. Scott (61) applied this method to the reconvictions of approved school boys, showing that although 64% were reconvicted in three years, 74% of their subsequent offences were very minor.

Further aspects of the criminal career came to light in the course of a study—originally for aftercare purposes—of a carefully stratified sample of 300 prisoners in three London prisons serving more than twenty-eight days (which excluded the 'drunks') (35). There was a great range, of course; 35% were aged under twenty-six, and 21% over forty. Since all were interviewed, information about juvenile offences (which are sometimes not recorded for adults with many convictions) were fairly reliably recorded; nevertheless only 36% had had convictions as juveniles and a further 22% under age twenty-one. A third had been in prison on three or more occasions; and 16% on six or more occasions.

In general the examinations and history supported the very broad generalization that the ex-juvenile delinquent who persists tends to have been more aggressive in attitude, and with poorer relationships, referred to as psychopathic; while the older offender with convictions only as an adult is more passive-inadequate, labelled as neurotic, from large, poor families with low expectations in life and delinquent parents or siblings.

Only 2% were considered psychotic, but 10% had a history of mental hospital admissions. There were a few schizophrenic defect states and subnormals, but half of the men with a mental history were alcoholic depressives; some had had clear-cut depressive illnesses, but most had had very short admissions to hospital for suicidal attempts.

This psychiatric group overlapped closely with the 20% who were first convicted after thirty, over half of whom were alcoholic, Usually some calamity, death or loss of supportive parents or wife, had precipitated depressions and drinking and thereafter they seemed unable to keep out of prison.

The problem of alcoholism, usually in the form of periodic or problem drinking rather than severe chronic alcoholism (found mainly among those serving twenty-eight days for drunken offences, which were excluded), seemed of paramount importance in chronic recidivism. For the whole group of prisoners, 40% had previous convictions for drunkenness or admitted problem drinking; but among those with six or more prison sentences or more than thirteen convictions the proportion was 69%, and follow-up showed that they were more often and more rapidly reconvicted in the year following release. Like other alcoholic populations they contained excessive numbers of Scots, Irish and Roman Catholics, were more often separated, divorced or unmarried, unemployed or out of touch with any relatives. They were heavily concentrated among those with two or more aggressive offences (usually minor drunken assaults on the police rather than major violent crimes), and if a prisoner had a mixed or poly-criminal record of property, sexual, and violent offences, he was almost invariably an excessive drinker.

Female crime

One of the cardinal features of criminal behaviour is that women are involved so much less than men. Nine men are convicted of offences of all types for every one woman, and among juveniles about six boys for every girl. The anti-social threat which they represent, which may be measured by the number in prison, is even lower; thirty-three men are sentenced to prison for every woman. In physical and psychiatric illnesses the sexes do not differ so greatly, and the difference might be taken as proof that the main causation of crime must be social. Yet there are biological, psychological, and social differences at all levels which suggest that the situation is far more complex and these differences provide a rich source of hypotheses about criminal behaviour. At least one would suppose that those women who do break the law with any persistence would be psychologically and psychiatrically more deviant than men, and all studies confirm that this is the case. Juvenile girls commit offences—especially shoplifting—with some frequency, but few are reconvicted as adults. When 350 girls of fifteen or sixteen who had been sent to a remand home for reports for offences or for being in need of care and control (a selection of the more disturbed girls) were followed for fifteen years, 25% received some conviction as an adult (usually once for theft), 6% had received a prison sentence and 10% a conviction for prostitution (largely the same group). Among a six-months total sample of all juvenile girls appearing before the London juvenile courts, 13% had convictions as adults, 2% had been in prison and 2% convicted of prostitution (36). Yet in a study of girls admitted to approved schools in 1958, Cowie, Cowie and Slater (37) considered that 32% showed abnormality of personality of a basic kind or oncoming mental illness, 20% had psychiatric symptoms of some severity, and only 48% were psychiatrically normal. When followed up, 8% were at some time admitted to mental hospitals and 4% attempted suicide. Although disorders may not be manifested in crime, the outlook for a reasonably happy life is not very favourable, according to Lee Robins' researches (38). She interviewed 115 girls seen in the child guidance clinic thirty years before for theft or running away, etc.: 10% were considered well adjusted, 22% 'undiagnosed but sick', 3% alcoholic, 9% psychotic, 44% neurotic, and 12% with multiple problems which she classed together as 'sociopathic'. Nearly all had married, but 70% had divorced. They had—perhaps fortunately—fewer children than average (47% were childless) but 65% of their children were showing behaviour disorders. The main effect of the maladjusted women is to help to produce the next generation's male delinquents.

There is a marked tendency for the small proportion of adolescent girls who do not stabilize, or at least avoid offences in the next few years, to enter a rapid downward spiral of social and personal maladjustment, convictions for theft, drunkenness, and prostitution, following in rapid succession. A few achieve a personally satisfying existence within an eccentric or underworld life. The choice of husbands becomes limited to male delinquents and it seems that few of these are successful enough to provide a stable home life. Among the few young adult women committed to Borstal the degree of psychiatric disturbance is quite marked; a third have been in mental hospitals (39).

A relatively new complication in the life of the adolescent girl has been the abuse of drugs, reflected in later admissions to Holloway prison. This has been investigated by Noble and his colleagues (19, 20). Among 227 girls in the remand home in 1966-68 who were taking non-narcotic drugs, 20% went on to take narcotic drugs in the next three years (a very similar figure was found among the boys), and 33 girls were already taking narcotics, compared with only 1% of a control group of remand home girls. Comparing three matched groups of thirty girls (those progressing to 'hard drugs', those not escalating, and those already on narcotics), the vulnerable group were taking a wider range of mixed soft drugs, and were more heavily involved in the drug culture. There was a more frequent history of mental hospital admissions, suicide, and depressive symptoms. Although half of the mothers in each group had abnormal personalities, those who went on to narcotic use had a more abnormal father. The girls came more often from a middle-class background with warring or separated parents with whom there was marked hostility. A Home Office study (39) has also confirmed that one of the few differentiating factors in the drug taker who goes on to taking hard drugs is the mental disturbance (including mental hospital admission) of parents of the teenagers. D'Orban (26, 40) studied sixty-six heroin-dependent young women admitted to Holloway prison in eighteen months in 1967-68, and has subsequently followed them. Twenty-four were no longer notified as addicted four years later. There was, however, no evidence that either hospital admission, prison sentences, or other measures were more successful than others in dealing with them.

In 1967 every fourth girl or woman admitted to Holloway prison (numbering 638) was studied (41). Holloway received half of all women sentenced to prison and 70% of those remanded for medical reports; the problem of sampling is much less difficult with women. One of the main objects of this study was to throw light on the legal and administrative aspects of the management of women offenders (see later). In the present context, however, the striking finding was the degree of psychiatric morbidity. Holloway is very largely a remand prison, some 80% of receptions being for investigation. Of the total intake, 20% are sentenced to prison (half having been remanded for enquiries beforehand) and 10% imprisoned in default of payment of a fine (usually for drunkenness). Yet in spite of the fact that fairly large numbers of young women aged under twenty-three are remanded for social enquiries without much evidence of serious maladjustment, the proportion of psychiatric abnormality is high in all the groups, whether remanded for social enquiries or for medical reports, imprisoned in default of a fine, or sentenced without enquiry. Major physical health problems were found in 15-20%, mental ill-health problems in 15-40% of different groups including inpatient treatment in the last three years in 14-26%, and a further 5-10% had such admissions more than three years before: 20-30% had attempted suicide at some time, 5-10% were alcoholic and 10-20% had sexually transmitted disease. A history of past or present prostitution was found in 25-35%. In the Special Hospitals for psychotic, subnormal, or psychopathic patients with violent tendencies, the proportion of women (one to three or four men) is ten times higher than in the prisons. They tend to be transferred there after proving unmanageable in prison rather than being committed directly by the courts. Tennent (42) has studied the sizeable group of arsonists in Special Hospitals. A minority have actually been convicted of arson; they tended to be psychotic women who had impulsively started fires in mental hospitals and were therefore regarded as especially dangerous.

That mental ill-health is not confined to those who are admitted to prison for investigation or on sentence is shown in a study of shoplifting (14). In 1959 all 500 women convicted of shoplifting in three inner and outer London courts were studied; only 4% were sent to prison and nearly all were merely fined. About 30% were foreign girls or women (the proportion of these foreigners convicted in the West End of London has now reached 65-70%) who rarely showed any mental abnormality. Among the British first offenders (about half of all) 2.5% were psychotic or mentally defective and 12% neurotic (among recidivists 9% and 11% respectively). Ten years later all these women were followed up with regard to subsequent convictions and also mental hospital admissions, though the latter could only be checked for the years 1965-70, i.e. starting five years after the offence (43). The criminal follow-up suggested four groups: (a) those convicted only once in their life in 1959 (70%); (b) those convicted before 1959 but not since (10%); (c) those convicted in 1958 and since but not before (10%); and (d) those convicted before and after 1959. One might expect the last group to be more unstable. The rate of mental hospital admissions over the five-year period for the general population of middle-aged women of this sort is about 2.5%. For the first group of sole offenders the rate was 5.8%, and for the others 2%, 12% and 20% respectively. For the whole group the admission rate was 8.5%—three times the national average. The majority of admissions were for depression, including suicidal attempts. There seemed some justification therefore for the clinical view that shoplifting in some middle-aged women marked the onset of depressive breakdowns, though in some it seemed that the loss of reputation accompanying arrest for impulsive shoplifting may have started a depressive trend. A group of cases sentenced to prison and seen in 1957 (all with several previous convictions) seemed to be almost equally divided into those who were quite level-headed professionals and those who were manifestly abnormal 'compulsive' shoplifters of objects of little or no value who had failed to respond to repeated attempts at medical treatment.

A psychological facet of some importance in the criminality of women is the wide occurrence of bisexuality or lesbianism. American authors (44) go so far as to state that while in men's prisons the social structure is largely determined by an anti-authoritarian and aggressive hierarchy, the social system in women's prisons is based upon a network of homosexual relationships. This is probably not so true in England, where women receive very much shorter sentences and at a later stage in life (45). Nevertheless, nearly half the series of narcotic dependent women described by D'Orban (26) showed homosexual orientation, and this was true of several other groups—especially prostitutes, among whom 16% were lesbian or markedly bisexual. In a society which is very largely controlled by men, there are considerable difficulties for girls with little education to achieve a satisfactory life which does not depend upon a sexual relationship with a man, and the adolescent whose experience has given her a deep distrust of male figures or an attitude of actual hostility, moves quickly into deviant groups.

Treatment

Research into the effectiveness of the varieties of treatment of delinquents has of course been a continuing pre-occupation. Treatment in this sense must include all that happens to an offender as a result of his arrest. The place of psychiatric treatment among these various influences presents a difficulty. A great many studies have been made of the results of particular 'treatments'—Borstal, detention centres, probation, etc. These may throw light upon the problems of these services, but their effectiveness can only be decided by comparison with a group not receiving this treatment. Yet a comparison of boys sent to detention centres with boys put on probation, for example, assumes that the court which made this discrimination did so at random, or on the basis of information which was quite irrelevant to treatment needs, which can hardly be assumed to be the case. Even when two groups are matched in relation to age, previous convictions and types of crime, for example, it is difficult to be sure that these are the only factors of importance, and that the two groups can be regarded as sufficiently similar.

One solution, especially in American studies, has been to take offenders committed to a particular form of institutional treatment and divide them at random into those who receive the standard or conventional form of treatment, and those exposed to some new method. This was adopted in the Highfields study (46) in which a randomly selected group of boys sent to institutional training was exposed to a shorter more intensive form of 'guided group interaction' using group therapy methods. The outcome of this study was that there was little difference in the outcome for white boys (except that the new treatment was shorter and possibly less expensive) but that there was a significant improvement in the response of Negro boys, perhaps because it was a more novel experience for them to be treated with individual care and concern. Random selection may be a valid method if the numbers involved are large enough to be able to presume that individual differences have been ironed out, but this is rarely possible.

Most of these studies have in fact been unable to show that it makes a great difference whether, for example, a boy is sentenced to three months in a detention centre or twelve to eighteen months in Borstal, or subjected to an alternative. A recent very detailed study of the consequence of adopting a more individual approach to the training of Borstal boys showed no significant difference in the rate of conviction in the first eighteen months of release, but this reconviction rate may not be a fair test (47). Since it is contrary to clinical and indeed human experience that offenders do not respond in varying ways to the treatment they receive—though it may of course be that the treatment is frequently insufficient—the theory was entertained that a form of treatment might be effective with some, but not only ineffective but actively harmful or confusing to others. This theory received some support in the Pico experiment (48), in which institutionalized boys were randomly allocated to either the standard care or a more intensive psychotherapeutically oriented type of treatment. Each group was however divided into those considered 'amenable' and 'non-amenable'. The amenables tended to be anxious, able to perceive they had problems and able to discuss them. Amenables subjected to the treatment did better than those without it. But though the results were somewhat inconclusive it seemed that non-amenables not only did not respond to the treatment, but did rather worse when subjected to it. In one of the few studies made in the UK, Craft (49) allocated psychopathic young offenders to either a mental hospital ward run on permissive self-governing lines, or a ward with a more conventional 'paternalistic' directive regime. The paternalistic regime appeared more successful for this type of boy with few inner resources.

It is clear that one has to consider types of offender in relation to different types of treatment, and both may be difficult to categorize. In a large recent study of the effectiveness of probation (50) the officers were invited to classify probationers into those who appeared to need support or control. The highest rate of success occurred in those who were rated as neither needing support nor control, suggesting that at least part of the very successful results were in relation to those who might not have needed probation at all, but might have been dealt with, for example, by conditional discharge or fines.

The most sophisticated of such studies has been in the massive Community Treatment Project of California, directed by Professor Warren (51). Unfortunately, many of the results are available only in privately circulated form. The first phase consisted of setting aside a group of boys aged fourteen to eighteen committed to the institutional care of the Youth Authority, leaving out a small proportion whose incorporation in the project would have caused public alarm. They were carefully classified into seven groups according to 'levels of immaturity in interpersonal relations'—a diagnostic approach of great clinical interest since it focused upon personality attributes which are almost certainly related to prognosis. Some in each group were left to continue institutional training while the experimental group were set at liberty at once, supervised very closely by officers with a case load of only eight to ten, and using methods of treatment devised separately for each type, with more directive and controlling methods for the more psychologically imma-ture and more stress on individual interpersonal relationships and conflict-resolution for the matured 'neurotic' boy. The first phase showed conclusively that the boys at liberty were treated more successfully than in institutions, a fact which led to general changes in public policy. In later phases the problem of matching the type of officer to the type of probationer has received close study. It has always been recognized that 'treatment' is closely related to the personality of the doctor or social worker dealing with the case, and success often seems to be dependent upon good 'matching'. Secondly, there is the problem of those who do not respond to treatment at liberty. As time has passed it has emerged that certain categories are much commoner than others, leading almost to a division into mature, and immature, and a demonstration that the immature may respond better to a preliminary period of institutional treatment. Also, although it may seem at first sight that treatment on probation is a substantial saving on institutional treatment, the long-term results have shown that this is not the case, if sufficiently concentrated supervision is provided. Economy is probably not a good argument for at least a great deal of penal reform; good treatment tends to be expensive.

The place of psychiatric treatment within this broad field of psychosocial treatment is difficult to define. It is probably generally accepted today that individualized psychiatric treatment is rarely sufficient for more than a small proportion of offenders, but that success depends upon the combination of psychological and social treatment in which the predominant importance of the roles of the psychiatrist and the probation officer or prison officer fluctuates.

The value of psychiatric treatment within the prison service is being investigated by J.C. Gunn and his colleagues in a large-scale study which combines some of the elements of 'treatment research' with what will be described as 'administrative research'. The latter consists in studying the means of making existing systems more effective rather than devising or testing new methods of treatment. In the prisons, those thought to be in need of psychiatric treatment may be transferred to Wormwood Scrubs prison (among other centres) where they receive individual 'outpatient' treatment (attending the hospital regularly from the main prison) or as inpatients in the hospital; other cases are selected with their agreement to go to Grendon psychiatric prison where treatment is not individual but on the basis of community therapy in which all levels of staff participate. Gunn has com-pared those referred for treatment to Wormwood Scrubs or to Grendon with a carefully matched group of controls in other prisons, and followed them up after release. Great care was taken to test the reliability of information by comparing the results of interviews by two observers. Much progress has also been made in recent years (52, 53), in testing the reliability of questionnaires relating to mental symptoms and relating these to standardized psychiatric interviews in which it can be shown that after some training psychiatrists can arrive at similar ratings of symptomatology and mental health. In Grendon, methods have also been found to assess changes in attitude during treatment. The final results are not available, but on the way it has been possible to delineate, for example, the characteristics of 20% of Grendon prisoners who turn out to be unsuitable in a relatively short time either because they ask to leave, are found unsutiable or enforce their transfer by breaking the few rules which they are told are fundamental (e.g. not trying to escape, importing alcohol and drugs, etc.). During the period of study a fortunate opportunity occurred to take part in a 10% census of the prison population in the South East of England undertaken by the Home Office. Mental Health question-naires were completed by about 80% of those prisoners in this sample, and a check on their reliability was made by arranging for a 10% sample of these (i.e. 1% of the whole) to be interviewed by a group of psychiatrists either experi-enced or trained in the standardized interveiw. Elaborated in many ways, these studies make progress with the vexed question of the variability in psychiatric opinion, and the infinitely more difficult question of what constitutes a 'psychiatric case' and 'who needs treatment'. It was concluded that the best criteria of a 'psychiatric case' were symptomatology, motivation, and previ-ous psychiatric treatment. Motivation for treatment may be absent in psychot-ics, but here symptoms are at their most obvious. Experience in Grendon and throughout the prison service tends to emphasize the cardinal importance of motivation to seek help. On this basis some 35% of the prison census population were thought to be 'psychiatric cases', a figure close to the 31% estimated by Bluglass (54) in the prison population of Perth. Difficulties occur of course in relation to the chronic nature of many of these abnormali-ties.

Administrative research

Nowadays there is much more interest in social and administrative processes affecting the treatment of offenders. This is of course particularly important in relation to criminology, where so many different processes are at work—the public who report crime, the police who investigate and arrest, the courts, the probation, penal and medical personnel—all with different attitudes and codes of practice. Deliberate decisions may have less effect on what happens than is often supposed.

Dr Gunn's study dealt not with the effectiveness of treatment, but with the processes by which an offender comes to receive treatment, and whether these procedures could be made more efficient. A second study by the Prison Medical Research Unit, supported by the Home Office, dealt with the machinery by which the courts obtained medical reports on offenders, which is often the first and most crucial step in obtaining psychiatric treatment in suitable cases. Between 1961 and 1971 the number of reports on offenders remanded in prison doubled, from 6366 to nearly 13,000. The total number of offenders coming before the courts increased by 30% in this time so the proportion has not increased so greatly, but nevertheless the work of the Prison Medical Service has doubled. Recent legislation has sought to reduce the number of offenders remanded in custody before sentence since the vast majority do not receive a prison sentence afterwards, but the need for a medical report is regarded in law and practice as a good reason for a custodial remand although facilities are increasingly available in the Health Service to obtain reports on bail. The research aimed to study the causes and consequences of this system as it has grown up. It needed quite elaborate procedures to find out how many offenders were dealt with on bail, which is not systematically recorded (55, 56).

All the medical reports requested, in custody or on bail, by the eighteen Inner London magistrates courts in 1969 were examined (about 4000, or one-third of the national total), and all the five hundred reports prepared in a Wessex Regional Hospital Board area as well as a more detailed clinical study of Wessex reports in 1970. The total 'turnover' of each of the courts by age, sex, offence and sentence was also obtained in order to show how the courts selected cases for reports; these are only requested for about 1-2% of all offenders, but for indictable offences the proportion reached 8% and for some offences (e.g. sex offences) about 20%. It was found that in London male cases only, about 10% of reports were prepared on bail compared with 35% in Wessex. This was associated with a very different proportion of recommendations for medical treatment. In London 8% obtained a medical disposal (3% probation with a condition of psychiatric treatment, Section 4, Criminal Justice Act, and 5% hospital orders, Section 60, Mental Health Act) but in Wessex 22% (14% Section 4 and 8% Section 60). The balance of probation or hospital admissions was clearly nearer to nature in Wessex, since milder cases suitable for outpatient treatment must necessarily be commoner than cases needing hospital admission. There was little to indicate that the population of offenders coming before the courts was very different, though London had a large proportion of down-and-out type offences and probably attracts the chronic psychotic vagrant. One of the main reasons why Wessex magistrates obtained a proportionately smaller but more accurately selected group of offenders is almost certainly that the Probation Service there interviews nearly all offenders and picks out those with a psychiatric history (21% of the men and no less than 40% of the women had had a mental hospital contact in the last year). In London the turnover of cases is so large that the Probation Services cannot see all cases and magistrates act on less information. There is also almost certainly a medical problem that in custody a prison medical officer must select cases and then send for a consultant to visit and agree to admit the patient or treat him as an outpatient. In serious cases this would always be done, but in lesser cases there may be more reluctance to arrange for outpatient treatment which involves asking the consultant to visit the prison. When the consultant sees the case himself on bail he is more likely to decide whom he feels he can help by outpatient treatment. More recently bail clinics have been set up at Brixton and Holloway prisons, but they are not greatly used; it seems that the traditional pattern of obtaining reports in custody tends to limit the amount of treatment offered to offenders.

Some 9% of those medically remanded are remanded a second time within a year for a medical report. Soothill (57) has looked at the characteristics of this group. Sometimes a court has no knowledge that a medical report has recently been prepared for another court, but in many cases it seems that the magistrates are pressing the doctors to suggest some non-penal solution to an almost insoluble social problem.

A large proportion of women remanded to Holloway prison are sent there partly or wholly for medical reports and about 80% do not subsequently receive a custodial sentence or hospital admission (58). Interviews suggested that about 39% were judged to be suitable for bail on general assessment, and this view was supported by using the American 'Vera System' by which criteria on a points system were experimentally evolved to establish suitability for bail; 34% were bailable on these criteria. Moreover in 29% the police or the courts themselves had previously bailed the offender before the decision had been made to remand in custody for a medical report. Among those remanded in custody were a number who had dependent children; Gibbs (59), working upon information from the survey, has examined the problem of what happens to the children of women in custody.

Similar studies are being made of the criteria which appeared to be used in practice rather than in theory for admission to the Special Hospitals for abnormal offenders who are violent or dangerous. Research of this kind, which can point to areas in which overstrained services can be improved without cost by pointing out unsuspected barriers to efficiency, may prove increasingly useful.

References

(1) Christies, N., Andenaes, J. and Skirkbekk, S. (1965) A study of self reported crime. In *Scand. Stud. Crim.*, Ed. K.O. Christiansen, *1*, 86-116. London, Tavistock.

(2) Elmhorn, K. (1965) Study on self reported delinquency among school children in Stockholm. In *Scand. Stud. Crim.*, Ed. K.O. Christiansen, *1*, 117-46. London, Tavistock.

(3) Belson, W.A. (1968) The extent of stealing by London boys and some of its origins. *Advances in Science, 25*, 171-84.

(4) West, D.J. (1973) *Who becomes Delinquent?* London, Heinemann.

(5) Power, M.J. (1965) An attempt to identify at first appearance before the courts those at risk of becoming persistent juvenile offenders. *Proc. R. Soc. Med., 58*, 704-5.

(6) Douglas, J.W.B. (1966) Delinquency and social class. *Br. J. Crim., 6*, 294-302.

(7) Wadsworth, M.E.J. (1972) See (4).

(8) Szasz, T. (1970) *The Manufacture of Madness.* London, Routledge.

(9) Taylor, I., Walton, P. and Young, J. (1973) *The New Criminology.* London, Routledge.

(10) Gibbens, T.C.N. (1956) *Cruel Parents.* London, Institute for the Study and Treatment of Delinquency.

(11) Shepherd, M. (1961) Morbid jealousy. *J. ment. Sci., 107*, 687-753.

(12) Mowat, R.R. (1966) *Morbid Jealousy and Murder.* London, Tavistock.

(13) Gibbens, T.C.N. (1958) Car thieves. *Br. J. Delinq., 8*, 257.

(14) Gibbens, T.C.N. and Prince, J. (1962) *Shoplifting.* London, Institute for the Study and Treatment of Delinquency.

(15) Scott, P.D. (1964) In *The Pathology and Treatment of Sexual Deviation*, Ed. I. Rosen. Oxford, Pergamon.

(16) Gibbens, T.C.N. (1957) Juvenile prostitution. *Br. J. Delinq., 8*, 3.

(17) Gibbens, T.C.N. (1957) Sexual behaviour of young criminals. *J. ment. Sci., 103*, 527-39.

(18) Noble, P.J. (1979) Drug-taking in delinquent boys. *Br. med. J., 1*, 102-5.

(19) Noble, P.J., and Gorell Barnes, G.M. (1971) Drug-taking in adolescent girls: factors associated with progression to narcotics use. *Br. med. J., 2*, 620-3.

(20) Noble, P.J., Hart, T. and Nation, R.R.N. (1972) Correlates and outcome of illicit drug use by teenage girls. *Br. J. Psychiat., 120*, 497-505.

(21) Skinner, A.E. and Castle, R.I., (1969) *78 Battered Children—a retrospective study.* Hoddesdon, Herts: Thomas Knight.

(22) Scott, P.D. (1973) Parents who kill their children. *Medicine, Science and the Law, 13*, 120-6.

(23) Scott, P.D. (1973) Memorandum on Battered Wives. Personal communication.

(24) Nichol, R., Gunn, J.C., Foggitt, R. and Gristwood, J. (1972) Quantitative assessment of violence in adult and young offenders. *Medicine, Science and the Law, 12*, 275-82.

(25) Schofield, M. (1965) *Sociological Aspects of Homosexuality.* London, Longman.

(26) d'Orban, P.T. (1970) Heroin dependence and delinquency in women—a study of heroin addicts in Holloway prison. *Br. J. Addict., 65*, 67-78.

(27) d'Orban, P.T. (1972) Baby stealing. *Br. med. J., 1,* 635-9.
(28) Soothill, K.L. and Pope, P.J. (1973) Arson: a twenty year cohort study. *Medicine, Science and the Law, 13,* 127-38.
(29) Hurley, W.P. and Monahan, T.M. (1969) Arson: the criminal and the crime. *Br. J. Crim., 9,* 4-21.
(30) Pichaud, M. (1958) *Bull. Int. Soc. Crim., 1,* 77.
(31) Gunn, J. (1974) Social factors and epileptics in prison. *Br. J. Psychiat., 124,* 509-17.
(32) Gunn, J. and Bonn, J. (1971) Criminality and violence in epileptic prisoners. *Br. J. Psychiat., 118,* 337-43.
(33) Gunn, J. and Fenton, G. (1971) Epilepsy, automatism and crime. *Lancet, 1,* 1173-6.
(34) Gunn, J. and Fenton, G. (1972) Epileptic prisoners and their drinking problems. *Epilepsia, 13,* 489-97.
(35) Gibbens, T.C.N. and Silberman, M. (1970) Alcoholism among prisoners. *Psychol. Med., 1,* 73-8.
(36) Gibbens, T.C.N. and Way, C.K. (1971) Follow-up of adolescent delinquent girls. Unpublished.
(37) Cowie, J., Cowie, V. and Slater, E. (1968) *Delinquency in Girls.* London, Heinemann.
(38) Robins, L.N. (1966) *Deviant Children Grown Up.* Baltimore, Williams and Wilkins.
(39) Goodman, N. (1967) *Studies of Female Offenders: a Home Office Research Unit Report.* London, HMSO.
(40) d'Orban, P.T. (1974) Court sentences in female narcotic addicts. *Br. J. Addict., 69,* 167-71.
(41) Gibbens, T.C.N. and Silberman, M. (1971) Female offenders. *British Journal of Hospital Medicine,* 279-86.
(42) Tennent, T.G., McQuaid, A., Loughnane, T. and Hands, N.J. (1971) Female arsonists. *Br. J. Psychiat., 119,* 497-502.
(43) Gibbens, T.C.N., Palmer, C. and Prince, J. (1971) Mental health aspects of shoplifting. *Br. med. J., 3,* 612-15.
(44) Ward, D.A. and Kassenbaum, G.G. (1966) *Women's Prison.* London, Weidenfeld.
(45) Kelley, J. (1967) *When the Gates Shut.* London, Longman.
(46) Weeks, A.H. (1958) *Youthful Offenders at Highfields.* University of Michigan Press.
(47) Bottoms, A.E. and McClintock, F.H. (1973) *Criminals Coming of Age.* London, Heinemann.
(48) Adams, S. (1961) *Interaction between individual interview therapy and treatment amenability in Youth Authority Wards.* Sacramento, California Board of Corrections.
(49) Craft, M.J. (1966) *Psychopathic Disorders and their Assessment.* Oxford, Pergamon Press.
(50) Folkard, S. (1966) *Probation Research. A Preliminary Report.* Home Office Research Unit Report, No. 7. London, HMSO.
(51) Warren, M.Q. (1972) Community Treatment Project. In *Sociology of Punishment and Correction,* Eds. N. Johnson, L. Savitz and M.E. Wolfgang. New York, Wiley.
(52) Goldberg, D. (1972) *The Detection of Psychiatric Illness by Questionnaire.* Maudsley Monograph, No. 21. London, Oxford University Press.
(53) Derogatis, L.R., Lipman, R.S. and Covi, L. (1973) SCL-90: an out-patient psychiatric rating scale. *Psychopharm. Bull., 9,* 13-28.
(54) Bluglass, R.S. (1966) A psychiatric study of Scottish convicted prisoners. M.D. thesis.
(55) Soothill, K.L. and Pope, P.J. (1974) *Medical remands in magistrates' courts.* London, Institute for the Study and Treatment of Delinquency.
(56) Gibbens, T.C.N., Soothill, K.L. and Pope, P.J. (1977) *Medical Remands.* Maudsley Monograph No. 25. London, Oxford University Press.
(57) Soothill, K.L. (1974) Repeated medical remands. *Medicine, Science and the Law, 14,* 189-99.
(58) Dell, S. and Gibbens, T.C.N. (1971) Remands of women offenders for medical reports. *Medicine, Science and the Law, 11,* 117-27.
(59) Gibbs, C. (1971) The effect of the imprisonment of women upon their children. *Br. J. Crim., 11,* 113-30.
(60) Sellin, T. and Wolfgang, M.E. (1964) *The Measurement of Delinquency.* New York, Wiley.
(61) Scott, P.D. (1964) Approved school success rates. *Br. J. Crim., 5,* 525-56.

4. Developments in research on the psychobiology of aggression

David A. Hamburg

Although there are obvious reasons for scientific interest in the evolutionary and developmental origins of human aggressive tendencies (1, 2, 3, 4), there has been little work on this subject. When the first version of this paper was in preparation for the Sir Geoffrey Vickers lecture of 1970, very little research on the psychobiology of aggression in humans or non-human primates was available. In the intervening years, an impressive upsurge of new work has become available. Major reviews cover evolutionary (5, 6), developmental (7, 8), endocrine (9, 10), adaptive (11), neurological (10. 12), and interdisciplinary approaches (13). Though beyond the scope of this paper, several excellent reviews of social science contributions have been published (14, 15, 16, 17, 18, 19). Moreover, an interdisciplinary research organization has been formed (International Society for Research on Aggression); and a new journal is making its appearance *(Aggressive Behavior)*. Here, a few of these lines of inquiry will be sketched, based in part on the work of my colleagues at Stanford University, especially those associated with the Laboratory of Stress and Conflict.

Aggressive behaviour of non-human primates in natural habitats

The first wave of scientific studies of non-human primates in their natural habitats occurred shortly before World War II. The war disrupted such studies and it was not until the late 1950s that they were resumed in earnest. Since then they have been burgeoning (20, 21, 22, 23, 24). These studies have the special advantage of providing insights into the adaptive properties of behaviour, including social behaviour. These animals, who biologically are relatively closely related to the human species, are observed as they meet their energy requirements, cope with dangers, reproduce, and assist their young in meeting environmental requirements. In this context it is possible to observe the forms and circumstances of aggressive behaviour, and to obtain clues regarding the adaptive significance of such behaviour.

The first two waves of primate field studies undertook a general description of major categories of behaviour, usually including aggression, but not sharply focusing on this kind of behaviour. Indeed, at the time of our initial field work, no study had been primarily directed toward the clarification of aggressive behaviour. Since then, much more attention has been directed toward these questions in primate field studies, including a major, long-term

A revised form of the Sir Geoffrey Vickers Lecture of 18 February 1970, an abridged version of which was published in *Nature* , 1971, *203*, 19-23.

effort in our collaborative programme with Dr Jane Goodall at the Gombe Stream Research Centre in Tanzania. These studies have mainly dealt with chimpanzees, the species most closely related of all living organisms to *Homo sapiens* (25). In recent years, the Gombe research has also dealt with baboons, largest of the old world monkeys. The observations of our group in many ways coincide with those of such pioneering workers as Hall, DeVore, Washburn, Altmann, Rowell and Ransom (26, 27, 28, 29, 30, 31, 32). The research directed by Goodall at the Gombe Stream Reserve in Tanzania (33, 34, 35, 36) has the advantage of detailed, systematic, close range, longitudinal observation with full recognition of individual animals and their habituation to human observers. Increasingly, other studies are moving in this direction.

Threat and attack patterns are most likely to occur among chimpanzees under the following conditions:

1. In daily transactions involving status or dominance;
2. In long-term changes of status or dominance, especially among males;
3. In frustration with animals of similar or higher status, precipitating aggression toward a lower status individual (re-direction);
4. In the protection of infants by adults of both sexes, but especially by females;
5. In defending against potential predators;
6. In killing and eating young animals of other species;
7. In terminating severe disputes among subordinate animals;
8. In association with a presumably painful injury;
9. In the exploration of strange or dangerous areas;
10. In meeting relatively unfamiliar animals;
11. In circumstances where highly valued resources are in short supply;
12. In circumstances where relatively strange animals are crowded in the presence of highly valued resources.

The crowding of strangers in the presence of valued resources appears to be a circumstance of practical significance that increases the probability of serious aggression among non-human primates (37), and may well provide a simple model of conditions fostering human aggression as well. This finding is illustrated by recent research at Gombe. In the early years of her study, Goodall arranged for the provision of bananas as a dietary supplement in a small cleared area of forest (38). This situation has now been systematically studied over a period of years during which the availability of bananas was raised to a higher level and then decreased to a low level at which it is at present maintained. Wrangham found that the attractiveness of the bananas drew unusually large aggregations of chimpanzees into this small area, some of whom probably had relatively little contact with each other in other circumstances (39). During this period, there was a high frequency of aggressive interactions among chimpanzees and also between chimpanzees and baboons. With the decline of banana feeding in the past few years, there is less crowding, two subgroups of adult males have largely withdrawn from each other, and aggressive interactions have become less frequent in the banana area. On a shorter time scale, similar observations have been made in other parts of the forest untouched by man—e.g. when fig trees are in season, since figs are another premium food. These observations are similar to several other studies of non-human primates (40).

In the past few years, the research on chimpanzee behaviour at Gombe has given detailed, systematic, and where possible, quantitative attention to chimpanzee aggressive behaviour. A series of studies under the direction of Goodall, Hinde and myself have been carried out by Bygott, Bauer, Halperin, Wrangham, Pusey and Riss. Most of these are still in progress.

The recently completed study by Bygott (41) adds much new information. He recorded attacks, behaviour patterns indicating that attack was imminent, and responses to both these kinds of behaviour. The often spectacular charging display is a vivid example of intimidating behaviour common among higher primates. Charging displays may be silent or noisy. The former are more dangerous. About 15% of non-vocal charging displays were accompanied by an attack, whereas less than 1% of vocal displays led to an attack, despite the fact that vocal and non-vocal displays were similar in form and occurred with equal frequency. The overwhelming preponderance of attacks were carried out by adult males. Attacks occurred most commonly when individuals encountered each other after a separation exceeding half an hour, often a matter of hours or days. Of 84 attacks by adult males observed in the forest (away from the banana feeding area), 42% occurred within five minutes of encounter between the attacker and his victim. This problem of behaviour upon reunion after separation is being studied in more detail by Bauer (42). It is especially interesting because, in addition to eliciting agonistic behaviour, the circumstance of reunion may elicit 'greeting' behaviour that shows remarkable resemblance to human behaviour in a similar context—e.g. touching, embracing, kissing, and patting one another. Thus, encounter after separation may elicit very different responses: aggression or affection. What are the factors governing this variability of response? Given the increasing evidence of enduring kinship bonds (43), it seems likely that kinship is one important factor here.

There is a tendency for chimpanzee attacks to occur in clusters. An aggressive animal may attack one or more others in rapid order. A screaming individual, having been attacked by one chimpanzee, may elicit another attack by a second animal who appears to be aroused by the screaming. About 30% of attacks occurred within five minutes of a previous attack.

Bygott and other workers at Gombe have found recently that members of different communities tend to avoid meeting each other. Nishida and Kawanaka (44), working elsewhere in Tanzania, have made essentially the same observation. In a valuable new paper, Nishida (45) gives an overview of years of research on wild chimpanzees. There is an impressive conjunction of findings between these investigators and the Gombe group. Increasing evidence at both locations indicates that communities of thirty to fifty individuals tend to be quite distinct from each other, though not totally impermeable. The members of different communities (called by the Japanese workers 'unit groups') tend to avoid each other, and smaller groups give way to larger groups when they meet. Relatively severe aggression tends to occur when members of different communities meet, mainly due to antagonism between adult males. Nishida describes these communities as having well delineated, traditional boundaries. In seven years of observation, none of the adult males and few of the adult females have crossed boundaries between communities.

Within the primary study community at Gombe, a fission has occurred during the past few years. Within each sub-community is a core of closely associated adult males who once were also close with the core males of the other sub-community; but now they are largely separate, wary of each other, and sometimes quite hostile when they meet. Riss (46) observed several episodes of this kind that led to extremely violent interactions between adult males of the two sub-communities.

Sometimes a group of males from one sub-community makes what appears to be a planned journey into the other's range, travelling directly and stopping little to feed until they locate members of the other sub-community (41). These encounters are characterized by vivid charging displays involving all the males of one group, and sometimes attacks as well; but this is often followed by a few hours in which the groups groom, feed and travel together, as they did regularly only a few years ago. Then the 'invading' group returns to its usual range.

These new observations of free-living chimpanzees by two independent groups of investigators conducting careful, longitudinal studies considerably strengthen the concept that stranger-contact is a powerful instigator of aggressive behaviour in higher primates (39, 40). The concept emcompasses relative strangeness involving individuals who have considerable familiarity with each other but are separated sufficiently in time or space to heighten the probability of aggression upon contact.

Bygott (41) has recently attempted a synthesis of information on chimpanzee aggressive behaviour in the context of their distinctive community structure in natural habitats. The following statement summarizes his view:

'The peculiar structure of a chimpanzee community may be in part an adaptation to life in a habitat where food varies seasonally in abundance and distribution. Such food resources can be used most efficiently if a number of chimps collectively inhabit and defend a large range, yet can form large or small parties depending on the type of food which is being eaten at any time of year. It is in the interest of individuals to prevent too many other chimps from sharing their range, and if food abundance is a limiting factor, it may be important for them to repel intruders who might place an additional burden on scarce resources. Territoriality may increase with population density. Certain physical specializations enable chimpanzees to give very loud calls ("pant-hoots") whose frequency increases with the size of a party. . . These may serve the dual function of informing scattered members of the community that a large party has collected (around a food source, or oestrus female), and warning "outsiders" that a large party is in the vicinity and should be avoided. There is a little evidence to suggest that repulsion between parties from different communities is effected through these calls, and may be reinforced by rare but severe gang attacks.'

'The environmental conditions which have brought about the dispersed social structure may not favor a fixed breeding season, as occurs in some primates. Anyway, non-lactating post-menarchal females cycle all year round, which means that adult males have to be in breeding condition all year round. This implies continual high levels of testosterone, and testosterone level in some primates is known to be correlated with dominance and with aggressive frequency. . . . This may explain why adult males display and attack more frequently than other age/sex classes. Such aggressive tendencies might be useful in defense of a communal range, but might hinder adult males from associating with males or females of their own community. The formation of temporary associations seems to be the time when aggressive tendencies are highest, yet one would expect selection to act against individuals who through their aggressiveness were severely hurt in fights, or endangered the life of their own offspring by attacking pregnant females or mothers with infants. Likewise, selection might favor females whose behaviour in such situations prevents accidental damage to their offspring. The "solution" seems to have been, not the elimination of aggressive tendencies in males (which may be an inevitable consequence of sex hormones or may be adaptive in territorial defense), but the evolution of species-specific displays—i.e. charging displays and pant-grunting—by which, respectively, aggressive tendencies may be "redirected" and non-aggressive tendencies expressed by individuals who have not yet come within contact distance.'

There are several reasons for studying baboons: (a) the adaptive success of the baboon-macaque group, having spread widely through Asia and Africa in various habitats; (b) the baboons are the largest monkeys; and (c) the relatively large extent of their ground-living capability, in a type of habitat (savanna) that was probably crucial in the emergence of early man. The species under consideration here is the common olive baboon of East Africa.

In certain circumstances the probability of overt threat behaviour and of fighting is higher than in the other contexts of baboon life (26, 27, 28, 29, 30, 31, 32). These include protection of the troop by adult males against predators; resolution of disputes within the troop by adult males; formation and maintenance of consort pairs at the peak of oestrus; attainment of preferred sleeping sites in the trees, particularly in the presence of predators; acquisition of premium foods such as figs, nuts, and bananas, especially when spatially concentrated rather than widely distributed; dominance interactions, especially in the presence of premium foods, scarcity of sleeping sites, or females in full oestrus; exploration of strange or manifestly dangerous areas, a function largely of adult males; and contact between different troops, especially if such contact is infrequent. But baboons, like chimpanzees, spend much of the day in peaceful activities, and there is abundant evidence of affectional systems, similar to those analysed by Harlow in rhesus macaque (47).

The list of situations eliciting threat-attack patterns in chimpanzees and baboons does not include the defence of a fixed territory (48). Although most higher primates do not live in permanently fixed territories which they defend rigorously, there is a behavioural distinction between currently familiar and relatively unfamiliar territory, as we have seen in the Bygott and Nishida studies. A savanna baboon troop may live in an area of about ten square miles for some months before moving to another nearby area. While it is living in a given area, the behaviour of its members tends to take on distinctive features at the fringes of this currently familiar space: they are highly vigilant, threaten readily, and some males move out a considerable distance beyond females and young in exploring the relatively unfamiliar area. An important topic for future research is the contact between groups in such circumstances. There is considerable caution, vigilance, and agonistic behaviour when groups meet, although usually they avoid serious fighting. Sometimes serious inter-group fighting does occur, for example, among rhesus macaque groups in cities in conditions of crowding, food shortage, and inter-species harassment (49). So too with chimpanzees and gorillas, the two species most closely related biologically to the human.

The observations of aggressive behaviour in higher primates deserve consideration in the framework of an adaptive evolutionary view of aggressive behaviour. Although we cannot be sure of the ways in which aggressive behaviour has functioned adaptively during the course of evolution, the following possibilities deserve serious consideration: (*a*) increasing the means of defence; (*b*) providing access to valued resources such as food, water and females in reproductive condition; (*c*) contributing to effective utilization of the habitat by distributing animals in relation to available resources—a spacing function of inter-group tension; (*d*) resolving serious disputes within the group; (*e*) providing a predictable social environment; (*f*) providing leadership for the group, particularly in dangerous circumstances; and (*g*) differential reproduction—it is plausible (though not proved) that relatively aggressive males are more likely to pass on their genes to subsequent generations than less aggressive males.

Some of these factors may have given selective advantage to aggressive primates, if they could effectively regulate their aggressive behaviour. Primates have well defined cues that usually terminate aggressive sequences, and an elaborate repertoire of submissive behaviour. Most of the time they have a stable dominance hierarchy that contributes to the predictability of the social environment, and they have clear sequences of aggression-submission-reassurance that have elements in common with the behaviour of man. Future research will profit from paying as much attention to the regulation and control of aggressive tendencies as to their sources and instigation.

Hormonal influences on the development of aggressive behaviour

If evolution is given serious consideration, it is difficult to overlook the likelihood that man has a vertebrate-mammalian-primate heritage predisposing him to aggressive behaviour. But what is known of the processes that govern the expression of such predispositions within the individual life cycle? Hormonal influences on brain organization early in life affect later aggressive and sexual behaviour (50, 51, 52). Even brief treatment of newborn female rats with testosterone produces lifelong abolition of female sexual behaviour and a tendency to male patterns of aggressive behaviour. Pregnant rhesus macaques given large doses of testosterone during the second quarter of gestation produced female offspring which were abnormal, with some anatomical and behavioural characteristics of the male type (53). One of the well documented behavioural characteristics of this species is a sex difference in the behaviour of infant monkeys, the males being more aggressive. This difference can be measured reliably in the first few months of life in the laboratory. Similar sex differences in aggressive behaviour have been observed in wild macaques and baboons.

Female infants of mothers given testosterone during pregnancy are more aggressive than normal females. They threaten other infant monkeys more often, initiate play more often, and engage in rough and tumble play more often than do normal females.

During growth and development, many influences can modify the expression of these aggressive patterns. For example, undue infant aggressiveness may be severely punished by larger and more powerful animals, leading to fearful inhibition later in life. In view of these possibilities for environmental influences during development, it is interesting that there is some tendency toward persistence of hyper-aggressive characteristics into adult life in females whose mothers are exposed to testosterone in pregnancy.

Is there any evidence that testosterone has similar effects on the development of behaviour in humans? We have been able to study a few cases of girls who had been exposed to androgens *in utero*, but much more extensive studies have been done in Baltimore and Buffalo. Money and Ehrhardt (54) studied girls in late childhood and adolescence whose brains had been exposed to high levels of early androgen. Those with striking anatomical abnormalities had undergone surgical treatment shortly after birth. By means of interviews and projective tests, information in each of several behavioural categories was obtained from each girl and from at least one parent. The research design undertook to control for observer bias. Results indicated that the early androgenized girls, in contrast with a control group, tended to be described by themselves and others as tomboys, to engage in outdoor sports requiring much energy and vigour, to prefer rough play, and to prefer toys ordinarily chosen by boys (such as guns). The results are at least compatible with the concept that testosterone is one of many influences which shape the development of aggressive behaviour in the human species (55).

The possibility that sex hormones play a role in mediating the development of human aggressive behaviour, especially rough-and-tumble play patterns, has been strengthened by two new studies. The first of these deals with the later effects of prenatal androgens. Ehrhardt, who collaborated with Money in the earlier work at Johns Hopkins, is conducting a new study with Baker on different patients. Their first paper on this study confirms and extends the previous work (56). They studied trends of childhood behaviour over many years through interviews with the children and their mothers, utilizing a semi-structured interview schedule covering general development, play behaviour, and sex-related behaviours such as toy preference, aggression, rehearsal of adult roles, and clothing preferences. Rating scales were developed to permit quantitative estimates of behavioural items. They were able to locate twenty-seven of the thirty-one patients who had been seen in the history of their clinic with the disease congenital adrenal hyperplasia. At the time of study, the age of the offspring ranged from four years to the early twenties; most were in middle childhood and early adolescence. For comparison, a sample of unaffected siblings consisting of eleven females and sixteen males with comparable age ranges was obtained. All children were receiving corrective hormonal therapy, most having begun this treatment very early in life. It had been effective.

The findings are based on comparison with same-sex siblings. In this disorder, the fetus is exposed to exceptionally large amounts of self-generated androgens during pregnancy. In childhood, these fetally androgenized girls showed a clear preference for vigorous, intense physical activity. From an early point in their lives, they sought rough outdoor play. However, there was no significant difference between the androgenized girls and their unaffected siblings in the frequency of starting fights, either verbal or physical. If given a choice of playmates during childhood, the androgenized girls more frequently preferred boys over girls in comparison with the unaffected siblings. The androgenized girls also showed a tendency to choose toys ordinarily associated with boys. Their interest in dolls was very low, and significantly more often than the unaffected siblings they showed indifference or aversion to small infants. A majority of the androgenized girls were regarded by themselves and others as 'tomboys' throughout their childhood, in marked contrast to the unaffected siblings. One of the principal findings is the difference in rough-and-tumble play. The preference for playing with boys and the toys associated with boys is probably secondary to the basic temperamental trait expressed in the enjoyment of rough-and-tumble play.

A new feature of this study is the inclusion of males. Thus, fetally hyper-androgenized males are compared with unaffected (normally androgenized) male siblings. The only significant difference between the two groups is that boys with a history of excess androgen show an exceptionally strong preference for vigorous, rough outdoor activities. This finding is similar to the fetally androgenized girls. Also, the excessively androgenized boys are more likely than their normal brothers to initiate fighting, both physically and verbally.

Another new study has examined the effects of intrauterine oestrogen and progesterone on psychosexual development in boys (57). They studied twenty sons of diabetic mothers who were given moderately high doses of oestrogen and progesterone during pregnancy. These boys were compared with two relevant groups: (a) sons of diabetic mothers who were not given exogenous oestrogen or progesterone; and (b) sons of non-diabetic mothers. Both comparison groups were matched as carefully as possible to the experimental group in several respects: age, social class, living in the same community, and attending the same schools. Behavioural assessment was undertaken on a double-blind basis to the maximum extent possible; it appears to have been successful in respect to boys who are assessed at six years of age, but only partially successful at the age of sixteen.

At age six, there is only a slight difference between the groups. According to the teachers' ratings (which were made without knowledge of prior conditions), the experimental boys were significantly less assertive than boys in the two comparison groups. They did not, however, differ in more dramatic variables of aggressive behaviour. It might be anticipated that such slight differences between the groups would be largely attenuated by age sixteen in the light of a decade's experience with all its cultural and subcultural influences. The finding is quite the contrary. At age sixteen, the experimental boys are not only less assertive than both comparison groups, but distinctly less aggressive over a broad range of situations. This applies to assessments of recent anger, history of anger intensity, physical toughness, fights, and adventuresome attributes. In other words, the boys exposed prenatally to female hormones showed fewer aggressive characteristics than the comparison boys, regardless of whether the estimates were derived from self-ratings, ratings by other people, systematic interviews, or a projective test. This is the first evidence derived from a specifically designed research study indicating that early exposure to female hormones may diminish aggressiveness in human males.

The hormonal changes of puberty, especially in males, may facilitate the learning of aggressive behaviour. In addition to the early effects of the female hormones on the developing brain, the nature of puberty may have been modified in the boys studied by Yalom et al. by prenatal exposure to large amounts of female sex hormones. The behavioural findings are more striking at age sixteen than at age six. It is possible that the upsurge of androgen that normally occurs in male adolescents may have been diminished by the early hormone exposure, or that the brain's response to such an upsurge was modified by the early exposure to female hormones.

In any event, these two new studies give some reason to believe that, even in the human species, the development of aggressive behaviour may be influenced by exposure of the fetal brain to sex hormones (58, 59). Such effects might well operate through the shaping of an early interest or preference of the developing organism, so that a slight bias toward the environment is established. This bias increases the probability that learning will proceed in certain directions; but it does not require it to happen and indeed environmental influences may overcome it.

Ease of learning aggressive patterns

The human species has a biological heritage of its vertebrate-mammalian-primate history (60). This heritage may include some predisposition toward aggressive behaviour, transmitted genetically yet requiring environmental stimulation for full development. The recent studies of chimpanzees referred to here show many similarities in basic elements of aggressive behaviour. These similarities include, among others: the forms of threat, attack, submission, and reassurance; the contexts and eliciting conditions of aggressive behaviour; the role of cooperation in facilitating aggression; the tendency to make status differentiations; the tendency to redirect aggression toward weaker or lower status individuals; the adolescent male aggression spurt; the sex difference in rough-and-tumble play. Such aggressive behaviour has been so prominent for so long in human societies—and in the pre-human societies that led to *Homo sapiens*—it is reasonable to consider the possibility that such behaviour may be transmitted by both social and biological mechanisms. One promising line of inquiry is to determine whether the human organism early in life is prepared to acquire certain elementary behaviour patterns with relative ease. There may well be a special facility for learning in spheres of activity that have been adaptively valuable for the species over a very long time in the course of its evolution. For any species, some patterns of behaviour are easier to learn than others (61). In the course of hominid evolution, learning in such adaptively-significant spheres as behaviour oriented to food, water, and reproduction must have had high biological priority; and aggression probably helped to implement these adaptive requirements over millions of years (62). Perhaps the inherited circuitry of the human brain manifests the long-term selective advantage of facility in learning such behaviour (63). A simple preference on the part of the infant, young child or adolescent might draw his attention to a certain class of stimuli or reward his engagement in a particular kind of activity. Once drawn in this direction early in life by an inherited preference, much learning could follow readily in accordance with the environmental conditions in which development occurs. Thus, future research on the ease-of-learning aggressive patterns will tend to integrate evolutionary and developmental approaches (64, 65, 66). This line of inquiry is amenable to experimental analysis in primates. Do some types of visual input elicit more sustained attention from infant monkeys than others? In one experiment, monkeys were raised in a total isolation chamber for the first nine months of life, during which they were exposed to various types of visual input from coloured slides (67). These slides depicted monkeys in various activities and also depicted various non-monkey stimuli. Monkey pictures elicited much more interest than non-monkey pictures, and moreover, pictures of monkeys showing a species-typical threat expression were especially potent in eliciting behavioural responses. Between two and a half and four months of age, threat pictures yielded a particularly high frequency of disturbance. Similar results were obtained with films in the same experimental design (personal communications from G.P. Sackett). This finding suggests that the infant rhesus has a built-in, special responsiveness to the threatening facial expression which is characteristic of its species. Given a responsiveness of this sort, it is not difficult to imagine how the infant in the natural environment would learn a great deal about threat and attack behaviour. Once the infant monkey's attention was powerfully drawn to threat stimuli, he would rapidly learn the conditions in which threat and attack patterns were likely to occur, and the actions likely to terminate aggressive sequences.

This brings us to a consideration of observational learning in primate adaptation (68). Traditionally, discussions of aggressive behaviour have associated unlearned responses with non-human creatures and learned responses with humans. Curiously, this linkage has persisted in spite of the enormous research literature on learning in non-human animals. One of the most interesting findings of the primate field studies in the past decade has been the recurring theme of observational learning in a social context (69). In many species and diverse habitats, the following sequence has been described: close observation of one animal by another; imitation by the observing animal of the behaviour of the observed animal; and practice of the observed behaviour, often for some hours after its occurrence, especially in the play group of young animals. This sequence of observation, imitation, and practice has been described in relation to several adaptive situations: food gathering, tool using and tool making (in chimpanzees), nest building, infant care, copulation and aggressive interactions. In essence, the young have access to virtually the full range of adult behaviour, and take advantage of it to learn patterns of behaviour that have been effective in adaptation. The motivation for such observational learning seems to be well established in the young primate. Observational learning in monkeys has also been studied experimentally. It has been demonstrated that one monkey readily learns from watching another in food choice situations. Moreover, the observing animal learns from incorrect as well as correct responses of the animal he is watching (70). In other words, he learns from the consequences of the operating animal's behaviour.

This line of inquiry is important for an understanding of the influence of the social environment on the development of aggressive behaviour. It provides another link between evolutionary and developmental views of the organism. Developmental psychologists have become increasingly interested in observational learning in young children (71). The child between one and two years of age is a devoted watcher. At this age, observation and imitation may well provide his principal mode of learning.

A remarkable set of findings has high-lighted the susceptibility of children to learn aggressive patterns by viewing models who act aggressively. For example, in one experiment pre-school children were exposed to an aggressive model attacking a target object for ten minutes in a laboratory situation, while a control group experience the same situation without an aggressive model. When the children were tested in the same situation six months later, the former were much more aggressive towards the target object than the latter—that is, a ten-minute exposure enhanced physical aggressiveness in the same situation six months later. This experiment is one of a series carried out by Bandura (72, 73) and his colleagues at Stanford, showing vividly how children can learn aggressive patterns by watching film or television and enact these patterns in their later play. They have shown that pre-school, middle-class children tend to imitate the aggressive behaviour of adults whether they observe it in person or depicted on film; moreover, the effect is obtained even with cartoon films. In short, aggressive patterns are imitated whether the dramatic presentation is realistic or fantasy-like. Imitation is increased if the aggressive model is rewarded in the drama, decreased if the aggressive model is punished. In general, these imitative acts are displayed spontaneously in the play of these young children, sometimes in remarkable fidelity to the model's original behaviour. The children are capable of performing imitatively many more aggressive acts than they show spontaneously, provided they are given an incentive for doing so. Thus, there is a tendency to restrain expression of aggressive patterns in spontaneous play; this is particularly true for girls and for patterns in which the model has been punished. But the patterns have been learned, and their performance can readily be elicited by a suitable incentive.

Thus, it seems that biological predispositions to learning aggressive patterns and exposure to specific social learning situations may interact to produce great individual differences in aggressiveness during later life (74, 75). In analysing such problems scientifically, the effective conjunction of biological and psychosocial disciplines, so far rarely achieved, holds much promise for future understanding. It hardly seems necessary to point out the aggressive tendencies of the human species today. Whatever adaptive functions such behaviour may have served in man's evolutionary past, there is serious doubt about its utility in contemporary society (76). The risks inherent in such behaviour have been greatly amplified within our lifetime. It is heartening that these problems are beginning to attract substantial attention in the scientific community. It is difficult to imagine a more important area for research in the future.

Summary

There is an upsurge of scientific interest in evolutionary and developmental origins of human aggressive tendencies. This paper describes several lines of inquiry: (a) aggressive behaviour of non-human primates in natural habitats; (b) hormonal influences on development of aggressive behaviour, and (c) ease of learning aggressive patterns.

Field studies of monkeys and apes in their natural habitats provide insights into adaptive properties of behaviour. These species, especially the chimpanzee, are closely related biologically to the human species. Recent studies have added much new information on the forms and circumstances of aggressive behaviour in primates.

Prominent among circumstances eliciting threat and attack patterns are those associated with: (*a*) defence; (*b*) access to valued resources; (*c*) contact among relative strangers.

Hormonal influences on brain organization early in life affect later aggressive behaviour in rodents and monkeys. Several recent studies indicate that this applies to humans as well. Prenatal exposure of human brain to androgens probably facilitates the acquisition of rough-and-tumble play patterns in childhood. Prenatal exposure to oestrogens and progesterone tends to diminish aggressiveness in later life. The hormonal changes of puberty are also relevant to the development of aggressive behaviour.

The human species has a long history of acquiring aggressive patterns— threat, intimidation, suspicion, hatred, attack—with remarkable ease. One important direction for future research is to clarify the factors that facilitate such learning. This includes an analysis of special interests and preferences in infancy, childhood and adolescence; hormonal influences on brain function; conditions of the social environment, including emotionally-charged customs and observation of aggressive models.

Biological predispositions and exposure to social learning situations interact to produce individual differences in aggressiveness. Clarification of such evolutionary and developmental roots of aggressiveness requires cooperative efforts of biological and social sciences.

Acknowledgements

The author is deeply indebted for support of the research referred to in this chapter to The Grant Foundation, The Commonwealth Fund and the H.F. Guggenheim Foundation.

References

(1) Hamburg, D.A. (Ed.) (1970) *Psychiatry as a Behavioral Science*, p. 103. Englewood Cliffs, Prentice-Hall.

(2) Garattini, S. and Sigg, E.B. (Eds.) (1969) *Aggressive Behavior*, p. 369. New York, Wiley.

(3) Daniels, D.N., Gilula, M.F. and Ochberg, F.M. (Eds.) (1970) *Violence and the Struggle for Existence*, p. 441. Boston, Little, Brown.

(4) Washburn, S.L. and Hamburg, D.A. (1968) Aggressive behavior in old-world monkeys and apes. In *Primates: Studies in Adaptation and Variability*, Ed. P.C. Jay, p. 458. New York, Holt, Rinehart and Winston.

(5) Hinde, R. (1974) *Biological Basis of Human Social Behavior*, p. 462. New York, McGraw-Hill.

(6) Hamburg, D.A. and van Lawick-Goodall, J. (1974) Factors facilitating development of aggressive behavior in chimpanzees and humans. In *Determinants and Origins of Aggressive Behavior*, Eds. W.W. Hartup and J. deWit, p. 57. The Hague, Mouton.

(7) Feshbach, N. and Feshbach, S. (1972) Children's aggression. In *The Young Child, Reviews of Research*, Ed. W. Hartup, Vol. 2, p. 284. Washington, National Association for the Education of Young Children.

(8) Feshbach, S. (1970) Aggression. In *Carmichael's Manual of Child Psychology*, Ed. P.H. Mussen, Vol. II, p. 159. New York, Wiley.

(9) Hamburg, D. (1971) Recent research on hormonal factors relevant to human aggressiveness. *International Social Science Journal*, *23*, 36-47.

(10)   Goldstein, M. (1974) Brain research and violent behavior. *Archs Neurol., 30*, 1.
(11)   Coelho, G.V., Hamburg, D.A. and Adams, J.E. (Eds.) (1974) *Coping and Adaptation*, p. 454. New York, Basic Books.
(12)   Clemente, C. and Chase, M.H. (1973) Neurological substrates of aggressive behavior. *Ann. Rev. Physiol., 35*, 329-56.
(13)   Lengyel, P. (Ed.) (1971) *Understanding Aggression. International Social Science Journal, 23*, 110. Paris, Unesco.
(14)   Smith, C.G. (Ed.) (1971) *Conflict Resolution: Contributions of the Behavioral Sciences*, p. 553. Notre Dame, University of Notre Dame Press.
(15)   Ehrlich, H. (1973) *The Social Psychology of Prejudice*, p. 208. New York, Wiley.
(16)   Levine, R. and Campbell, D. (1972) *Ethnocentrism, Theories of Conflict, Ethnic Attitudes and Group Behavior*, p. 310. New York, Wiley.
(17)   Holsti, O. (1972) *Crisis, Escalation, War*, p. 290. Montreal, McGill-Queen's University Press.
(18)   Deutsch, M. (1973) *The Resolution of Conflict: Constructive and Destructive Processes*, p. 420. New Haven, Yale University Press.
(19)   Alcock, N. (1972) *The War Disease*, p. 238. Oakville, Canadian Peace Research Institute.
(20)   Washburn, S.L. and Jay, P.C. (Eds.) (1968) *Perspectives on Human Evolution*, Vol. 1, p. 287. New York, Holt, Rinehart and Winston.
(21)   DeVore, I. (Ed.) (1965) *Primate Behavior: Field Studies of Monkeys and Apes*, p. 629. New York, Holt, Rinehart and Winston.
(22)   Jay, P.C. (Ed.) (1968) *Primates: Studies in Adaptation and Variability*, p. 503. New York, Holt, Rinehart and Winston.
(23)   Rowell, T.E. (1967) Social organization of primates. In *Primate Ethology*, Ed. D. Morris, p. 219. Chicago, Aldine.
(24)   Washburn, S.L. and Hamburg, D.A. (1965) The implications of primate research. In *Primate Behavior: Field Studies of Monkeys and Apes*, Ed. I. DeVore, p. 607. New York, Holt, Rinehart and Winston.
(25)   Sarich, V.M. (1968) The origin of the hominids: An immunological approach. In *Perspectives on Human Evolution*, Eds. S.L. Washburn and P.C. Jay, p. 94. New York, Holt, Rinehart and Winston.
(26)   Hall, K.R.L. and DeVore, I. (1965) Baboon social behavior. In *Primate Behavior: Field Studies of Monkeys and Apes*, Ed. I. DeVore, p. 53. New York, Holt, Rinehart and Winston.
(27)   DeVore, I. and Hall, K.R.L. (1965) Baboon ecology. In *Primate Behavior: Field Studies of Monkeys and Apes*, Ed. I. DeVore, p. 20. New York, Holt, Rinehart and Winston.
(28)   DeVore, I. (1965) Male dominance and mating behavior in baboons. In *Sex and Behavior*, Ed. F.A. Beach, p. 266. New York, Wiley.
(29)   Hall, K.R.L. (1964) Aggression in monkey and ape societies. In *The Natural History of Aggression*, Eds. J.D. Carthy and F.J. Ebling, p. 51. New York, Academic Press.
(30)   Rowell, T.E. (1967) A quantitative comparison of the behavior of a wild and a caged baboon group. *Anim. Behav., 15*, 499-509.
(31)   Altmann, S.A. (Ed.) (1967) *Social Communication Among Primates*, p. 392. Chicago, University of Chicago Press.
(32)   Ransom, T. (1972) Ecology and social behavior of baboons in the Gombe National Park. Unpublished doctoral dissertation, University of California, Berkeley.
(33)   van Lawick-Goodall, J. (1968) Behaviour of free-living chimpanzees of the Gombe Stream Area. In *Animal Behaviour Monographs*, Eds. J.M. Cullen and C.G. Beer, p. 165. London, Bailliere, Tindall and Cassell.
(34)   van Lawick-Goodall, J. (1968) A preliminary report on expressive movements and communication in the Gombe Stream chimpanzees. In *Primates: Studies in Adaptation and Variability*, Ed. P.C. Jay, p. 313. New York, Holt, Rinehart and Winston.
(35)   Goodall, J. (1965) Chimpanzees of the Gombe Stream Reserve. In *Primate Behavior: Field Studies of Monkeys and Apes*, Ed. I. DeVore, p. 425. New York, Holt, Rinehart and Winston.
(36)   Goodall, J. (1964) Tool-using and aimed throwing in a community of free-living chimpanzees. *Nature, 201*, 1264-6.
(37)   Hamburg, D. (1971) Crowding, stranger contact, and aggressive behavior. In *Stress, Society and Disease*, Ed. L. Levi, p. 209. New York, Oxford University Press.
(38)   van Lawick-Goodall, J. (1971) Some aspects of aggressive behaviour in a group of free-living chimpanzees. *International Social Science Journal, 23*, 89-97.

(39) Wrangham, R.W. (1974) Artificial feeding of chimpanzees and baboons in their natural habitat. *Anim. Behav., 22*, 83-93.

(40) Southwick, C.H. (1972) Aggression among nonhuman primates. *Addison-Wesley Module in Anthropology, 23*, 1-23.

(41) Bygott, J.D. (in press) Agonistic behavior and dominance among wild chimpanzees. In *Behavior of Great Apes*, Eds. D.A. Hamburg, E. McCown and J. Goodall. Menlo Park, W.A. Benjamin.

(42) Bauer, H. (1974) *Behavioral changes about the time of reunion in groups of chimpanzees in the Gombe Stream National Park*. Presented at the Fifth International Congress of Primatology, Nagoya, Japan, August.

(43) van Lawick-Goodall, J. (1973) The behavior of chimpanzees in their natural habitat. *Am. J. Psychiat., 130*, 1-12.

(44) Nishida, T. and Kawanaka, K. (1972) Inter-group relationships among wild chimpanzees of the Mahali mountains. *Kyoto University African Studies, 7*, 131-69.

(45) Nishida, T. (in press) The social structure of chimpanzees of the Mahali mountains. In *Behavior of Great Apes*, Eds. D.A. Hamburg, E. McCown and J. Goodall. Menlo Park, W.A. Benjamin.

(46) Riss, D. (1974) Observations of aggressive behavior among free-living male chimpanzees. Personal communication.

(47) Harlow, H.F. and Harlow, M.K. (1965) The affectional systems. In *Behavior of Nonhuman Primates*, Eds. A.M. Schrier, H.F. Harlow and F. Stollnitz, Vol. II, p. 287. New York, Academic Press.

(48) Crook, J.H. (1968) The nature and function of territorial aggression. In *Man and Aggression*, Ed. M.F.A. Montagu, p. 141. New York, Oxford University Press.

(49) Southwick, C.H., Beg, M.A. and Siddiqi, M.R. (1965) Rhesus monkeys in north India. In *Primate Behavior: Field Studies of Monkeys and Apes*, Ed. I. DeVore, p. 111. New York, Holt, Rinehart and Winston.

(50) Harris, G. (1964) Sex hormones, brain development and brain function. *Endocrinology, 75*, 627-48.

(51) Levine, S. and Mullins, R.F., Jr. (1966) Hormonal influences on brain organization in infant rats. *Science, 152*, 1585-92.

(52) Young, W.C., Goy, R.W. and Phoenix, C.H. (1964) Hormones and sexual behavior. *Science, 143*, 212-18.

(53) Goy, R.W. (1968) Organizing effects of androgen on the behavior of rhesus monkeys. In *Endocrinology and Human Behavior*, Ed. R.P. Michael, p. 12. London, Oxford University Press.

(54) Money, J. and Ehrhardt, A.A. (1968) Prenatal hormonal exposure: Possible effects on behavior in man. In *Endocrinology and Human Behavior*, Ed. R.P. Michael, p. 32. London, Oxford University Press.

(55) Hamburg, D. (1969) A combined biological and psychosocial approach to the study of behavioral development. In *Stimulation in Early Infancy*, Ed. A. Ambrose, p. 269. New York, Academic Press.

(56) Ehrhardt, A.A. and Baker, S.W. (1973) *Hormonal aberrations and their implications for the understanding of normal sex differentiation*. Presented at the Society for Research in Child Development, Philadelphia, March.

(57) Yalom, I.D., Green, R. and Fisk, N. (1973) Prenatal exposure to female hormones: Effect on psychosexual development in boys. *Archs gen. Psychiat., 28*, 554-61.

(58) Clayton, R.B., Kogura, J. and Kraemer, H.C. (1970) Sexual differentiation of the brain: Effects of testosterone on brain RNA metabolism in newborn female rats. *Nature, 226*, 810-12.

(59) Hamburg, D.A. and Lunde, D.T. (1966) Sex hormones in development of sex differences in human behavior. In *Development of Sex Differences*, Ed. E. Maccoby, p. 1. Stanford, Stanford University Press.

(60) Young, J.Z. (1971) *An Introduction to the Study of Man*. London, Oxford University Press.

(61) Seligman, M.E.P. (1970) On the generality of the laws of learning. *Psychol. Rev., 77*, 406-18.

(62) Hamburg, D.A. (1963) Emotions in the perspective of human evolution. In *Expressions of the Emotions in Man*, Ed. P. Knapp, p. 300. New York, International Universities Press.

(63) Hamburg, D. (1968) Evolution of emotional responses: Evidence from recent research on nonhuman primates. In *Animal and Human*, Ed. J. Masserman, p. 39. New York, Grune and Stratton.

(64) Bruner, J.S. (1972) Nature and uses of immaturity. *Am. Psychol., 27*, 1-22.
(65) Bruner, J.S. (1973) Organization of early skilled action. *Child Dev., 44*, 1-11.
(66) Hinde, R. (1972) Aggression. In *Biology and the Human Sciences*, Ed. J.W.S. Pringle, p. 139. Oxford, Clarendon Press.
(67) Sackett, G.P. (1966) Monkeys reared in isolation with pictures as visual input: Evidence for an innate releasing mechanism. *Science, 154*, 1468-72.
(68) Hall, K.R.L. (1968) Aggression in monkey and ape societies. In *Primates: Studies in Adaptation and Variability*, Ed. P.C. Jay, p. 149. New York, Holt, Rinehart and Winston.
(69) Hamburg, D.A. (1969) Observations of mother-infant interactions in primate field studies. In *Determinants of Infant Behaviour*, Ed. B.M. Foss, Vol. IV, p. 271. London, Methuen.
(70) Riopelle, A.J. (1960) Complex processes. In *Principles of Comparative Psychology*, Ed. R.H. Waters, D.A.Rethlingshafer and W.E. Caldwell, p. 208. New York, McGraw-Hill.
(71) Siegel, A.E. (1970) Violence in the mass media. In *Violence and the Struggle for Existence*, Eds. D.N. Daniels, M.F. Gilula and F.M. Ochberg, p. 193. Boston, Little, Brown.
(72) Bandura, A. (1965) Vicarious processes: A case of no-trial learning. In *Advances in Experimental Social Psychology*, Ed. L. Berkowitz, Vol. 2, p. 1. New York, Academic Press.
(73) Bandura, A. (1973) *Aggression: A Social Learning Analysis*, p. 390. Englewood Cliffs, Prentice-Hall.
(74) Boelkins, R.C., and Heiser, J.F. (1970) Biological bases of aggression. In *Violence and the Struggle for Existence*, Eds. D.N. Daniels, M.F. Gilula and F.M. Ochberg, p. 15. Boston, Little, Brown.
(75) Daniels, D.N., and Gilula, M.F. (1970) Violence and the struggle for existence. In *Violence and the Struggle for Existence*, Eds. D.N. Daniels, M.F. Gilula and F.M. Ochberg, p. 405. Boston, Little, Brown.
(76) Hinde, R.A. (1971) The nature and control of aggressive behaviour. *International Social Science Journal, 23*, 48-52.

5. The purposes and organization of psychiatric research

Denis Hill

Research, of course, is practised in the humanities no less than in the sciences. While one purpose shared by all research is to increase knowledge, scientific research is said to be that which increases knowledge of the phenomena of nature. It is therefore knowledge of a certain kind, arrived at in certain ways. Throughout most of history man organized himself according to what he believed to be true, rather than what he knew to be so. He now understands that belief and knowledge are different things. For centuries the advance of medical science was held up because its knowledge was derived from beliefs— from religious ideas, authoritative opinion or inspiration. The development of psychiatry was delayed even longer for the same reason. Knowledge which is called scientific can be described as the awareness and understanding of the theoretical and practical relationships which exist in nature, by which it is organized and functions. Knowledge of this kind can only be acquired by methods of science and in no other way. But if scientific knowledge is only about natural events, it is necessary to define what these are. 'Natural knowledge is knowledge of material things. Apart from this it has no meaning' (1). Man, of course, is a material thing, and knowledge of the relationships between material things is part of scientific knowledge. The term 'human nature' has particularly difficult connotations. Some think we could do without it; some think it of the essence of things. By tradition human nature is that aspect of man which is provided by what is inherent and innate, by his biological constitution, an aspect of himself he shares with all others and by which he is recognized as being one of the same species with them. But if human nature is a function of biological constitution it is also subject to biological variation. The biologically determined differences between individuals are certainly relevant to psychiatry, but compared with twenty-five years ago there are few now who look to greater knowledge of these differences to explain and to provide control over the majority of mental disorders. The account they provide of the variety of human nature is inadequate. However, using this concept of human nature, scientific knowledge indeed has been acquired, for the study of it is concerned with the theoretical and practical relationships between the materials of which man is constituted. For a long time there existed a strongly held opinion that the scientific study of psychiatry should be based on the natural sciences, and on the natural sciences alone. Indeed, in the opening sentence of that well known British textbook of clinical psychiatry, Slater and Roth (2) state that their 'book is based on the

A revised form of the Sir Geoffrey Vickers Lecture of 23 February 1972, the original version of which was published in the *British Journal of Medical Psychology*, 1973, *46*, conviction of the authors that the foundations of psychiatry have to be laid on the ground of the natural sciences'.

Without disregarding or underestimating the contributions of biological science, social scientists now lay claim that their theoretical conceptions, their models of human nature and their methods of investigation promise much. They can point to some achievements, but, as in many fields of human controversy, biological and sociological issues are discussed as if one or the other had a right of primacy. There are those who believe that only biological research will reveal knowledge of the essential causes of the functional psychoses. Social scientists pursue their research with the same objective in view.

Some who have investigated the nature of scientific knowledge have pointed to issues which have prejudiced those who have attempted to promote it (1, 3). Himsworth (1) has discussed the familiar and traditional model to describe the interrelatedness and development of the sciences: that of the analogy of the tree of knowledge. The model gives structure to the belief that all scientific knowledge has a common root or trunk which is basic; from this trunk all other sciences sprout, develop and diverge, one growing from another. Applied to the sciences of man such a model describes the inorganic proceeding to the organic. The common root is physics growing into chemistry, and chemistry into biochemistry, and hence into physiology and structure. From knowledge of the cell we proceed to knowledge of tissues, and hence to organs, and through organs to organisms and thus to man himself. Logically, therefore, biology should lead to anthropology; and the greater knowledge of the normal should provide us with knowledge of the abnormal. Pathology should be derived from physiology, and the social sciences from the biological ones. Knowledge of the roots, the trunk and then the branches should lead to knowledge of the most peripheral parts of the tree. From this model we would have to conclude that only a deeper understanding of the biological nature of man in the physical sense will lead to the solution of the problems of psychiatry. We have often acted on this and there have been a few noteworthy advances. Because of the prejudicial influence of the model it has usually been agreed that biological research in psychiatry is more 'basic' or 'fundamental' than psychological or sociological research. The conviction has led in the past to a preference for supporting biological research even in areas of inquiry where the relevance to psychiatry could not be discerned. Moreover, because of the general acceptance of the conceptual thinking in the model by many medical scientists of great distinction, it has delayed the entry into medical and psychiatric research of social scientists. Further, it has had, until quite recently, serious effects on medical education, both undergraduate and postgraduate.

The traditional model of the tree of knowledge is perhaps outmoded. Himsworth (1) believes it to be entirely mistaken and has drawn attention to the danger of 'concealing from ourselves the influence such models have upon our conceptual thinking'. Indeed, those whose conceptual framework of science is determined by the tree of knowledge analogy are in an intellectual straitjacket from which there is usually no escape. The model which Himsworth proposes is diametrically opposite and carries no interpretation of the interrelatedness of the hierarchy of the sciences according to some natural order. Knowledge does not necessarily extend from the centre to the periphery: more often quite the reverse. We are confronted with 'a vast globe of primitive ignorance round the periphery of which there are a whole series of problems prompting men to seek knowledge'. Among these are the problems of health and sickness.

Even accepting, as we must, the interrelatedness of those sciences which deal with the universe of materials, the continuity of physical structure from the inorganic to the organic, from the cell to the organism, the traditional model contains a serious defect. At each level of organization the integration is subject to its own laws which are different from those at other levels. The laws of physics are different from those of genetics, and these are different from those governing the integration of functions within the nervous system; these again are different from those governing the social behaviour of man. Although each level or system is superimposed upon the one lower than it, the properties of the higher or superimposed integration are *not* contained in any of its components. The higher system is not reducible to its elements (4). At each level of organization the data refer to a different and unique aspect of reality. We cannot deal with one in terms of another or derive one from another.

If man, as both a biological and psychosocial animal, can best be conceived as a complex organization with different levels of integration, each operating within its own laws, then two important consequences follow. The first, as Lorenz (4) has pointed out, is that: 'as a living system it possesses all the systematic properties of the subsystems of which it is composed and that none of the natural laws, down to those of physics and chemistry which prevail in its components, suffer any infraction in the functioning of the whole'. Moreover, although the higher levels of integration cannot be understood or explained by reduction to their elements, a 'level by level analysis of the component subsystems and their structure can be undertaken', thus providing *one sort of explanation* of the higher levels. But only to a certain point. For the second consequence is that at the highest level of human organization, man's social behaviour, we cannot detect a system of natural laws which govern it. We are confronted by the fact that man behaves not according to *laws* but according to *rules,* which have to be learnt. They are imposed more by the social milieu than by the biological heritage. At the level of social adaptation, man is currently seen as acquiring roles which he has to play. They are complex, numerous, applicable to one situation, not another, and they are learned unconsciously. We know more about them in other societies than in our own; more about them in other people than in ourselves.

The distinction between 'laws' and 'rules' governing different levels in living systems is of the greatest importance. We must conclude that we shall never be able to predict human behaviour with the expectation of any mathematical certainty; the best we can expect when knowledge has greatly increased, is to do so in terms of probability. Explanations of human behaviour as given by the social sciences will lack the precision and assurance we find in natural scientific explanations (5). Moreover, we cannot examine the structure of rules as if they were laws, or in the same terms as those governing other integrations such as reflex, response to stimulus or endocrine secretion, in which laws operate. Rather, we find that the rules of role-playing are related to human interests and needs, to value systems incorporating attitudes—what is felt to be desirable or undesirable, the meaning of events, what is right or wrong, good or bad.

Those who research into mental illness at the psychosocial level of integration are confronted by the fact, which is difficult to ignore, that human behaviour has an essentially teleological or, as Lorenz (4) prefers, a 'teleonomic' element in it. Clinical psychiatry operates from a basis of theories about human behaviour which implicitly accept that the meaning of any human situation, including mental illness, can only be interpreted in terms of the interests of the person or persons involved. All such theories have therefore a teleological form. Social scientists, investigating mental illness, cannot as yet with few exceptions operate with such theories, because of their subjectivity and the lack of suitable methodology. They are therefore constrained to ignore the persons involved and their interests, and to examine clinical events as if they were events determined by laws rather than by rules, and which do not behave teleologically. For this reason there is a disjunction between the theoretical positions of most clinical psychiatrists and those social scientists who endeavour to increase our knowledge of the subject. The clinical position provides the psychiatrist with what he believes is 'insight' into his patient's needs, attitudes and stresses. From this the patient may be helped. But knowledge of the individual rarely contributes to scientific knowledge of the disorder from which he suffers. It is important to distinguish between the need on the one hand to understand the meaning of pathological behaviour, and on the other to provide an explanation of the mechanisms which bring it about (6). It can be said, of course, that the psychiatrist's need to interpret behaviour according to his understanding of the meaning of it merely distinguishes psychiatry as an immature branch of medicine, equivalent in development to that of general medicine at the beginning of the last century. The model of GPI (general paresis) has inspired many to adopt this position. Given certain knowledge of aetiological agents, of the mechanisms of pathogenesis and provided with sure therapeutics, the psychiatrist would have no need to study the 'meaning' of his patient's symptoms. But the problems of psychiatry are inherently more complex, more difficult to tackle, than were those of general medicine.

The nature of mental disorder

What is the nature of mental disorder? Regrettably there is no simple answer. Is mental disorder a unitary phenomenon, having one set of causes but different manifestations, or are there many mental disorders, each being a distinct syndrome or disease entity with its own causation, manifestation, and natural history? At what level or levels of integration or faulty integration is any particular manifestation dependent—either molecular, neurophysiological, or at the psychological level? Even if mental disorder is unitary, which of its different manifestations are due on the one hand more to biologically given differences in structural subsystems, or on the other to cultural or other differences in the superimposed social system? These are familiar questions but they express the contrasting theoretical positions of American and European psychiatrists and research workers as a distinguished sociologist,

David Mechanic (7), pointed out. We have to admit that across the broad spectrum of major mental disorders and incapacitating neuroses and personality disorders, we do not know the answers to these questions. If the purposes of psychiatric research are to meet public needs, should we not be as much concerned with research into the causes of human distress, methods of alleviating the effects of emotional crisis due to life problems, as with research into manifest psychosis? Moreover, lying between the clinical consequences of simple unhappiness, social and personal plight on the one hand, and manifest madness on the other, there is the vast problem of neurotic anxiety and disability and personality deviation with its associated risks of alcoholism, drug addiction, and a host of other maladaptive social consequences. Psychiatric epidemiologists are well aware of the implication of these problems for their work and of the difficulty of determining when a case is a case. A well known American study (8), based on the unitary or continuum hypothesis and using comprehensive criteria of mental disorder, suggested that less than 20% of the population are mentally well, while various European workers following the syndrome hypothesis based on the medical model find that between 2 and 14% of the population are mentally ill. It is conceded, of course, that there are many discrete syndromes or disease entities in the medical sense within the total morbidity, having a known causation. There are the rare conditions due to specific biochemical defects and there are also metabolic disorders and other diseases of inflammatory or degenerative nature, affecting the brain and hence affecting behaviour. These are well known and there are certainly more discoveries to be made. For the majority of the mentally sick, however, the aetiological issues are more complex. It is now generally conceded that the great majority of mental illnesses have a multifactorial causation. But this does not imply that many causes only operate at one level of integration. There may have been infringements of biological laws as well as errors of social rule learning. To what extent the latter is related to the former, whether there is any causal relationship between them, is often obscure.

Aetiological research

If these arguments about the nature of scientific knowledge related to behaviour can be sustained, a simple conclusion is justified. When confronted with a particular aspect of pathological behaviour—a recognizable common type of mental disorder—we have to ask ourselves at what level of integration in the living system can we most usefully and successfully examine it. Since there are many types of explanation available for any behaviour, which type of explanation is, in the particular instance, appropriate, and is the research which might illuminate it feasible?

The answer to the first question, in respect of any particular syndrome or manifestation of mental disorder, is given when we know what the primary data of the disorder are. The question must be answered, what are the observable, even if at present unmeasurable yet specific and relevant, data which cannot be reduced to the level of a subsystem of integration without loss of identity or meaningful character? As knowledge increases, so no doubt will the strategic position change, but two examples will serve to illustrate.

The clinical aspects of that form of mental subnormality known as phenylketonuria have very little specificity. This means that there are no primary clinical data. From them alone there is difficulty in distinguishing this form of mental subnormality from many others. The discovery of abnormal substances in the urine of some defectives indicated a disturbance at the biochemical level of integration, which of itself was far more specific than the clinical symptoms, but it did not reveal the causes. The discovery that this defect at the biochemical level was associated with a specific type of inheritance demonstrated that causation lay in an infringement of natural law. But this knowledge that failure to utilize a single amino acid in protein synthesis is associated with failure to develop normal intelligence can be exploited by strategic research. On the one hand, it has led to an examination of amino acid metabolism in other forms of mental subnormality and mental illness; on the other to the realization that disturbances of protein synthesis in the brain are important in determining intelligence.

We can contrast this situation with that of schizophrenia. Despite much argument among experts, the condition is recognized throughout the world by its clinical specificity, and by this alone. There is no unique abnormality of bodily structure or function. The condition is recognized by the overt behaviour of patients over a period of time and by the disordered verbal communications and subjective experiences. If schizophrenia is a disorder specifically human, true animal analogues could not exist. Despite worldwide efforts for more than thirty years to demonstrate a specific heredity, none has been found, although a substantial degree of vulnerability of genetic origin is proven. Moreover, the clinical phenomena of schizophrenia have no similarity with those of metabolic diseases of either genetic or acquired origin. It is becoming unlikely that a specific, essential cause at the biochemical level of integration will be found. Yet if any new lead is given, we cannot afford not to explore it. If a biochemical marker which identified the genetic vulnerability was discovered, it would be a great advance. Thus viewed, the primary data of the disorder in the present state of knowledge are unique and are at the level of psychosocial integration, and it is at this level that the strategic research effort should be directed. There are many approaches to this. Psychological research into the mechanisms of disordered thinking is promising. It remains to be seen how far social science research examining clinical events as if they were determined by laws rather than by rules, and forced by the methodological limitations to ignore patients as persons, in the teleological frame of reference, can provide relevant knowledge of this disorder. This approach to the problems of schizophrenia does not deny that there are disordered functions at biological levels of integration, for indeed there are, certainly at neurophysiological and psychophysiological levels. But it is to assert the belief that they will prove to be more correlational than aetiological. Study of them may throw great light on the pathogenesis, may explain some symptoms, and may provide instruments for measuring therapeutic change. What can be said about schizophrenia applies with even greater force to the problems of neurosis and personality disorder.

Neurobiological research

The impact on psychiatry of the successful development of psychotropic drugs has been profound, and the implications for research are far reaching. Some have suggested that they are aetiological. It is important to discover the method of action of these drugs, for in this way their therapeutic effect can be elucidated. As a result there is hope that the disturbed functions in the nervous system which accompany or underlie mental illness will be discovered. There is a large new field of research where knowledge about psychiatric disorders is being developed and it is most relevant to the clinical data. It is concerned with the many functional changes, at different levels of integration which accompany mental illness. They are detectable at the psychological, the neurophysiological, and at times the biochemical level of integration. While their existence has been known for many years, only recently have technological advances been made by which they can be accurately detected and measured. In this, modern computer technology has played a leading role. Their importance lies in the fact that not only may their study throw light on pathogenesis, but also the measurement of these correlates provides a great opportunity for the study and evaluation of any clinical changes which occur in patients, either spontaneously or as a result of therapeutic intervention. They may also provide knowledge of the processes underlying that intervention. This is applicable even to the processes of psychotherapy as it is to the new subjects of psychopharmacology and behaviour therapy, both of great importance and potential. Much of this research, whether psychological, psychophysiological, or neurophysiological in nature, is still at the level of devising new instruments, new techniques and methods. University departments of psychiatry are now fostering such research as far as they can, supported by the Medical Research Council (MRC) and the Foundations, generally on a short-term project basis.

Clinical research

Since the War there has been a great increase in clinical research, much of it of a classifying, codifying or 'tidying up' nature, or concerned with drug trials. Yet, across the broad spectrum of psychiatry the irreducible data with which the researcher must work are behavioural, i.e. clinical, data. These are the patient's verbal communications, his psychophysical posture and motility, his conduct and the way he behaves in several identifiable contexts—sex, occupation, social, marital and family relationships. These lose their identity and specificity when we attempt to reduce them to the lower level of integration than the psychosocial one. If we accord primacy to the behavioural data of psychiatry, we have to admit the present limitations of the scientific method. We cannot by it investigate, except with a few techniques, the phenomena of subjective experience, the so-called psychic or internal reality which many clinicians hold to be of primary importance. The scientific method has hitherto limited research to those aspects of behaviour which are perceptually observable. Yet the limitation should not be overemphasized for there is abundant evidence that clinical research is now entering a new phase.

Arthur Koestler (9) has remarked that one of the most spectacularly successful aspects of science in the last three centuries has been the reduction of qualities in nature into measurable quantities. Psychiatry is now in fact trying to order its observations, to increase their exactitude and then to measure them, to transform things essentially qualitative into things quantitative. As this is being done, we become aware how inexact are our clinical observations and how much depends upon the observer as upon the observed. This process, applied both to the clinical phenomenology of individuals and to the epidemiology of different disorders, has made it necessary to devise new methods of examination and measurement, a process again made possible by the new computer technology. Given adequate resources of manpower and educational opportunities, many believe we can look forward to a great increase in clinical research of a quality and relevance which we have not seen before.

A joint working party of the Department of Health and Social Security (DHSS) and the Medical Research Council have reviewed the progress of the scheme for decentralized clinical research which has been in operation since 1958. The purposes were to foster the research spirit in medicine and to facilitate the discovery and encouragement of local talent. A broad view has been taken of what clinical research is, for it includes 'research into the mechanism and causation of disease, including its prevention and cure . . . [as well as] field studies in epidemiology and social medicine and observations in general practice'. The scheme is regarded as a success, and 'not only useful but in many ways vital at the local level'. Expenditure is now running at £1,200,000 a year. Psychiatry has had its full share in this scheme. There can be no doubt that clinical research in the subject has been stimulated and has greatly benefited from it.

Organization

The organizational framework in which research should be promoted and funded should be designed to meet the needs of the subject as well as the needs of the customer. If we do not look after the former we shall not be able to meet the latter. In the case of the subject, there is research designed to increase knowledge of it, and this must include provision for those who can increase it, to provide them with security and a career structure, as well as to promote the education and training of clinicians and scientists who can take part in the endeavour. Three developments now seem to threaten the future realization of these requirements. The first is the changed public attitudes to postgraduate education and research; the second is the loss of autonomy of the statutory bodies responsible for it (the University Grants Committee and the Research Councils) and their subjection to the executive departments of Government; and the third, particularly affecting medicine, the financial restrictions and the manpower shortage.

Public attitudes

The idea is now being challenged that, as a part of postgraduate education, a full-time period of research leading to a higher degree is beneficial either to the individual or to society. It is questioned whether it justifies the expense involved. The Expenditure Committee of the House of Commons reports (10) that it does not think so, has evidence that those acquiring a PhD are not much wanted in industry, commerce or the Civil Service, and strangely deplores the fact that three groups of occupations—teachers, professional scientists and doctors (13%)—account for nearly three-quarters of higher degree holders in employment. It is suggested that the universities mistakenly encourage postgraduates to take higher degree courses, and that they are responsible for the increasing demand.

'... ambitious professors may seek to add to their prestige by accepting postgraduate research students for projects of little intrinsic value or social benefit and by using them as though they were research assistants. To some extent also, it (the increased demand) must have reflected the reluctance of some students to face the world of work outside the cosy academic atmosphere; study for a higher degree at government expense is sometimes a comfortable way of postponing the choice of a career' (para. 59).

The Expenditure Committee considers that postgraduate education 'should be shaped by the needs of the economy and of society as a whole, and not be mainly a means of training more teachers and more research workers'. But the main argument would appear to be a moral one. The Committee asks:

'Is it socially just that, when only just over 10% of young people are able to enjoy full-time higher education at all, more than a quarter of public expenditure on universities should be devoted to the postgraduate education of a small minority, little more than 2% of the age group? Is it fair to spend several thousands of pounds training one postgraduate to acquire the skills which enable him to earn a higher income when more resources are urgently needed in primary schools?' (para. 75).

It is suggested by the Committee that this problem can be solved in one of two ways, but preferably the second. Either the UGC could limit the number of postgraduate research students in universities, allowing sufficient to take care of teacher vacancies, or all postgraduate students who had not had experience of employment should be excluded from postgraduate research.

The research councils

The publication of the Rothschild (11) and Dainton reports in 1971 (12) provoked intense controversy throughout the scientific community at the national level. Despite widespread misgiving, the Government implemented Lord Rothschild's proposals in 1972. The customer-contractor principle which will determine the way in which public money will be spent on applied research once again raised the question of what is basic and what applied in medical research. Himsworth's model of the nature of knowledge reduces the sharpness of any distinction between them. There is no such thing as basic knowledge; only knowledge which is unspecialized and that which is specialized and specific. Unspecialized knowledge may have wide application, or at a given time none at all. Specialized knowledge has utility as specific as the problem from whose solution it was derived. The departments of government are quite naturally only interested in specialized knowledge. Basic research is to increase knowledge but has no practical objective; applied research on the other hand has an 'end-product'—a practical objective—and is determined by the needs of the customer. Yet, as the Dainton Report (12) made clear, there is another important distinction, often drawn in the past between basic and applied research on the one hand and research which is *strategic* in character on the other. 'Development' is the administrative application of scientific knowledge about a particular clinical problem to the public benefit; it may require operational research to determine how best to do it effectively and cheaply. Applied research uses the technologies of the sciences, from knowledge which, in Himsworth's term, is less specialized to elucidate problems about which specialized knowledge is required. Strategic research is different. It prepares the way both for knowledge which is least specialized, and for knowledge which is specialized. It prepares the way therefore for tactical or applied research. It is essentially technological, and there is no immediate 'end-product'.

It is too early to assess the consequences for medical or psychiatric research of the new organization and new structure of the Government's administration. It is clear that large financial resources have been made available to the Department of Health and Social Security and that the financial resources of the MRC have been diminished. The influence of the DHSS in promoting practical and applied research upon the activities of the MRC has greatly increased. At the same time the Department has now available to it either through its own advisory machinery under the control of the Chief Scientist, or indirectly through full access and participation in the advisory machinery of the MRC to the range and depth of scientific knowledge and expertise which formerly were only available to the MRC itself. Senior clinical scientists and research workers will in future have an opportunity to play a much more significant role in policy decisions concerning medical research. For psychiatry, these changes have been evident and propitious. A substantial increase in research in social psychiatry had already occurred (13), support for research in the underdeveloped areas of psychiatry—child psychiatry, forensic psychiatry and subnormality may well be forthcoming, but the shortage of scientifically trained manpower is serious. University departments, following the customer-contractor principle, have contracted in a number of projects to answer problems of practical importance to the health and well-being of the community.

The MRC have attempted to reassure university departments that the Council's support for them will continue, and that the Government, as stated in the White Paper (para. 54), attach great importance to the support which they give. Nevertheless there will 'have to be some changes in the balance and distribution of the Council's research programmes'. It is evident, however, that it will still fall to the Research Councils with their restricted resources and the charitable bodies providing funds for psychiatric research not only to support the university departments in their training role for research workers, but also to support research whether it is called 'basic', fundamental or strategic, which cannot claim to meet society's immediate needs. It is upon such research that future advances in knowledge leading to control over mental disorder should come. Moreover the new arrangements for applied research have not included as yet any increased provision for careers in psychiatric research. Young science postgraduates entering a research team for a short or long-term project, undertaken at the request of the Department, can see no career prospects ahead of them. There is the danger that the Government through their new arrangements may, to use Sir Geoffrey Vickers' phrase (14), kill the goose that alone can lay the golden eggs.

Manpower

Yet, overshadowing the research scene for the next decades is the medical manpower shortage. We must anticipate that as academically-minded young psychiatrists complete their training, or even before, they will be called upon to take up posts where clinical service is given the first priority. The emerging university departments of psychiatry must be staffed, and with parsimonious provisions for establishments both in them and in the mental health services as a whole (15), those trained and able to develop clinical research will be forced, whatever their inclinations, to give it a low priority. The greatly increased demands of undergraduate and postgraduate teaching must be met if the nation's need for many more doctors is to be realized. It is a particular misfortune for psychiatry and psychiatric research, still emerging and undeveloped, that Government, through all its executive departments, has decided that iron rations should be imposed upon medicine as a whole.

In this restricted situation university departments of psychiatry are unlikely not to respond positively to requests to undertake contractual research to solve problems which are immediate, practical and important. Indeed they have a social responsibility to try to do so, and if support for more fundamental work is not to be forthcoming, it is practically certain that they will accede. A situation could however be envisaged in which a significantly large proportion of all the resources, intellectual and physical, of small departments could be used for contractual research, and this obviously could have profoundly adverse effects, not only upon the university staff concerned, but also for the future of psychiatry itself. University departments therefore have a responsibility to preserve the academic base for psychiatry, to husband essential resources so that, when the economic position has improved, the growth of scientific knowledge in psychiatry may continue in this country.

The short-term future of social science research in psychiatry would seem to be assured. There are less grounds for optimism in the whole field of biological research, for this is unspecialized and is concerned usually with theoretical issues related to pathogenesis. There is no immediate practical problem to solve, no immediate application, and Lord Rothschild (11) has warned the customers against research which is open-ended, unspecific and having unduly general objectives. It is the research into the unspecialized areas of knowledge, whether biological or psychological, which others would call 'basic', which is likely to go unsupported for lack of funds and because there will be no customers.

If psychiatric research which has already acquired some momentum is to maintain it during the lean years which lie ahead, it will do so only if those who feel responsibility for it plan together a strategic campaign to ensure that no significant area is lost. This applies as much to the education, training and support of research workers as it does to the range of knowledge required, particularly to its less specialized aspects. Priorities will of course have to be decided and no doubt difficult decisions will have to be taken. If knowledge is to be increased, as well as its applications exploited, the role of the Trusts and charitable bodies supporting research may acquire an even greater importance.

References

(1) Himsworth, H. (1970) *The Development and Organization of Scientific Knowledge.* London, Heinemann.
(2) Slater, E. and Roth, M. (1969) *Clinical Psychiatry.* London, Bailliere, Tindall and Cassell.
(3) Medawar, P.B. (1967) *The Art of the Soluble.* London, Methuen.
(4) Lorenz, K. (1969) Innate bases of learning. In *On the Biology of Learning,* Ed. K.H. Pribram. New York, Harcourt, Brace and World.
(5) Beck, I..W. and Holmes, R.Z. (1968) *Philosophic Inquiry,* 2nd ed. Englewood Cliffs, N.J., Prentice Hall.
(6) Hill, D. (1970) On the contributions of psychoanalysis to psychiatry: mechanism and meaning. *Br. J. Psychiat., 117,* 609-15.
(7) Mechanic, D. (1970) Problems and prospects in psychiatric epidemiology. In *Psychiatric Epidemiology,* Eds. E.H. Hare and J.K. Wing, London, Oxford University Press.
(8) Srole, L. *et al.* (1962) *Mental Health in the Metropolis: the Midtown Manhattan Study.* New York, McGraw-Hill.
(9) Koestler, A. (1964) *The Act of Creation.* London, Hutchinson.
(10) Third Report from the Expenditure Committee (1973) *Postgraduate Education,* Vol. 1. London, HMSO.
(11) Rothschild, Lord (1971) The organization and management of Government R & D. In *Framework for Government Research and Development.* London, HMSO.
(12) *Framework of Government Research and Development* (1972). London, HMSO.
(13) McLachlan, G. (Ed.) (1971) *Portfolio for Health.* London, Oxford University Press.
(14) Vickers, G. (1968) The promotion of psychiatric research. *Br. J. Psychiat., 114,* 925-34.
(15) Department of Health and Social Security (1971) *Hospital Services for the Mentally Ill.* London, HMSO.

6. Biochemistry and mental function

Seymour S. Kety

If we are ever to understand and rationally meliorate the disturbed processes which underlie mental illness, it will be by investigation of the clinical problems themselves and examination of the mental, social, neural and biological elements which comprise behaviour. It is all of these which the Americans call 'psychiatric research', and in Great Britain, the Mental Health Trust and Research Fund has added much to its vigour for more than a decade.

Although they are not alone in their importance to psychiatry (1), the biological sciences have a significance which is not attenuated by community with the social psychological sciences, nor is their power less real by having been only partially demonstrated. It is the area, tentative as yet, between biology and human psychology that I have chosen to dwell on, and I shall do so largely in terms of the work of my associates and myself in the Laboratory of Clinical Science at the National Institutes of Health, Bethesda, without any pretension that this will constitute an adequate review of a growing field.

The time is not yet at hand, if in fact it will ever be reached, when one can speak meaningfully of the biochemistry of mental state. There are, however, a few areas where one can see the beginnings of correlations and significant interrelationships and these include consciousness, intellectual function and affect.

My interest in consciousness goes back to the Science and Philosophy Club at the Central High School in Philadelphia, a club which bore the brave motto *'Felix qui potuit rerum cognoscere causas'*, and in which a great teacher, Edwin Landis, introduced us to Berkeley, Mach, Eddington and the fathomless problem of the nature of consciousness. Many years later I was introduced to the cerebral circulation by Carl Schmidt, through his definitive work in the rhesus monkey, and began to feel how much might be learned from measurements in man, whose brain, with its subjective wealth, and whose diseases could not be replicated in animals. Making use of some fundamental principles of inert gas exchange, the Fick principle, and a little calculus, we were eventually able to make what still appear to be satisfactory measurements of blood flow, oxygen and glucose consumption in the conscious human brain under a variety of physiological and pathological conditions. In Table 1 are presented some normal values representing the average of the first investigations of healthy volunteers of about twenty-five years of age (2). Measurement of glucose consumption followed later, con-

A revised form of the Sir Geoffrey Vickers Lecture of 26 February 1965, the original version of which was published in *Nature*, 1965, *208*, 1252-7. Added paragraphs are indented and enclosed in brackets.

TABLE 1   Overall blood flow and energy metabolism of the normal human brain

Blood flow ml/100g/min	54
Oxygen consumption ml/100g/min	3.3
Respiratory quotient (CO_2/O_2)	0.99
Glucose consumption mg/100g/min	4.9

firming the thesis that the major substrate for oxidative energy in the brain is glucose, the utilization of which represented an almost stoichiometric equivalent of the oxygen consumed. From these measurements it was possible to compute the rate of energy utilization by the human brain which turned out to be close to 20 W. In comparison with the enormous expenditure of energy which modern computers require, this represents a remarkable degree of efficiency and miniaturization.

[Recent studies have demonstrated that there are certain conditions in which the brain can shift partially from the utilization of glucose to the utilization of other substrates, in particular ketone bodies. In complete, prolonged starvation, as much as 50% of the oxygen consumption of the brain can be accounted for by the oxidation of ketone bodies (44). It has also been learned that in ketosis of any type (starvation, fat feeding, ketone body infusion), the brain will tend to utilize ketone bodies sparing a certain part of its glucose metabolism (45). It is interesting to note that the enzymes for the utilization of ketone bodies in brain follow a natural pattern of postnatal development paralleling the nutritional history of the organism. In the neonate during suckling and the ingestion of a diet rich in fat, the brain utilizes ketone bodies more effectively because of higher levels of the enzymes necessary for their metabolism (46, 47). After weaning and the assumption of a normal diet, the enzymes decline to low levels but are available for augmented use in the adult whenever the concentration of their substrates may increase].

We were anxious to examine states markedly different from the normal in functional level and chose states of altered consciousness (Table 2). It was quite apparent that there was a rough correlation between level of consciousness and over-all oxygen and energy utilization by the brain (3). In anaesthesia, for example, where the cerebral oxygen consumption was reduced by 40%, there appeared to be support *in vivo* for the earlier *in vitro* investigations of Quastel (4), who has shown that anaesthetics interfere with the oxygen consumption of brain slices. But all these data merely tell us that the oxygen

TABLE 2   Cerebral oxygen consumption in the states of depressed consciousness (expressed as percentage of the value in healthy young men)

Senile psychosis	82
Diabetic acidosis	82
Insulin hypoglycaemia	79
Surgical anaesthesia	64
Insulin coma	58
Diabetic coma	52

consumption and energy-level of the brain are reduced in states of depressed consciousness; they do not explain the coupling between function and metabolism which is one of the most interesting topics of present concern. One could argue that the primary effect in any of these conditions was on the metabolic 'power supply' of the brain necessary for the maintenance of consciousness. An alternative hypothesis, however, would be that the primary site of interference was in the interaction between neurons at the synapses, which, once inhibited, depressed both the functional activity and the energy requirements of the system. This interesting problem of the coupling between function and metabolism must await clarification by the work of those like McIlwain, Rodnight, Larrabee and Chance, among others.

[A week long conference was recently held on the topic of the coupling of function, metabolism and blood flow in the brain (48).]

There are states of altered consciousness, however, in which such a neat correlation with total cerebral metabolism and energy does not exist (Table 3).

TABLE 3   Cerebral oxygen consumption in various mental states (expressed as percentage of the value in normal control states)

Normal sleep	97
Schizophrenia	100
LSD psychosis	101
Mental arithmetic	102

Normal sleep is one such state; the poetic description of the wakening brain by Sir Charles Sherrington in *Man on His Nature* is well known:

'Suppose we choose the hour of deep sleep. Then only in some sparse and out of the way places are nodes flashing and trains of light-points running . . . the great knotted headpiece of the whole sleeping system lies for the most part dark . . . Should we continue to watch the scheme we should observe after a time an impressive change which suddenly accrues. In the great head end . . . spring up myriads of twinkling stationary lights and myriads of trains of moving lights of many different directions. . . . the great topmost sheet of the mass, that where hardly a light had twinkled or moved, becomes now a sparkling field of rhythmic flashing points with trains of travelling sparks hurrying hither and thither. The brain is waking and with it the mind is returning.'

Not only did our results (5) force the rejection of a simple cerebral ischaemic theory for sleep which dated back to Alcmaeon; they challenged as well the generally accepted 'Sherringtonian' notion which equated sleep with neuronal activity. More recent neurophysiological findings are more consonant with what we learned about the nature of sleep. Evarts (6), in very elegant investigations of the activity of individual neurons which he has observed through microelectrodes permanently implanted in the cortex of unanaesthetized cats, has found no net decrease in cortical neuronal activity during natural sleep. He has, on the other hand, demonstrated characteristic alterations in the activity of individual neurons or groups of neurons, some showing inhibition when the animal sleeps, but others coming into greater activity at that time.

[More recent studies in the cat by Reivich, Isaacs, Evarts and Kety (49) have revealed a moderate increase in blood flow throughout the brain during slow wave sleep and a marked increase, almost a doubling of that function, during REM sleep. It is likely that these measured changes in blood flow reflect comparable increases in energy metabolism.]

The results in schizophrenia (7), during LSD psychosis (8) or in mental arithmetic (9) all reinforce the concept that the brain, unlike the heart or the liver or kidney, is an organ for computation and communication. In such functions there is no necessary correlation between the energy utilized and the efficiency of the process or the quality of the output. To differentiate these alterations of consciousness in terms of the cerebral oxygen consumption would be like trying to correlate the nature of a radio programme with the power used.

Some of our more recent investigations have attempted to examine the energy utilization of many structures within the living brain. The first approach to measurement of oxygen consumption is in defining the local perfusion rates. Using basic principles similar to those of the nitrous oxide method, we have related the quantity of an inert diffusible substance taken up by a small tissue region to its perfusion (10). If the tracer is radioactive, one can measure its uptake during a standard time interval in the various structures of the brain by autoradiography. In the autoradiogram, density is related to the concentration of tracer which in turn can be related to the blood flow during the physiological state just prior to the abrupt killing of the animal. Under most physiological conditions there is reason to believe that the blood flow is determined by the oxygen consumption, so that in a rough way the autoradiographic density gives information on the differential energy utilization in various structures of the brain. Such investigations have revealed a remarkable differentiation of cortical blood flow in the unanaesthetized brain with the primary sensory areas showing far greater activity (11). This differentiation does not appear to be present in the brain of the fetus or the neonate. Anaesthesia obscures this differentiation, reducing the areas of greater cortical oxygen consumption to a relatively homogeneous average value, while there is evidence that sensory stimulation results in a recognizable increase in blood flow and, presumably, oxygen consumption along the appropriate sensory pathways (12).

[Sokoloff and his associates have developed a technique for the measurement of regional glucose utilization in the brain which employs ^{14}C-deoxyglucose (50). This has made it possible to demonstrate that in normal and anaesthetized states, local glucose utilization correlates very closely with blood flow in the brain (51). Autoradiograms produced by the labelled deoxyglucose give a pictorial representation of the metabolic activity in the various regions of the brain and can be used to map the increased metabolism which accompanies functional activity. Thus, it has been possible to localize the representation of the retinal blind spot in the striate cortex and to demonstrate the alternating vertical columns of high and low activity in that cortex in unilaterally enucleated monkeys, which appear to correspond to the patterns of optical dominance described by Hubel and Wiesel. These results clearly confirm a correlation between glucose utilization and functional activity (52).]

The maturation of intellectual function and its mal-development depends on many processes in addition to oxygen consumption. In 1949, when

Sokoloff first became associated with us, we undertook an investigation of cerebral blood flow and oxygen consumption in patients with hyperthyroidism. This resulted in the quite surprising finding that although the total oxygen consumption of such patients was markedly elevated, there was no significant increase in the oxygen consumption of the brain (13). These results demonstrated that the effects of thyroid hormone were not uniformly applied to the metabolism of all cells in the body. A finding such as this requires an explanation and Sokoloff set about to find one. Using radioactive thyroxine he learned that the hormone crossed the blood-brain barrier and was available to the cells of the brain. He knew also that the brain was peculiar, in that its oxidative processes were almost entirely confined to a single substrate, glucose, and that, although Richter, Waelsch and others had demonstrated an active protein synthesis in the mature brain, that process was still considerably slower in brain than in liver and could scarcely account for a significant fraction of the cerebral oxygen consumption. These considerations led him to the hypothesis that thyroxine neither stimulated oxidative metabolism directly nor uncoupled it from phosphorylation (which were the prevailing concepts) but acted on some specialized process such as protein synthesis.

In 1954 he came to the National Institute of Mental Health and began a highly productive collaboration with Kaufman. In 1959 they were able to report that l-thyroxine, administered to normal animals *in vivo* or added directly to the incubation medium *in vitro*, stimulated the rate of amino acid incorporation into protein in cell-free, rat liver homogenates. This stimulation of protein synthesis *in vitro* occurred in the absence of changes in oxygen consumption or oxidative phosphorylation. They further suggested that the characteristic effects of thyroxine on energy metabolism were secondary to the stimulation of reactions which required energy such as protein biosynthesis (14).

[Although the thyroxine effect on protein synthesis is localized at the step involving the transfer of tRNA-bound amino acid into microsomal protein (16), mitochondria are clearly involved in the mechanism of action of thyroid hormones in this process (15, 53). When added *in vitro* to cell-free systems from thyroxine-sensitive tissues, thyroxine stimulates protein synthesis only if mitochondria are present in the incubation medium. When administered *in vivo*, thyroid hormones also have effects on a variety of cellular processes and properties, such as nucleic acid synthesis and ribosomal content, but these effects occur hours after and probably secondary to an earlier mitochondria-dependent hormonal stimulation of protein synthetic activity. There are, therefore, two components to the effects of thyroid hormones on protein synthesis *in vivo*. There is first a mitochondria-dependent stimulation of the activity of the existing cellular machinery for protein synthesis followed in intact cells capable of regulation and adaptation by a secondary increase in the cellular content of protein synthetic machinery. The site for the initial action of the hormonal molecule appears to be in the mitochondria. Only the first effect is seen *in vitro* in the cell-free system, and this system has been used to define the nature of the mitochondrial involvement. These studies have shown that thyroxine interacts with mitochondria in an ATP-requiring reaction to produce a soluble, small, dialysable, heat-stable substance which in turn stimulates ribosomal translational activity and accelerates the elongation, completion and release of the nascent polypeptide chains (54). The identity of this substance is still unknown, but it is clearly not cyclic AMP or cyclic GMP, cyclic nucleotides which participate in the mechanism of actions of a number of other hormones.]

Klee and Sokoloff (18) examined the effects of thyroid hormones on protein synthesis in brain. Thyroxine does not stimulate protein synthesis in mature brain, explaining its failure to increase cerebral oxygen consumption in hyperthyroid adult man. In contrast, thyroxine stimulates both protein synthesis and oxygen consumption in neonatal brain. The basis for the difference in thyroxine sensitivities of adult and neonatal brain has been found to reside in the nature of their mitochondria. Mitochondria of immature brain are capable of reacting with thyroxine in the initial interaction necessary to stimulate protein synthesis. This mitochondrial capability is apparently lost in the course of postnatal development because mitochondria of mature brain are incapable of participating in this reaction.

These findings help to explain the well-known clinical effects of the thyroid hormone on the development of the brain and of intellectual function in infants compared with its relatively minor effects on these functions in the adult. They corroborate and offer a mechanism for Eayrs's finding of the requirement for thyroxine in the dendritic proliferation of immature cerebral cortex. Thus, this work forms a crucial link between the absence of thyroid hormone and the retarded cerebral development in cretinism.

In 1956, soon after the Laboratory of Clinical Science, National Institute of Mental Health, was organized, some of us became interested in the cluster of thought disorders which is called schizophrenia, and gave attention to the hypothesis which attempted to explain many of the mental symptoms of schizophrenia on the basis of an abnormal degradation of circulating epinephrine to abnormal oxidation products such as adrenochrome or adrenolutin (19). That hypothesis seemed especially plausible because it took cognisance of the evidence for genetic factors as well as the importance of stressful life experiences in the pathogenesis of the mental disorder. The difficulty in testing the hypothesis lay in the lack of knowledge concerning the normal metabolism of epinephrine, let alone its possible abnormality in schizophrenia. In 1956 one could account for some 5% of administered epinephrine which was excreted unchanged in the urine, while the remaining 95% was disposed of by unknown mechanisms.

Isotopic techniques, which had been so valuable in the tracing of other metabolic pathways, were not readily applied to this problem because the pharmacological potency of epinephrine prevented the administration of enough of the hormone labelled with carbon-14 which was then available to permit characterization of its products. It was apparent that to use isotopic techniques to advantage for studies of the metabolism of epinephrine, especially in man, would require an isotopically labelled epinephrine of unheard-of specific activity. We were finally successful in having a few millicuries of 7-[^{3}H]-epinephrine synthesized. The tritium label made possible the high specific activities required, while its position at C7 met our expectation that the label would be retained through the various possible metabolic degradations.

In 1957, Armstrong, McMillan and Shaw identified the first major metabolite of epinephrine (vanillylmandelic acid, VMA, or 3-methoxy-4-hydroxymandelic acid) in the urine of a patient with phaeochromocytoma and in normal urine (20).

A few years before, Julius Axelrod had joined the Laboratory, bringing with him great interest and competence in the catecholamines. Although the metabolism of adrenaline to VMA was generally regarded as involving first deamination by monoamine oxidase and then O-methylation, Axelrod, on the basis of pharmacological and biochemical evidence, postulated the existence of an alternative pathway with O-methylation as the first step followed by deamination. He then proceeded to demonstrate in the urine the existence of that hypothetical compound which he designated 'O-methylepinephrine' or 'metanephrine', a second major metabolite of epinephrine (21). He described and characterized the enzyme responsible for this conversion (catechol-O-methyl-transferase) and the requirement of S-adenosylmethionine as the methyl donor (22). He suggested that O-methylation rather than deamination was the principal enzymatic process involved in the inactivation of circulating epinephrine and later went on to show that norepinephrine was metabolized through completely analogous pathways by the same enzymes (23). Figure 1 shows the present state of knowledge of the metabolism of these two catecholamines with a number of additional minor metabolites which Axelrod et al. have identified. Together all these metabolic products account for some 98% of administered epinephrine or norepinephrine and, presumably, a similar accountability would hold for these substances when they are released into circulation under physiological conditions.

With the background of information on the normal degradation of the hormone which was thus provided, it was then possible to examine the metabolism of epinephrine in schizophrenic patients and normal volunteers using the tritium-labelled substance (24, 25). We were unable to find any evidence for a significant abnormality in the metabolism of intravenously administered epinephrine among the schizophrenics either qualitatively or quantitatively, the four normal metabolites and the unchanged hormone accounting for 98% of the tritium in the urine in both groups of subjects.

The synthesis of tritiated epinephrine which was stimulated by that hypothesis, and in particular the work of Axelrod and his colleagues, have had important implications for psychiatry. The identification of the metabolites of epinephrine and the development of methods for their estimation in urine make it possible to obtain information on the secretion of this hormone in a variety of physiological and pathological states and in response to drugs. Investigations by Axelrod and Kopin, among others, with norepinephrine were a logically related step, and in the past few years the storage and release of norepinephrine at the sympathetic nerve endings and the factors which control these processes have become one of the most exciting fields of pharmacology (26). The insights which such investigations have given us into the possible actions of drugs which affect mood will be discussed later.

[In 1970, Axelrod, together with von Euler and Katz, received the Nobel Award in Physiology and Medicine for his elucidation of the biochemical and physiological processes of metabolism and inactivation of noradrenal-

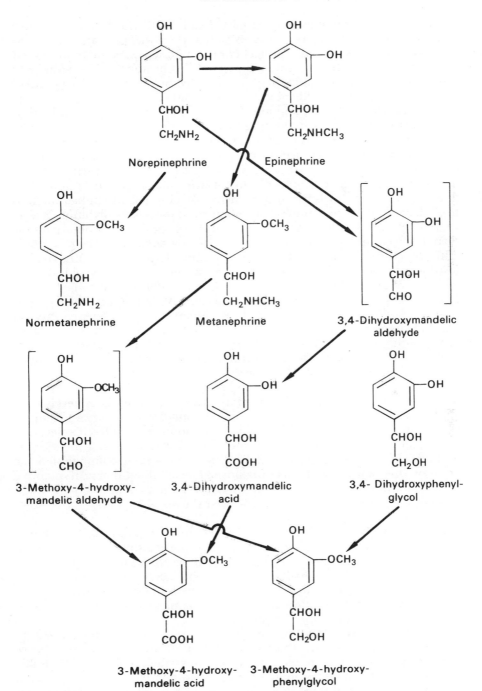

Figure 1 Present knowledge of the metabolism of epinephrine and norepinephrine (after Axelrod and Kopin).

ine at synaptic endings. In the past decade, evidence has accumulated indicating that the antipsychotic as well as the antidepressant drugs have important effects on central catecholaminergic synapses, suggesting their involvement in schizophrenia (55), as well as the affective disorders. The development and examination of heuristic hypothesis in that area is one of the most important fields of current psychiatric research.]

Thirteen years ago Osmond and Smythies, in conjunction with Harley-Mason (27), advanced the interesting hypothesis that there was an accumulation of an abnormal methylated compound with hallucinogenic properties in schizophrenia. They were led to this possibility by the fact that the potent psychotomimetic drug, mescaline, was almost identical with trimethylated dopamine. In the same communication Harley-Mason pointed out that the dimethyl derivative (3,4-dimethoxy-phenylethylamine), which had interesting behavioural effects, could possibly be formed by transmethylation *in vivo*. In 1961, Pollin, Cardon and I (28) tested this hypothesis by observing the mental effects of methionine given orally to a small number of chronic schizophrenic patients who had been maintained on a monoamine oxidase inhibitor. We reasoned that under those conditions it was conceivable that the levels of S-adenosylmethionine, which Cantoni (29) had shown to be an important methyl donor, could be increased and the biological transmethylation of amines facilitated. In some of the patients there was a temporary but quite obvious exacerbation of psychotic symptoms associated with methionine administration. These observations have now been confirmed by several other groups (30-32); in addition, Brune and Himwich found similar effects with betaine, another methyl donor (30).

Further work by investigators in our laboratory has tended to support some of this reasoning. The absence of information regarding tissue levels of S-adenosylmethionine led Baldessarini and Kopin (33) to devise an ingenious assay of high specificity. By means of this they found a considerable elevation of S-adenosylmethionine in brain and liver of rats following methionine feeding. Axelrod (34) demonstrated the presence in normal mammalian tissue of an enzyme capable of methylating normal metabolites, that is, tryptamine and serotonin, to their dimethyl derivatives in the presence of S-adenosylmethionine. Dimethyltryptamine has been shown to be a potent psychotomimetic agent (35).

In 1962, Friedhoff and Van Winkle (36) detected a substance which behaved like 3,4-dimethoxyphenylethylamine in the urine of a substantial fraction of schizophrenic patients and which appeared to be absent from normal urine. That finding which has had substantial confirmation by Bourdillon and Ridges (37) lends further support to the hypothesis of Osmond, Smythies and Harley-Mason, especially since it was that compound to which Harley-Mason had directed attention ten years previously.

Our observations of the effect of methionine in schizophrenic patients as well as the findings of Friedhoff and Van Winkle are open to a number of explanations which have not been ruled out. Nevertheless, the hypothesis that the accumulation of one or more methylated compounds plays a significant part in some forms of schizophrenia remains a plausible and parsimonious explanation of a number of different and independent observations and seems worthy of further evaluation.

[During the past decade, a number of serious challenges have been made to the inference that 3,4-dimethoxyphenylethylamine of endogenous origin appears in the urine and that it is characteristically related to schizophrenia. Metabolites of the phenothiazine drugs confound the chromatographic identification of the compound and the confirmatory reports have been criticized because drug ingestion was not satisfactorily controlled. Although the compound has been identified in normal urine with mass-spectographic techniques, it has not, with that technique, been shown to be elevated in the urine of schizophrenics. Attention has been focused on the hallucinogenic methylated indoleamines and the presence of the appropriate methylating enzymes in the brain. A methyl donor (methyltetra-hydrofolic acid) which is capable of mediating N- and O-methylation of biogenic amines (56) is of interest because of its possible implications to transmethylation and schizophrenia (57).]

The possible interrelationships between the biogenic amines and affective states have become a subject of lively interest and productive investigations in the relatively few years which have elapsed since the pioneering studies of Gaddum and Vogt in Great Britain, Erspamer in Italy, Rapoport and Woolley in the United States. Interest centred at first on serotonin after the remarkable demonstration by Shore *et al.* (38) of a depletion of that amine from the brain during reserpine-induced depression and its elevation following the antidepressant monoamine oxidase inhibitors. As evidence accumulated, however, it was learned that these drugs also affected noradrenaline and dopamine levels in the brain and that the catecholamine precursor, dopa, promptly and effectively reversed the depressant actions of reserpine in animals, suggesting to some an equally important role for catecholamines in the action of these drugs and possibly in affective states. It has been difficult to explain, however, the action of two effective antidepressant drugs in terms of the central biogenic amines. These agents, amphetamine and imipramine, are not especially active as monoamine oxidase inhibitors and have not been shown to elevate the levels of norepinephrine or serotonin in the brain.

Recently, Kopin was able to demonstrate, in the isolated, perfused heart, a differential metabolism of tritiated noradrenaline released under different circumstances (39). When the catecholamine was liberated in a manner which did not provoke its characteristic effects on the heart, that is, by reserpine, it appeared largely as deaminated products in the perfusate. On the other hand, when its release was accompanied by cardiac stimulation as with stimulation of the cardiac sympathetic nerves or by tyramine, O-methylated products appeared in the perfusate. These observations have suggested the generalization that catechol-O-methyl transferase is the enzyme normally involved in the degradation of norepinephrine which is released physiologically and perhaps its O-methylated metabolites are indicative of adrenergic activation, at least in the periphery.

The release and metabolism of noradrenaline in the brain, however, remained quite a mystery, since the blood-brain barrier prevented the uptake by the brain of radio-active norepinephrine and the amount of label which could be applied through synthesis from tagged tyrosine was hardly enough for fractionation. In 1964, Glowinski, who had applied Feldberg's technique to injection into the lateral ventricles of rats, joined Axelrod and Kopin and succeeded in developing what appears to be a valid technique for labelling, at a high specific activity, the norepinephrine stores within the brain by injecting the tritiated form intraventricularly (40). The label distributes itself quite rapidly in a pattern similar to that of endogenous norepinephrine and shows the same intracellular localization. Furthermore, it follows a curve of disappearance from the brain similar to that of ^{14}C-norepinephrine endogenously produced from ^{14}C-tyrosine.

With convincing evidence that they were studying the metabolism of endogenous norepinephrine in the brain, they examined the effects of a number of psychoactive drugs. Reserpine caused a rapid depletion and the predominant formation of deaminated products as it did in the heart. On the other hand, monoamine oxidase inhibitors, amphetamine and imipramine, all of which are antidepressant or euphoriant drugs, were followed by an increase in O-methylated norepinephrine products in the brain (41). If one may generalize from Kopin's findings in the heart and infer physiological activity from an increase in norepinephrine O-methylation, these findings are compatible with the thesis that the drugs which induce depression or elevation of mood do so by depressing or facilitating the release of physiologically active norepinephrine in the brain or altering its availability at effector sites.

Such a hypothesis as well as the possibility that normal and abnormal changes in mood are dependent on alterations of catecholamines in the brain remain to be validated. The possibility of labelling norepinephrine in the brain has overcome a major obstacle in the way of elucidating its physiological role there. The role of central catecholaminergic synapses in behaviour and mood has been the subject of extensive investigation both in animals and in man. Although the field is in considerable ferment, and it appears likely that the catecholamines, in conjunction with other neurotransmitters, operate in pathways mediating affective and appetitive states, there is no general agreement upon their specific role in particular types of behaviour or clinical psychopathological states.

Another recent development in this laboratory has some clear-cut implications, this time for cardiology. Despite the expectation that monoamine oxidase inhibitors should elevate the levels of the sympathetic neurotransmitter, these agents are found to have hypotensive and other sympatholytic effects which, though undesirable in psychiatry, have been found useful in the treatment of hypertensive disease and angina pectoris. An explanation of this paradoxical effect has been advanced by Kopin et al. (42), who presented evidence for the normal synthesis and accumulation of octopamine, the β-hydroxylated derivative of tyramine, in the region of the sympathetic nerve endings, its enhancement by monoamine oxidase inhibitors and its release by sympathetic stimulation. Their hypothesis that this relatively inactive amine may replace norepinephrine and act as a false neurochemical transmitter appears capable of explaining the partial sympathetic blockade observed after chronic inhibition of monoamine oxidase.

Much of what I have outlined is illustrative of an important generalization from the history of science, a principle which, though taken for granted by most scientists, nevertheless requires reinforcement today. The most practical way to attack a major medical problem or to bridge a great hiatus is not usually head-on, but by strengthening and extending the foundations on both sides and narrowing the gap which lies between. This is best accomplished when the scientists themselves choose their logical next steps, which each will do from his knowledge of the state of the field, the feasibility of an approach, the likelihood and significance of its being successful.

Nearly a hundred years ago in England, Thudichum, whom many regard as the father of modern neurochemistry, advanced a hypothesis that many forms of insanity were the result of toxic substances produced within the brain by faulty metabolism. But, more important, he went on to suggest that these processes, then quite obscure, would be obvious when we understood the biochemistry of the brain to its utmost detail (43). It was in the latter area that he spent the next ten years in what was to become the classical isolation, description and characterization of the chemical constituents of the brain.

It is not difficult to predict what would have resulted had Thudichum spent those years and the funds made available to him by the Privy Council in a premature search for the toxins of insanity. With the tools, techniques and knowledge available to him at that time, it is extremely unlikely that he would have found any of those hypothetical substances; it is equally unlikely that he would have made his fundamental contributions to our present knowledge of the biochemistry of the brain.

References

(1)   Kety, S.S. (1960) *Science, 132*, 1861.
(2)   Kety, S.S. and Schmidt, C.F. (1948) *J. clin. Invest., 27*, 476.
(3)   Kety, S.S. (1957) in *Metabolism of the Nervous System*, Ed. D. Richter, p. 221. Oxford, Pergamon.
(4)   Quastel, J.H. (1952) *Anaesthesia and Analgesia, 31*, 151.
(5)   Mangold, R., Sokoloff, L., Conner, E., Kleinerman, J., Therman, P,G. and Kety, S.S. (1955) *J. clin. Invest, 34*, 1092.
(6)   Evarts, E.V., Bental, E., Bihari, B. and Huttlenlocher, P.R. (1962) *Science, 135*, 726.
(7)   Kety, S.S., Woodford, R.B., Harmel, M.H., Freyhan, F.A., Appel, K.E. and Schmidt, C.F. (1948) *Am. J. Psychiat., 104*, 765.
(8)   Sokoloff, L., Perlin, S., Kornetsky, C. and Kety, S.S. (1957) *Annals of the New York Academy of Sciences, 66*, 468.
(9)   Sokoloff, L., Mangold, R., Wechsler, R.L., Kennedy, C. and Kety, S.S. (1955) *J. clin. Invest., 34*, 1101.
(10) Kety, S.S. (1960) In *Methods in Medical Research*, Ed. H.D. Bruner, *8*, 228. Chicago, Year Book Publishers.
(11) Landau, W.M., Freygang, W.H., Rowland, L.P., Sokoloff, L. and Kety, S.S. (1955) *Transactions of the American Neurological Association, 80*, 125.
(12) Sokoloff, L. (1961) In *Regional Neurochemistry*, Eds. S.S. Kety and J. Elkes, p. 107. Oxford, Pergamon Press.
(13) Sokoloff, L., Wechsler, R.L., Mangold, R., Balls, K. and Kety, S.S. (1953) *J. clin. Invest, 32*, 202.
(14) Sokoloff, L. and Kaufman, S. (1959) *Science, 129*, 569.
(15) Sokoloff, L. and Kaufman, S. (1961) *J. biol. Chem., 236*, 795.
(16) Sokoloff, L., Kaufman, S., Campbell, P.L., Francis, C.M. and Gelboin, H.V. (1963) *J. biol. Chem., 238*, 1432.
(17) Sokoloff, L. (1964) The action of thyroid hormones on protein synthesis, as studied in isolated preparations and in the whole rat. *Proceedings of the Second International Congress on Endocrinology*, London, 17 Aug. 1964. Amsterdam, Elsevier.
(18) Klee, C.B. and Sokoloff, L. (1964) *J. Neurochem., 11*, 709.
(19) Hoffer, A., Osmond, H. and Smythies, J. (1954) *J. ment. Sci., 100*, 29.

(20) Armstrong, M.D., McMillan, A. and Shaw, K.N.F. (1957) *Biochimica et Biophysica Acta*, *25*, 422.
(21) Axelrod, J. (1957) *Science*, *126*, 400.
(22) Axelrod, J. and Tomchick, R. (1958) *J. biol. Chem.*, *233*, 702.
(23) Axelrod, J. (1959) *Physiol. Rev.*, *39*, 651.
(24) LaBrosse, E.H., Axelrod, J. and Kety, S.S. (1958) *Science*, *128*, 593.
(25) LaBrosse, E.H., Mann, J.D. and Kety, S.S. (1961) *J. psychiat. Res.*, *1*, 68.
(26) Kopin, I.J. (1964) *Pharmac. Rev.*, *16*, 179.
(27) Osmond, H. and Smythies, J. (1952) *J. ment. Sci.*, *98*, 309.
(28) Pollin, W., Cardon, P.V. and Kety, S.S. (1961) *Science*, *133*, 104.
(29) Cantoni, G.L. (1953) *J. biol. Chem.*, *204*, 403.
(30) Brune, G.G. and Himwich, H.E. (1963) In *Recent Advances in Biological Psychiatry*, *5*, 144. New York, Plenum Press.
(31) Alexander, F., Curtis, G.C., Sprince, H. and Crosley, A.P. (1963) *J. nerv. ment. Dis.*, *137*, 135.
(32) Park, L.C., Baldessarini, R.J. and Kety, S.S. (1965) *Archs gen. Psychiat.*, *12*, 346.
(33) Baldessarini, R.J. and Kopin, I.J. (1963) *Anal. Biochem.*, *6*, 289.
(34) Axelrod, J. (1964) *Science*, *134*, 343.
(35) Szara, S. (1961) *Federation Proceedings*, *20*, 855.
(36) Friedhoff, A.J. and Van Winkle, E. (1962) *J. nerv. ment. Dis.*, *135*, 550.
(37) Bourdillon, R.E. and Ridges, A.P. (1967) In *Amines and Schizophrenia*, Eds. H.E. Himwich, S.S. Kety and J.R. Smythies. Oxford, Pergamon.
(38) Shore, P.A., Pletscher, A., Tomich, E.G., Carlsson, A., Kuntzman, R. and Brodie, B.B. (1957) *Annals of the New York Academy of Sciences*, *66*, 609.
(39) Kopin, I.J. and Gordon, E. (1963) *J. Pharmac.*, *140*, 207.
(40) Glowinski, J., Kopin, I.J. and Axelrod, J. (1965) *J. Neurochem.*, *12*, 25.
(41) Glowinski, J. and Axelrod, J. (1966) *Pharmac. Rev.*, *18*, 775-85.
(42) Kopin, I.J., Fischer, J.E., Musacchio, J.M., Horst, W.D. and Weise, V.K. (1965) *J. Pharmac.*, *147*, 186.
(43) Thudichum, J.L.W. (1884) *A Treatise on the Chemical Constitution of the Brain*. London, Bailliere, Tindall and Cox.
(44) Owen, O.E., Morgan, A.P., Kemp, H.G., Sullivan, J.M., Herrera, M.G. and Cahill, G.F. (1967) *J. clin. Invest*, *46*, 1589.
(45) Sokoloff, L. (1974) In *The Neurosciences: Third Study Program*, Eds. F.O. Schmitt and F.G. Worden. Cambridge, Mass., MIT Press.
(46) Klee, C.B. and Sokoloff, L. (1967) *J. biol. Chem,*, *242*, 3880.
(47) Krebs, H.A., Williamson, D.H., Bates, M.W., Page, M.A., and Hawkins, R.A. (1971) *Advances in Enzyme Regulation*, *9*, 387.
(48) Ingvar, D.H. and Lassen, N.A. (Eds.) (1975) *The Working Brain: The Coupling of Function, Metabolism and Blood Flow in the Brain*. Copenhagen, Munksgaard.
(49) Reivich, M., Isaacs, G., Evarts, E. and Kety, S.S. (1968) *J. Neurochem.*, *15*, 301.
(50) Sokoloff, L., Reivich, M., Patlak, C.S., Pettigrew, K.D., DesRosiers, M.H. and Kennedy, C. (1974) *Transactions of the American Society of Neurochemists*, *5*, 85.
(51) DesRosiers, M.H., Kennedy, C., Patlak, C.S., Pettigrew, K.D., Sokoloff, L. and Reivich, M. (1974) *Neurology*, *4*, 389.
(52) Sokoloff, L. (1975) In *The Working Brain: The Coupling of Function, Metabolism and Blood Flow in the Brain*, Eds. D.H. Ingvar and N.A. Lassen. Copenhagen, Munksgaard.
(53) Sokoloff, L. (1968) In *Regulatory Mechanisms for Protein Synthesis in Mammalian Cells*, Eds. A. Pietro, M.R. Lamborg and F.T. Kenney. New York, Academic Press.
(54) Krause, R.L. and Sokoloff, L. (1967) *J. biol. Chem.*, *242*, 1431.
(55) Matthysse, S. and Kety, S.S. (Eds.) (1974) *The Catecholamines and Their Enzymes in the Neuropathology of Schizophrenia*. Oxford, Pergamon.
(56) Banerjee, S.R. and Snyder, S.H. (1973) *Science*, *182*, 74.
(57) Laduron, P. (1974) In *The Catecholamines and Their Enzymes in the Neuropathology of Schizophrenia*, Eds. S. Matthysse and S.S. Kety. Oxford, Pergamon.

7. Abnormal sex chromosomes, behaviour and mental disorder

Paul E. Polani

Incidence of chromosome anomalies

Major chromosome anomalies of number or structure affect a high proportion of human conceptions. Conservatively, I had estimated this at 3 to 4% of recognizable pregnancies from about eight weeks of gestation (1, 2), and more recent estimates suggest that possibly 10% may be a correct value for chromosome anomalies in recognizable pregnancies from the fourth week of gestation (3). This estimate is based on the known frequencies of spontaneous abortions in the population of pregnant women and the high frequency of chromosome anomalies in spontaneous abortions, particularly the early ones, of which 50% or more may be chromosomally abnormal (4, 5).

TABLE 1   Estimated frequencies % of chromosome anomalies and variants among one hundred conceptions from the fourth week of gestation onwards

	Chromosome variants	Major chromosome anomalies	
		Balanced	Unbalanced
Spontaneous abortions: 20	5%	0.15%	>40%
Perinatal deaths: 2	5%	0.15%	>5%
Survivors: 78	5%	0.15%	0.5%
All Pregnancies: 100	5%	0.15%	>8.5%

Granted the assumptions that have to be made in estimating the frequency of chromosome anomalies in human conceptions, and disregarding pre-implantation losses in these calculations, one may estimate that only about one in twenty embryos with unbalanced chromosome complements survives beyond the neonatal period, the rest dying mostly as spontaneous abortions or in the perinatal period (6, 7, 8). However, the high prenatal mortality is not

A revised form of the Sir Geoffrey Vickers Lecture of 19 February 1969, an earlier version of which was published in *Nature*, 1969, *223*, 680-6. The additional material was used in the Kenneth Craik Award Lecture at St. John's College, Cambridge, on 29 November 1974.

evenly distributed among all types of chromosome anomalies with imbalance. For example, it involves a good proportion of trisomic 18 fetuses, particularly perinatally, some two-thirds of 21 trisomics (9, 10), over 97% of 45,Xs* (the single commonest chromosome anomaly in man) and nearly all triploids. Conversely, seemingly only a few of the sex chromosome trisomics, XXY, XYY and XXX, die prenatally.

In about 5 to 10% of cases the chromosome error is balanced and apparently harmless to the individual who carries it; and the 'variants' are also assumed to be innocuous. Morphological 'variants' of human chromosomes were recognized early in the history of human cytogenetics. Using conventional methods of staining it has proved difficult to decide and define what constitutes a variant so that the estimate of frequency in human populations has ranged, for example, from about 1.5 (11, 12) to 30% (13). The variability in males is greater than in females due to the length variation of the long arm of the Y chromosome. The recently developed fluorescent (14) and other chromosome banding techniques, particularly C and related methods of staining (15, 16, 17, 18), have made possible the detection of yet other morphological variants (19, 20), some of which, like that of the centric region of chromosomes Numbers 16 and especially 9, are particularly interesting and not infrequent (21).

Balanced chromosome anomalies (22), such as reciprocal translocation, centric fusions and inversions, are relatively common in survivors and probably somewhere between one in ten and almost half of them are *de novo* mutations, the remainder being inherited from a carrier parent. Specific mutation rates for individual chromosomes and specific events are, of course, considerably smaller (23). Direct information on these finer points is only just coming to hand and the numbers on which these estimates are based are relatively small. On the other hand, for the commoner chromosome anomalies, mostly numerical changes, data are quite good in the aggregate. For example, the incidence of X chromosome anomalies is known from X-nuclear sexing studies on amnion or oral mucosa cells and direct chromosome studies done on nearly 160,000 infants, the deviant results having generally been validated by chromosome studies where these were not the primary investigation (24, 25).

The more time-consuming, direct chromosome investigations which alone

TABLE 2   Frequency of sex chromosome anomalies in surviving neonates

47,XYY	1/650 — 1/700 males
47,XXY	1/700 — 1/850 males
46,XY/47,XXY *et al.*	1/1400 males
47,XXX	1/1200 females
45,X	1/2500 — 1/5000 females
Others	? 1/3000 females

*45,X means that the subject has forty-five chromosomes with only one sex chromosome, which is X. By the same token 47,XXY describes a subject with forty-seven chromosomes of which the sex chromosomes are X, X and Y.

can detect balanced structural anomalies and, until three years ago, numerical anomalies of the Y chromosome, are now also quite substantial. When the studies done in Canada, the USA and Scotland were reviewed in 1972 (26) more than 24,000 infants had been studied and to these we can add at least some 10,000 from Denmark, Russia and Scotland (12, 27, 28). Unfortunately, because of the small numbers of cells analysed in these studies, no estimates are possible of the frequency of mosaicism which, however, evidence suggests, is not too uncommon (29). From these studies one may conclude that, conservatively, more than one in two hundred newborn surviving infants has a major chromosome anomaly, but this seems to be an underestimate. A possible figure for Northern Europe, at least, is between one in 120 and one in 140 (12, 27). In over one-third of the abnormal complements the anomaly is a *balanced* translocation or a centric fusion, and in about one in twenty the translocation is unbalanced. All the structural changes involve, almost exclusively, the autosomes of which they might represent over half of the abnormalities. Among the survivors with major chromosome anomalies *with imbalance,* developmental disorders affect brain, body or sex, simply or, more often, in combination, and about 60% of the abnormalities are of the auto-somes and 40% of the sex chromosomes. We can estimate that in Britain more than 4000 infants a year are born with an unbalanced chromosome anomaly and that there may be in the population some 100,000 affected persons, making allowance for the high mortality of the autosome anomalies and assuming that in this respect the bulk of the sex chromosome anomalies are not much less viable than average. The former strikingly affect somatic development and result in serious disorders of mentation and, generally in gross brain maldevelopment (reviewed in 30). Sex chromosome anomalies seldom, except in the 45,X condition and in the rare sex chromosome polysomies with more than three sex chromosomes, affect somatic develop-ment, though they may affect sex development. On the whole they result in less drastic changes and more subtle distortions of brain function.

Two lines of evidence associate sex chromosome anomalies with mental disorder: first, anecdotal descriptions or the detection of chromosome anoma-lies in loosely defined populations, but this information is incomplete and biased; and second, the prevalence of chromosome anomalies in special groups compared with the general population. Special groups are usually adults or older children, whereas the control population is usually newborn infants with few exceptions (14, 15, 31, 32).

In what follows I shall consider the sex chromosome anomalies grouped into four main classes of brain dysfunction, and adaptation and behaviour disorder: subnormality, mental illness, criminal behaviour and borderline defects. General trends link these categories with specific major sex chromo-some abnormalities. For each major chromosome disorder within each class I shall try to discuss aspects of cognition, behaviour and personality. In the last part of this review I shall discuss possible mechanisms of action of sex chromosome imbalance.

The borderlines of brain dysfunction and intellectual impairment

Although ultimately one would wish to describe, categorize and quantify the

TABLE 3   Chromosome findings in 461 patients with dysgenetic ovaries

| | Normal chromosome structure | | | | | Abnormal chromosome structure | | |
| | Non-mosaics | | Mosaics | | | | | |
Type	No.	%	Type	No.	%	Type	No.	%
45,X	236	51.19%	45,X/46,XX	49	10.63%	i(Xq) {Mosaic / Non mos.	53 / 19 }72	11.50% / 4.12% }15.62%
46,XX	19	4.12%	45,X/47,XXX etc.	11	2.39%	Xp— / Xq—;i(Xp)	8 / 9 }17	3.69%
46,XY	10	2.17%	45,X/46,XY, etc.	21	4.56%	r(X)	10	2.17%
						Others	3	0.65%
	265	57.48%		81	17.58%		102	22.13%
						Y's and ?Y's	13	2.82%
				346	75.06%		115	24.95%

Note: The 461 patients whose chromosome findings are listed are described in nine surveys (references in 33) including an unpublished study by Polani and Angell. Fifty-nine patients had Pure Gonadal Dysgenesis and thirty-nine of these had apparently normal sex chromosomes, 46,XX or XY, but the rest were mosaics and four were 45,X. The symbols of the structural anomalies of the X chromosome are: Xp— or q—, deletions of the short (p) or long (q) arm of the X; i(Xp) or i(Xq), isochromosomes of the respective arm and r(X) ring chromosome following double, short and long arm deletions.

effects of sex chromosome anomalies on detailed cognition, personality and social behaviour and to analyse the influence of these attributes on the adaptation of the affected persons, initially the simplest way to consider these effects is through the global influence of the anomalies on some characteristic which, in the nature of things, has to be relatively gross but quantifiable such as 'measured intelligence' (IQ). In the specific case of the more common sex chromosome anomalies the effect on IQ is not as profound as in autosome anomalies with imbalance such as Down's syndrome. The result is a greater or lesser shift to the left of IQ means without much alteration of the variation. On the whole, different sex chromosome anomalies result in different degrees of shift, though when shifts and numbers are small, statistical significance of comparisons may not be achieved. The result of the IQ shifts is that variable proportions of subjects from each homogeneous chromosomal group fall into such more or less discontinuous categories as borderline, educationally subnormal or severely subnormal and therefore may be disproportionately represented, compared with the general population, in one or more of these educational/clinical groups. However, this simple view of matters disregards the complications which derive from the more specific, as opposed to the global, alterations of brain function and which result in a variety of behavioural and adaptive profiles. These, considered together, tend to impart a note of specificity to the brain dysfunction produced by a given sex chromosome anomaly, irrespective of whether the dysfunction is the direct result of the chromosome anomaly or is secondarily triggered by it in a complex interplay of constitution and environment. Therefore, placement of an individual in a clinical, educational or behavioural class is not simply a matter of his IQ or other coarse aspect of brain function, but often rests on effects which may be quite subtle. Ultimately his placement may depend more on social than biological factors, on provisions for remedial or custodial care in the given environment and society, and the tolerant or otherwise attitudes of the latter as determined by its customs and laws. This calls for special caution in pooling results or in comparing biological parameters where the comparisons are derived from studies and surveys conducted in diverse environmental settings. The complexity of the situation is not surprising when we consider the great variability of individuals which, it is difficult to imagine, would be reduced to a simple stereotype by a chromosome anomaly. It is this complexity which is responsible for the difficulties of quantifying behavioural and personality traits, an essential prerequisite for a rigorous analysis.

The first group of subjects requiring consideration is that which clinically presents with one of the syndromes of dysgenetic ovaries (33). The two clinical types of special interest are the patients with Turner's syndrome and those with Ovarian Dysgenesis, a distinction worth retaining (see below) if for no other reason than because the latter, apart from their ovarian malfunction, often expressed only at puberty, and the short stature, are somatically normal. Practically all the former and almost half of the latter have an XO sex chromosome complement (45,X) (Table 3). Of the latter about half of those who are not 45,X carry an isochromosome for the long arm of the X.

In general, brain function in 45,X subjects and other chromosomally abnormal women with dysgenetic, sterile ovaries is not very deviant. A small but probably excessive proportion of these subjects have been found with an

IQ in the educationally subnormal (ESN) range, i.e. with an IQ of less than 70 (34, 35, 36). By pooling the published data from X-sexing surveys of patients seen in general hospital clinics, in whom somatic anomalies had also been recorded, it was found that the intellectual impairment tended to be more common in patients with webbing of the neck—Turner's syndrome in a strict sense—than in those with Ovarian Dysgenesis (37), but later studies failed to substantiate this (38, 39). Our data still show that among the 45,X subjects with Turner's syndrome there are slightly more (five out of forty-two) with an IQ of less than 70, than among the patients with Ovarian Dysgenesis (one in nineteen), but the numbers are exiguous. As Bekker and van Gemund (40) remark, it is still considered an open question whether in these patients as a group there is evidence of intellectual impairment and there is also a belief that a degree of intellectual impairment cannot be considered a characteristic of the group because a proportion of 45,X subjects have normal or superior measured intelligence. Our data on fifty-one patients, all referred from general paediatric or endocrine clinics and tested on standard tests, show that six (12%) have an IQ below 70.

By pooling this information with the original and reviewed data of Bekker and van Gemund (40), seventeen out of 169 45,X subjects test with an IQ of below 70 (i.e. 10%, with 95% confidence limits of 6% to 16%) which, compared with the general population, would appear to be an excess in the educationally subnormal range. Furthermore, few subjects are found towards the upper end of the IQ scale (39).

In 1962 Cohen (41) and Shaffer (42) noticed a consistent discrepancy when comparing subsets of the Wechsler scale. In Shaffer's sample of fifteen patients with dysgenetic ovaries there was a significantly higher verbal than performance IQ with a difference of about eighteen points, and this finding was confirmed by other (43, 44, 45), but not all, studies (40). Furthermore, on test factor analysis (46) there was an associated lowering of another factor, perceptual organization, compared with verbal comprehension. This was observed in other 45,X subjects but only in those older than thirteen (40).

Results of our tests, mostly done by M. Dicks-Mireaux, are summarized in Table 4. Two clinical groups of 45,X subjects are contrasted with a group with mosaicism and structurally normal sex chromosomes, and another group with structurally abnormal chromosomes. The mosaics tend to a higher total score than the 45,X subjects. In the three major groups combined, there is a significantly better verbal than performance score, but in the 45,X patients with Ovarian Dysgenesis the effect is small and not significant compared with the 45,X patients with Turner's syndrome.

The overall interpretation of these findings on verbal compared with performance tests and on impaired perceptual organization and arithmetic score and digit span (indices of distractability) in the face of normal verbal comprehension, was that there was a specific defect of a cognitive component, interpreted as a 'space-form blindness' (47, 48). The existence of a special defect was supported by other tests (40) and analyses of test results (44), and by poor abstract or human-figure drawing ability (41, 42, 49), by impaired constructional and directional tests involving right-left discrimination (48), coupled with normal reading ability (50). These findings have suggested the presence of a developmental parietal lobe syndrome of the Gerstmann type

TABLE 4 Results of intelligence testing of females with dysgenetic ovaries

	No.	Mean verbal score ± standard error of mean	Mean performance score ± standard error of mean	Total IQ ± standard error of mean
45,X { Turner's syndrome Ovarian Dysgenesis	32 19	96.2 ± 2.5 96.6 ± 5.0	84.2 ± 2.3 92.3 ± 4.5	90.4 ± 2.4 94.6 ± 4.8
Mosaics, normal structure	14	107.3 ± 4.0	98.7 ± 4.2	102.2 ± 4.4
Mosaics, abnormal structure	25	102.2 ± 4.0	95.9 ± 3.9	98.4 ± 3.5

Tested on WAIS, WISC, WBI

involving extrapersonal space (51). Garron and Vander Stoep (39) have questioned the theoretical interpretation of these findings, which they prefer to consider at their face value as the observed fact that 45,X females are poor at non-verbal but normal at verbal tasks. This fact is clearly the major, or possibly the only, contributor to the depressed global IQ, the moderate retardation and the increased proportion of educational subnormality which are found in this group of persons. This is yet another expression of the difficulty of knowing what 'intelligence tests' measure. Conveniently, the assumption is often made that there is, and that one can measure in each subject, a quantity of general intelligence, and that this is an indicator of his place on the scale of mental achievement, all the way from highest to defective. What truly happens is that we have very individual abilities on each of the tasks set in a test, and these can be expressed as objective and factual scores. These tasks are specific, they can be fixed and inheritably selected in experimental situations, but may not correlate with other tasks nor necessarily can they be validly considered as proofs of the existence of something unitary, described as general intelligence.

There is another facet to the reported space-form difficulties of 45,X subjects. Spatial visualization, as an ability to visualize relations of objects in space and to handle visual images, has been known for some thirty years to be a faculty more obvious in males than females, and has been attributed to the action of a recessive X-linked allele (52). Recent work (53, 54, 55) has added support to this hypothesis by family studies and comparisons based on correlations between parents and children, according to classical theory of the inheritance of quantitative characters (56, 57, 58). Based on the size of the correlations, the allele in question would have a frequency of about 0.5 in the population (55). However, it is pointed out (59) that the poor spatial ability of the 45,X subjects contrasts with expectation unless the relationship between the hemizygous state of the hypothetical recessive allele and its manifestation is complex as indeed seems to be the case (55, 60). Also on the grounds of experience with the (46,XY) testicular feminization syndrome of androgen target organ resistance, it has been postulated that proficiency in spatial tasks is subject to androgenic hormonal influences. Inadequacy of such influences might explain the poor spatial ability of the 45,X subjects and others with dysgenetic ovaries and does not necessarily clash with the idea that spatial visualization rests on X-linked genes and on alleles with high population frequencies.

Yet a different effect on brain function may be seen in the frequency with which anosmia and abnormalities of taste can be detected in 45,X patients (61). There are other aspects of the make-up of patients with dysgenetic ovaries that have received attention, particularly their sexual adaptation and more generally their personality. It seems clear that these subjects react adversely to their often odd appearances, their short stature and their physiological dysfunctions by which they are considerably disturbed (62), though not as gravely as they might be. They have been invariably found to orient and identify in a feminine way (63, 64), including marrying, the wish to have children and adopting (65). Sexually they seem to have a low erotic potential and in general they display passivity and a certain emotional blunting which can be considered not detrimental to their personality and to their family and social adaptation (47, 62, 63, 65, 66). Consequently there appears to be little psychopathology arising. These aspects have been reviewed (39, 67).

Among the higher cerebral functions which are essential to most of man's activities and interactions, are those which underlie communication and especially expressive speech and manipulation of symbols, in reading, for example. Disturbance of these functions is often part of general retardation particularly when severe, but there exist selective communication disorders. These, together with disorders of memory functions, are among the behavioural phenotypes of man that seem particularly worthy of investigation from the viewpoint of genetic variation (68). Particularly, specific reading disability has been, and continues to be, a useful subject for genetic investigation. By contrast, less attention has been paid to specific and selective language disorders. A recent study has shown that hyperdiploid sex chromosome anomalies, especially with mosaicism which includes a normal cell line, might be at the origin of a not indifferent proportion of expressive speech disorders in children (69).

Subnormality

Intellectual subnormality is found particularly in 47,XXY males with Klinefelter's syndrome, in triple X females and in the rarer cases with more than three sex chromosomes. The more extra sex chromosomes there are, the greater seems to be the intellectual impairment (70, 71, 72). In the 45,X condition the degree of total intellectual impairment as measured by IQ is slight, as we have seen.

Züblin (73) and Pasqualini (74) noted a childishness, shyness, lack of drive and a degree of intellectual impairment in patients with Klinefelter's syndrome. Males with this syndrome seemed to have subnormal intelligence and there was possibly a direct relationship between variability of chromosome counts and degrees of intellectual impairment (75). In a general sense, if the variability of the counts reflects cases with mosaicism and if one of the cell lines is normal, mosaics would be expected to function more normally, at least in straight intelligence tests.

These mostly clinical studies indicate an association between X-chromatin positive Klinefelter's syndrome and mental subnormality, and prevalence

TABLE 5   X-nuclear sexing and chromosome results in surveys of severely subnormal and educationally subnormal males

Group	Total no.	X-chromatin positive		47,XXY	
		No.	Proportion	No.	Proportion
Severely subnormal	14,231	103	1 in 138 (0.72%)	79	1 in 180 (0.56%)
Educationally subnormal	4111	34	1 in 120 (0.82%)	29	1 in 142 (0.71%)

(Sources, see refs. 30, 32, 76-84)

studies confirm it. The information is derived from males in mental subnormality hospitals or from special schools for educationally subnormal children (30, 32, 76-84).

The overall prevalence among the severely subnormal patients in hospitals of one in 140 is lower than among less severely affected subjects in special schools. Maclean *et al.* (84) found a prevalence of X-chromatin positive males of 5.4 per 1000 and in published data it varied inversely with the degree of intellectual impairment (85-7). This confirms that the degree of intellectual impairment in X-chromatin positive males with a single mass tends to be relatively mild; at the same time the presence of many of these subjects in institutions for the severely subnormal must reflect the fact that their admission is also determined by additional factors, perhaps biological in origin, but more clearly social in practice (see below). However, it is clear that at the present time all inferences about the cerebral malfunction and other behaviour aspects of 47,XXY males are based on cross-sectional data and on prevalence comparison, and that we have hardly any information of the natural history of this and other sex chromosome disorders. Considerable time will have to pass before a substantial body of information becomes available from longitudinal follow-up studies of sex-chromosomally abnormal neonates detected in the course of routine cytological studies. Their follow-up, when they have no obvious somatic stigmata, introduces problems in relation to patient, parents and physicians, and to the hopefully unbiased nature of the observations towards a natural history of their chromosome aberrations. Nevertheless, some interesting results are beginning to emerge which seem not to clash with the inferences so far drawn from cross-sectional comparisons (29, 88). Be this as it may, the proportion of 47,XXY males in subnormality hospitals is four times, and that among the educationally subnormal boys five times, the proportion of 47,XXY males at birth, and this information is based on data from more than 83,000 males. It is probable that the excess of 47,XXYs in the deviant groups is in fact greater than shown by a comparison with birth frequency, due to their mortality in infancy and childhood (25). The X-nuclear sexing survey of Fujita *et al.* in 1972 (32) is especially informative as it gathered control data over three years from 2500 schoolboys, a one in eight random sample in the primary schools of Osaka. The test cases were 805 educationally subnormal children in special classes in Osaka and 515 institutionalized severely subnormal children from the same area. Among the normal boys there were two mosaics (46,XY/47,XXY) and one non-mosaic (47,XXY). Among the educationally subnormal there were five 47,XXYs and there were two such subjects among the severely subnormal. Thus there were five times as many aneuploid children among the former and three times among the latter, compared with the controls. Excluding the mosaics, however, there were fifteen and ten times as many 47,XXYs among the subnormal compared with the normal children. Only one of the ten aneuploid children (nine of them tested on the WISC) had an IQ of 50, all the rest had a higher IQ and the 47,XXY in an ordinary school had an IQ of 133. It is clear that these data support the findings from the other surveys. They also emphasize how global IQ is only one of the factors which lead to institutionalization. In other studies, for example, it was found that almost one third of 47,XXY males in mental hospitals had been admitted for antisocial activities such as larceny, arson, or indecent exposure or other sexual offences, more common among the chromosomally abnormal institutionalized males than among comparable controls (89, 90).

Mosaics 46,XY/47,XXY may be between five and six times more common in subnormality hospitals than among newborn males and normal school children in whom the prevalence is in keeping with their estimated incidence at birth, as the survey by Fujita *et al.* (32) shows. While chromosome mosaics in general tend to a higher IQ than chromosomally abnormal non-mosaic subjects (25), it might be that the admixture of cells within the brain has an adverse effect on its more subtle functions and on the social adaptations of mosaic individuals, which might explain their relative frequency in subnormality hospitals. However, other explanations are possible; for example, selective early mortality of the non-mosaic subjects, for which there is evidence from two studies (29, 89). Apart from epidemiological studies on incidence and prevalence, following the pattern of the earlier studies on intelligence and behaviour of males with X-chromatin positive Klinefelter's syndrome, a number of recent psychological and psychiatric studies have led to considerable information on brain function and behaviour in the 47,XXY male (45, 91, 92, 93). The main work is a comparison between thirty-four 47,XXY and sixteen 46,XY hypogonadal males. The chromosomally abnormal males were out-patients attending a general hospital and their mean IQ of 103 was lower than that of the chromosomally normal controls (IQ of 115). The latter had a somewhat higher verbal than performance score while in the former the reverse was true and this shift, albeit slight, to the advantage of the performance score has been observed also by other workers (93). The poorer verbal ability of X-chromatin positive males seems to be a real feature of the brain dysfunction profile of these subjects in view also of the evidence which is being marshalled (69) about their generally poor speech development in childhood, sometimes in the face of otherwise normal general cognitive attributes. All in all, the aneuploid patients were observed to have a 'global' unpliable pattern of perception and to have a rather passive cognitive functioning devoid of analytical subtleties. Although the 46,XY patients also showed a low score on the subtests which sort out the attention factors, the 47,XXY males were significantly more distractable. Equally their performance was significantly poorer in the Verbal Comprehension subtests. Their body image, too, proved defective and poorly organized and they generally lacked vigour, displayed anxiety and had feelings of inadequacy and insecurity, an infantile, dependent and labile emotionality, and a limited repertoire of defence mechanisms. Particularly striking was their weakness in speech and verbalization, which permeated all their test responses. They lacked verbal precision, constructed sentences poorly and left them incomplete, used words inappropriately, had difficulty in finding words, often used circumlocutions and were generally imprecise in articulation and in sentence structure.

Presumably not directly related to their subnormality, other peculiarities of the personality of 47,XXY males are those of their sexual adaptations and their insecure male gender role (47, 93, 94) which have already been touched upon in relation to reasons for their hospitalization. It is presumably this gender uncertainty which is responsible for the fact that among homosexuals they are found in excessive, though small, proportions. They figure, too, in statistics of the chromosome make-up of male (to female) transsexuals, among whom they may represent more than 6% of karyotypes (95, 96), a fact which warrants further study towards a better understanding of the origin of this disease.

The proportional frequency in mental subnormality hospitals of females with two X-chromatin masses in the nuclei of their oral mucosa (out of almost 14,000 women) is one in 255. These are presumptive and generally chromosomally proved 47,XXX (46,XX/47,XXX mosaics have been excluded). The overall prevalence is five times their incidence at birth. There is little doubt that the 47,XXX condition, which incidentally has a somatically indistinct phenotype, predisposes to retardation, and that the other behavioural attributes (see below) and the general cognitive malfunctioning are the factors which lead to relatively frequent institutionalization. The impression is that these females are in general more retarded than 47,XXY males (see also 72), and prospective data (29), though numerically small, support this impression. This receives further support by the slightly lower frequency of 47,XXX among the educationally subnormal in schools compared with the severely subnormal in institutions, in contrast with the opposite trend in 47,XXY males.

TABLE 6 Sex chromosome anomalies in surveys of severely subnormal females in institutions

	Total	47,XXX	45,X	Others*
Number	13,791	54	4	9
Proportion		1 in 255 (0.39%)	1 in 3448 (0.03%)	1 in 1532 (0.07%)

*Excluding two 46,XX/47,XXX and one higher polysomic subjects.

Note: The data are derived from a number of X-nuclear sexing surveys (refs. 30, 32, 77, 79, 84, the study of Barr *et al.* (165) and some surveys referred to by these authors), but only women in institutions have been included.

While 47,XXX females are more prevalent among the severely subnormal than among neonates, the prevalence of 45,X females in the same sample is a little lower than their incidence at birth. This suggests that there is no tendency for 45,X women to be admitted to subnormality hospitals. However, the prevalence of 45,X women in the population from which the patients in hospital were drawn is unknown. 45,X infants are often seriously malformed and, though some of them may die in the perinatal period (6), others survive only to die in later infancy or childhood (25, 84), with the consequence that prevalence estimates in older subjects, based on newborn incidence, are likely to be unduly high.

By contrast with 45,X females, those with sex chromosome mosaicism and a 45,X line have been found in mental subnormality hospitals with a frequency of one in 1500, and this is likely to be an underestimate. There are no reliable data on the prevalence of these mosaics in the general population, but there may be a true excess of such patients in subnormality hospitals; this may parallel the 47,XXY condition and its mosaics.

As the degree of global intellectual impairment of 45,X subjects seems very slight, so that the curve of distribution of their IQs is only slightly shifted to the left, it would be interesting to know what proportion of such children attend schools for the educationally subnormal. One study (97) gives direct information on this point and two other studies (78, 87), which also included some girls in subnormality hospitals, can be used, together with the results of other surveys (quoted in 32, 165). Between them, these surveys have indicated a prevalence of 45,X of about one in 700, or four or five times the newborn incidence which overestimates the prevalence in older children. In these studies, 47,XXX females were about three or four times more common than among the newborn, but less prevalent than among the severely subnormal.

There is some information about the effect on intelligence of more than three sex chromosomes and the more sex chromosomes there are, the greater the depression of intellectual level, as will be discussed below (70, 71, 72). The prevalence of 48,XXXY males in hospitals for the subnormal is of the order of one in 1200. The newborn incidence of these males is certainly very low—no case was detected in more than 83,000 male births (24).

The prevalence of 48,XXYY males in mental subnormality hospitals could exceed by more than twenty-fold their incidence at birth. Clinical data on 49,XXXXY males show that they are all severely mentally subnormal (99). As for the females, only one 48,XXXX has been found in nearly 10,000 women in mental subnormality hospitals and apparently none among nearly 75,000 newborn girls. Those described clinically were seriously subnormal (100). Two 49,XXXXX infants were severely retarded (101, 102).

Mental illness

It is difficult to investigate specific diagnostic categories of patients in institutions. It would be ideal to have information on clinically homogeneous groups admitted on uniform criteria, but this is seldom available. In 974 chronic psychotic patients (103), we found more 47,XXY males and 47,XXX females than would have been expected in the general population. Ninety-five per cent of the patients had been diagnosed as schizophrenic and our principal results are compared with those from other surveys of a similar type and shown in Table 2. As in our survey, most of the other chromosome studies were done on the indication of the X-nuclear sexing findings, I have selected those, or those parts, that concern patients with schizophrenia or a

TABLE 7 X-nuclear-sexing results in 'schizophrenic' patients

	Males		Females	
	Total	X-chromatin positive	Total	X-chromatin positive with double masses
Number	4806	28	7658	28
Proportion		1 in 172		1 in 274
		(0.58%)		(0.37%)

Refs. 30, 84, 104-10

schizophrenia-like illness; mentally subnormal patients with schizophrenia were classified as schizophrenic. Therefore some data (for example, ref. 84) were adjusted and there may have been a slight overestimate of the prevalence of abnormal X-chromatin and sex chromosome findings.

The overall prevalence of X-chromatin positive males—three-quarters of whom may be 47,XXY without evidence of mosaicism and the rest mosaics with a 47,XXY line—from all studies combined was one in 172. This is near the frequency in mental subnormality hospitals and in schools for the educationally subnormal, and is more than double the incidence of X-chromatin positive males at birth. Primary diagnosis and inclusion or rejection of cases on diagnostic grounds can affect the distribution of sex chromosome anomalies and their overall frequency (for example, 84, 85) and factors like the level of IQ of patients admitted to hospital, or the inclusion or exclusion of subjects with epilepsy, are important (84, 111).

These observations on X-chromatin positive males with Klinefelter's syndrome tend to confirm earlier observations and conjectures on their tendency to bizarre and deviant psychological functioning. Forssman and Hambert (112), surveying males in mental hospitals, concluded that in these males certain features of mental illness were common, including schizophreniform disturbances, paranoid reactions, and even typical cyclothymia. Nielsen and Fischer (98) found similar features of mental illness in Klinefelter's syndrome males with sex chromosome anomalies among mental hospital patients. The propriety of making a diagnosis of schizophrenia in a proportion of mentally ill X-chromatin positive males, even if the term is used in a purely descriptive sense, has been questioned by Hambert (111) in his study of 6265 males in Swedish mental hospitals, and Nielsen (91, 106) also comments on the atypical features of their disease. Nevertheless it would seem useful at the present time to apply this diagnostic label, when appropriate, and, if possible, to categorize the clinical variant of the illness which the chromosomally deviant subjects show (106). The type of schizo-affective psychosis of most of these patients is discussed, in relation to the work of Hambert, by Vartanyan and Gindilis (107, see also 113).

In addition to subnormality and a degree of proneness to mental illness, there is other evidence of brain dysfunction in X-chromatin positive males. Neurological abnormalities have been observed (114) and an association with Parkinsonism has been noted (76). Electroencephalogram (EEG) abnormalities in Klinefelter's syndrome have been described with a certain frequency, though they generally lack specificity (91, 111, 115, 116).

By comparison with studies in adults, few cytological studies of schizophrenic children have been done, but the results have been negative (see 84) though a recent report has discussed four patients with a 47,XXY chromosome complement and a childhood or adolescent onset of the illness among 350 schizophrenic males (117).

Considering the surveys that included females diagnosed as schizophrenic, the prevalence of women with two X-chromatin masses, about half to three-quarters of whom may be 47,XXX without evidence of mosaicism, is one in 274; it is therefore about five times the newborn incidence and of the same order as among females in mental subnormality hospitals.

In a study (118) not included in Table 2 (but see 119), a high proportion of mosaics was detected and a further report stresses this finding (120). Of the 1061 female patients screened by X-nuclear sexing of the oral cells, eleven mosaics were found in cultures of the peripheral blood and in eight this was of the 45,X/46,XX type and, interestingly, it was related to a doubtful X-negative oral smear. Others (107) also lay stress on mosaicism in cultured lymphocytes. It should not be assumed that all mosaics are of developmental as opposed to proliferative origin, and that mosaicism is necessarily present in other tissues than in the blood. This mixoploidy is possibly part of, or related to, aneuploidy of ageing (103), as is the finding in chronic schizophrenics of an excessive proportion of cells with acentric fragments (103, 110, 120), but this matter requires further study. In a Swedish survey of over 1500 women in mental hospitals, in some way a parallel to Hambert's (111) survey in males, Olanders (121) found one in 265 with two X-chromatin bodies. None of the hospitals surveyed admitted patients with uncomplicated mental deficiency. Although no specific diagnoses are given for the patients in the survey, five of the six patients with abnormal X-chromatin were psychotic or had had serious psychotic episodes. In general these women had early difficulties, for instance, at school, but their more serious and overt mental illnesses started in their late twenties. The psychotic nature of the mental state of 47,XXX women is brought out clearly by a survey of twenty-two known patients in six mental subnormality and five mental hospitals in Scotland, compared with suitably matched controls (122); and, for example, Nielsen (106) is impressed by the typical schizophrenic features of their psychotic illnesses.

A negative finding from the many studies listed in Table 7 is that only exceptionally is a 45,X patient found among schizophrenic women (119). Neuropsychiatric disorders, with or without EEG changes, have been recorded in presumptive 45,X subjects (115, 123), but there is no evidence that the incidence of these disorders is unduly high in them.

So far I have discussed, in relation to mental illness, specific and easily documented aneuploid sex chromosome changes. There are, however, other findings, as yet of tentative significance, which may turn out to be of importance (103). Although it is quite possible that none of the 'minor' variants is relevant to mental illness, the finding may be of potential interest in this respect, and warrants investigation.

Criminal behaviour

The proneness to outbursts of aggression and violence of subjects with Klinefelter's syndrome was noted in the pre-chromosomal and nuclear sexing era (73, 74). It was suggested (124) that antisocial behaviour may be a feature of sex chromosome anomalies in males, a view supported by some later findings (89). A small survey of juvenile delinquents and felons revealed a low prevalence of X-chromatin positive males (125) but, in a group of Swedish criminals and difficult-to-manage males admitted to hospitals for the mentally subnormal, Forssman and Hambert (112) found ten times the expected population incidence of X-chromatin positive males. In 1966, a survey by Casey and his collaborators (126), conducted in two English special hospitals for patients under special security because of persistent violent or aggressive behaviour (Moss-side and Rampton), yielded a proportion of X-chromatin positive males almost identical to that found by Forssman and Hambert. However, in Casey's survey, one in three of these males was 48,XXYY, compared with one in ten to one in thirty in mental subnormality hospitals. An investigation by direct chromosome methods of males in the Scottish State Hospital of Carstairs (127, 128), carried out in the light of these findings (86), yielded an almost double overall proportion of sex chromosome anomalies, due to a large proportion of 47,XYY males whose presence could not be detected by the X-nuclear sex screening of Casey. By comparison, in the Scottish study, there was a low proportion of 48,XXYYs and 47,XXYs. Subsequent findings suggested also that at Rampton and Moss-side there might be a high proportion of 47,XYY males (129). Findings in similar institutions in France were in keeping with the British results (130). At this stage the conclusion was that these males were very much more common (2.9%) among the institutionalized violent patients than among newborn males—twenty times more common, given the present data on birth incidence of one in 650-700 males. However, the overall proportional frequency with which X-chromatin positive males have been found in the three special security institutions screened in Great Britain is almost 2%, almost twice the prevalence in males in mental subnormality and mental hospitals, and nearly ten times the incidence in newborn males; so the fact that 47,XXY and 48,XXYY males may also be 'at risk in respect to criminality' was put into relief and was supported by other data (126, 131, 132).

Little is known about the prevalence of 47,XYYs in mental subnormality hospitals, though they appear to be infrequent among the severely retarded (85, 86, 132). As for 47,XYYs in mental hospitals where a low prevalence was suggested (129), the data of Nielsen (133) might indirectly suggest a figure around 0.30 to 0.40% and those of Åkesson (134) a similar figure— considerably less than in the special security institutions, but higher than in the population at large (see below).

It is worth considering the chief characteristics of the 47,XYY males in prison. Compared with an average height of 170 cm for the inmates in general, the 47,XYY males were on average 15 cm taller, and two-thirds (135) or perhaps three-quarters of them exceeded 183 cm compared with just over 10% of men in the general population. The association between height and XYY sex chromosomes is further highlighted by the facts that abnormal males tended to differ significantly from their parents and siblings (86) and that chromosome studies of the taller males, 183 cm and more, in special security hospitals detected about 25 to 30% of 47,XYYs (127, 136). A lower proportion—about 10%—has been found by Wiener and his co-workers (132) in a multi-purpose establishment in Melbourne, but the height selected for chromosome studies was 175 cm and over. Different proportions have been found in some prison establishments in the USA (137, 138, 139), and the same can be said for Danish data on tall criminal psychopaths in institutions (140). In ordinary prisons, for which data are as yet scanty, about 7% of tall males are 47,XYY (129, 141) and in boys in approved schools with heights at above the 90th percentile for age, 10% have an XYY sex chromosome complement (142). In relation to the total number of boys, a minimum estimate of the prevalence of 47,XYY in this group is three per thousand.

Other types of 'delinquent populations' have also been studied. For example, Nielsen (143) reports on 211 males referred by the courts to a regional psychiatric observation and treatment clinic in Jutland. He detected four 47,XYYs (1.9%) and one 47,XXY (0.5%) and noted also a significantly higher proportion of males with an excessively long arm of the Y chromosome compared with a sample of newborn infants and with data from other studies of normal adults, in confirmation of the findings of Kahn (144) in remand homes in England.

Many of the studies done before 1970 on various populations of delinquents, mostly prison, are reviewed in the report of a conference on the XYY sex chromosome anomaly addressed especially at the behavioural, criminal and legal aspects of the condition (145). Among 1786 subjects not selected for height, seventeen 47,XYYs were detected (0.95%), whereas among the 3556 'tall' males (mostly 183 cm or taller) there were 86 (2.42%), a significant difference.

The different types of populations sampled, the relatively small size of the individual surveys, the lack of uniform sampling criteria and the different countries where the surveys originated (with their different customs, legal systems and social structures and services) must be stressed when considering the studies on 47,XYYs and the overall bearing which the findings have on the interpretations of the behavioural and somatic aspects of the XYY sex chromosome anomaly.

It has been suggested that the high frequency of 47,XYYs in special prison hospitals is entirely due to selection by height of these criminals, whose committal would be influenced by their formidable appearance (146), and that the 47,XYY anomaly is common generally among tall males, though pilot studies have failed to show this (129, 147). However, the investigation by Zeuthen and colleagues (148) is informative on this point and also relevant to assessing prevalence findings of 47,XYYs in deviant populations screened on a height basis. In the course of compulsory examination for military service in Denmark, out of 3840 representative recruits, Zeuthen selected 1021 using as criteria a height of 181 cm or over and good testes size, and a further 94 males who had small testes or might for other reasons repay chromosome studies. Twenty refused chromosome studies, but among the 1021 tall males, five 47,XYYs, or one in 204, were found. On the assumption that these were the only males with this anomaly in the total group of recruits, the normal adult male population prevalence should be near one in 768, which agrees well with the results of the Danish (12) and other newborn surveys. Incidentally the chromosomally abnormal recruits were essentially normal though with abnormal spermatogenesis, a well documented feature of the condition. Studies in several groups of normal adult males in Scotland, totalling over 9000, give a prevalence of 47,XYY or about one in a thousand (145).

Analysis of the criminal acts and records showed that 47,XYY males, compared with the other males, in special security hospitals tended to come from families in which there was less crime; in spite of their physique they committed unskilful crimes, significantly more often against property than people, and their gain was small. From a Danish comparison of eleven 47,XYYs, thirty-four males with Klinefelter's syndrome who had been charged with criminal acts, and other delinquent groups, and in the light of national statistics, the impression is derived that arson was a frequent charge in the 47,XYYs and that sexual crimes, especially towards children, were a feature of the two sex chromosome trisomies (149). Males with XYY sex chromosomes in special security hospitals inclined towards an earlier start, at puberty or even before, to their criminal activities, as the findings among boys in approved schools also suggest (150). Retrospective findings support this suggestion (136), 47,XYYs being convicted, on average, 4½ years earlier than males with Klinefelter's syndrome and six years earlier than the other offenders (151); and in isolated reports of the condition in young children there is evidence, albeit anecdotal, of behaviour difficulties before puberty (152, 153).

The intelligence level of 47,XYYs was estimated to be borderline and in this way they did not differ from their fellow prisoners (149, 154), but data on their cognitive functions are inadequate (71). It is possible that on average they may not be intellectually impaired to any very great degree, but, as with 47,XXY males, the results of the performance tests are better than those of the verbal tests.

It has been suggested that the 47,XYY anomaly is responsible for a progressive illness, not only in terms of ingravescent social maladjustment, but also as a true organic deterioration (132, 155), and there is evidence of a variety of distinct neurological abnormalities, with intention tremor, and of a high prevalence, almost 7%, of overt seizures, about six or more times that in the population at large (156). In keeping with this it appears that EEG changes, which, however, tend to be non-specific, may be frequent in 47,XYY males and may be relevant to their behavioural abnormalities (138, 157, 158).

By temperament, 47,XYY males are said to be violent and aggressive, though this judgment is based almost entirely on those in prison. Actually the impression of their behaviour is perhaps more one of impulsiveness. Their personality seems to be obsessive and introverted and they are slow and cautious in deciding. In a questionnaire comparison of 47,XYY males with their fellow patients in a State mental hospital, there were apparently marked differences in the structure of 'defensiveness' (or its concept) of the two groups as well as, possibly, in those of 'hostility' and 'aggression' (159). Indeed, the chromosomally normal controls were, in hospital at least, more overtly aggressive and hostile (150).

The strength of the association between certain sex chromosome anomalies in males and social maladaptation is unknown, but only a few of the 47,XYY males at risk seem to have been traced among the abnormal groups that have been screened, and the fate of the rest is unknown (31, 86). Indeed a Scottish study of 2608 males, many in Approved Schools, a number of new entrants into Borstals, some in Prisons, some in Allocation and in Detention Centres and a few young offenders, has failed to show an excessive concentration of chromosomal abnormalities (160). It is clear that this requires confirmation. It is also clear that the previous findings stand, but that accumulation of 47,XYY males in certain institutions may reflect differences in their turnover, as well as in risk of their admission. There obviously are differences between institutions which may operate a selection of their inmates. Furthermore, there are differences in the legal systems and in the practical application of the law between countries, and sometimes regions, as there is variation of standards of prison, hospital and clinical facilities, and of the practice of forensic psychiatric assessment. Delinquency and crime are not capable of precise definition: many are the behaviour patterns which are interpreted as breaches of the law; many who commit such breaches are not discovered, fewer are charged and fewer still are committed, and at each level the process is likely to be non-random (145). The overall feeling at the present time is that chromosomally deviant males, and particularly, but not only, the 47,XYYs, *are* at risk of behavioural difficulties which *may* put them on a collision course with the law; that the risk is not unequivocally correlated with the abnormal chromosome complement, the effect of which on general behaviour may be circuitous; that the size of the risk is difficult to assess and is clearly not automatically determined by the chromosome anomaly. These points raise important theoretical issues which require further and accurate studies (145), both epidemiological and more directly biological, while the practical implications of abnormal chromosome complements in respect to criminality remain literally *sub judice* at the present time.

Particularly important is the systematic collection of unbiased and preferably prospective information, though the latter is bound to accumulate at a slow rate. Nevertheless, the seventeen 47,XYY infants identified among about 11,000 newborns by four routine chromosome surveys of neonates, and those that are gradually swelling their ranks, already give some interesting results in terms of developmental trends (pooled data of Jacobs *et al.*, 161).

Nothing accurate can be said about the effect of more than two Y chromosomes, because few reports are available (162, 163).

At Rampton and Moss-side, Casey *et al.* (126) found two women with double X-chromatin masses, alleged 47,XXX, among 410 whom they tested, a prevalence similar to that found among institutionalized mentally subnormal or psychotic women, and about six times that found among newborn females; but Berg (164) found none among 109 mentally ill women admitted for criminal reasons to Broadmoor Hospital. Kaplan (119) reports on an X-nuclear sexing survey of women offenders and of juvenile delinquent females in Ohio prisons. Among the former, he found two out of 200 with two X-chromatin masses, presumptive 47,XXX. Among the latter, he detected four X-chromatin negative subjects, presumptive 45,X in 379, a ratio of one in 95 compared with population incidence at birth of one per 2500 or so females, an unexpected result.

In summary: sex chromosome anomalies are found to correlate, but neither uniformly nor unequivocally, with cognitive and personality deviations. They appear to be a factor in psychopathic development in a proportion of chromosomally unbalanced subjects, who thus seem to be at special risk for these behavioural mishaps. Triple-X women may be at greater cognitive disadvantage compared with the other common anomalies and at some risk of mental illness; 47,XXY males may be at a slightly lesser cognitive risk, but at similar risk of psychotic disorders; the risk of the individual 47,XYY male of criminal behaviour and commitment seems greater than average; 45,X females have only slightly deviant global cognitive skills, but demonstrate a seemingly specific brain dysfunction.

continues overleaf

The mechanism of sex chromosome imbalance

Considering together autosome and sex chromosome anomalies, one or more extra chromosomes—and it is simpler to consider first this form of imbalance—can have three types of effect which can be termed specific, semi-specific and non-specific (166). Specific effects may be attributed to the presence in abnormal numbers (for example, in triplicate) of alleles, the gene loci of which are on the extra chromosome (or chromosomes). In the case of structural major genes it is likely that different products are manufactured in the cells in response to each gene locus. But protein and enzyme synthesis in complex cells is a carefully regulated and adjusted process, so that no simple quantitive rule can be given as to the result. Specifically, given three doses of the same allele of a structural gene, a 50% increase of the gene products should not necessarily be expected. However, in view of what is known of dose effects in heterozygotes for some metabolic errors, trisomics (or other polysomics) should reveal some dose effects. On the other hand, if each locus were occupied by a different allele of the gene under consideration, each gene product should be easily detected. Now that gene loci for some enzyme proteins have been assigned to specific human autosomes, the effect of trisomy can be selectively tested and evidence suggests that some genes on some trisomic autosomes can show a dose effect of the gene product (167). Where an excess of regulator genes is concerned, a decrease of structural gene products might be expected. Regulators seem to influence negatively the rate at which structural genes are copied, because their products can reversibly bind to specific sites on the chromosome, whence the copying of structural genes proceeds, so that the structural gene is temporarily blocked. Such a mechanism, demonstrated in bacteria (168), has been postulated for human autosomal trisomies (169). As most chromosomes will carry a mixture of controlling genes and factors, and of structural genes, one general approach is to study the 'protein profile' of a given trisomy, compared with that produced by the disomic state and with the trisomies for other chromosomes. This method has shown the chemical specificity, for example, of the different trisomies of barley (170).

Semi-specific effects may be attributed to those special chromosomes in the human set which carry nucleolar-organiser regions, the acrocentric autosomes responsible for two of the three major autosomal trisomic syndromes. The presence of the ribosomal genes in the SAT region—the satellite stalk—of these chromosomes has been inferred from morphological criteria and has recently been demonstrated by the technique of *in situ* RNA-DNA hybridization (171). This could successfully be applied because of the repetitive nature of the ribosomal genes, of which man may possess some 450. An extra acrocentric autosome should add a set of these genes, say fifty, to the cells, as is now known to be the case in trisomy 21 (172), particularly if the ribosomal genes of the different acrocentrics were not all identical, as is just possible. This addition might affect cellular metabolism through excessive production of special RNA species, and consequently of nucleolar material, with effects on protein-enzyme synthesis by the cells as a whole.

With respect to human sex chromosome anomalies, a semi-specific effect, as defined, can be disregarded and, for reasons that will be detailed below, specific effects are highly improbable, with the odd exception. By contrast, non-specific chromosome imbalance effects seem to be particularly relevant. These seem to be due to whole chromosomes, or entire chromosome segments, and may be unrelated to the specific gene content of these chromosomes or chromosome parts. Some of these effects may pertain to some autosome segments and I think it probable that some of the so-called minor 'variants' (for example near the centromeres, or in the short arms of acrocentric chromosomes) have a phenotypic effect, perhaps on fertility or on some of the subtle functions of the nervous system. These effects can be broadly called 'heterochromatic' and thus attributed to the 'heterochromatin' of the chromosomes. It is thought that especially the human sex chromosomes, like those of other mammals, may *be*, or may *become* at some stage of development, largely or completely heterochromatic in the somatic cells. The former applies to the Y, the latter to the X chromosome.

Heterochromatin

I shall deal rather more fully with the generalities about heterochromatin and with the ideas often derived from the study of other organisms than man, because they constitute a necessary background against which to consider the complexities and uncertainties of heterochromatin and its properties.

The story is complex and the subject controversial, particularly in respect to its implications, but it is relevant to the action of unbalanced chromosomes, particularly the X and the Y.

Heterochromatin was originally described and named by Heitz in 1928 (reviewed in 173) as a component of chromosomes and exclusively as a cytological feature. What set it apart was its staining character, which differed from that of the rest of the chromatin, the euchromatin. While the euchromatic portion of the chromosomes became unstainable and invisible because decondensed, the heterochromatin was highly stainable and condensed, forming in the so-called resting nucleus one or several masses or chromocentres. In a series of careful observations Heitz showed that parts of individual chromosomes changed gradually as mitosis proceeded, from the condensed metaphase condition to a diffuse, practically unstainable state, while other parts, the heterochromatic regions, remained condensed. From this cytological and descriptive starting point, aspects of the behaviour of heterochromatin were observed which led to speculations about its *raison d'être*, and its function. The most important observation concerns the genetic, or better genic, inertness of the heterochromatin, which stems from the study of heterochromatin in *Drosophila*. There was evidence that the fruit-fly's heterochromatic Y chromosome was inert; its X chromosome revealed a section, homologous to parts of the Y, largely devoid of mappable genes (see 174) while, in addition, in the rest of the chromosome complement there was correspondence between heterochromatin and inertness. Another property of heterochromatin relates to gene inactivity: there is evidence that heterochromatin in mammals, man included, 'makes' RNA less profusely than the euchromatic parts of the chromosomes (175-7), which suggests a diminished or absent activity of gene transcription. Two other important aspects of the behaviour of heterochromatin, which are especially relevant to development and give a clue to some of its functions, are, first, that different cells show differences in the quantity and distribution of heterochromatin, so that the chromosomes and their segments have special characteristics which are related to the type of cell in which they operate; and, second, that heterochromatin has an inhibitory effect on the action of genes transposed close to it which, however, does not alter the basic make-up of these genes, as can be shown by the fact that they resume normal reactivity when they are returned to their original sites (position effect) (178, 179). A further property of heterochromatin, especially important in respect to the mammalian X chromosome, was the discovery of its late DNA synthesis during the course of chromosome replication. These observations that heterochromatin represents cyclical physiological states of chromosome segments (180), that it is not a 'permanent' characteristic and may not be seen at certain stages in development and thus that its formation is variable, and that what is true for one stage, cell type or sex may not be valid for other situations (181), led to a shift of emphasis from heterochromatin as a *substance* to heterochromatin as a *state*. From the concept that heterochromatin was chromosome material devoid of genes, the idea emerged that it was a substance containing genes, but that they are masked and inactivated. That there can be standard genes in heterochromatin, a view once refuted, is clear from studies of experimental organisms and from a simple consideration of the human X chromosome when it forms the X-chromatin mass, or Barr body. Among the former, evidence has come from *Drosophila* (181), but especially from the Mealy bugs in which a whole set of genically active chromosomes can be inactivated in transmission between one generation and the next (174). As for the X chromosome and its derived heterochromatic X-chromatin (which fits the criteria of 'heterochromatin', see below), its content of major standard genes requires no comment. Consequently heterochromatin can be redefined as a state of chromosomes, or of sections of chromosomes, which are often and regularly heterochromatic when circumstances are similar. In line with this, new terms have been introduced to distinguish the more 'classical' heterochromatin devoid of standard genes, the *constitutive* heterochromatin, from that which, though rich in standard major genes, in the course of development becomes genically inert, the *facultative* heterochromatin (174).

Recent new knowledge has accrued concerning the distribution and qualities of different types of heterochromatin within the genome; and a principal reason for considering these regional, and presumably functional, differences of heterochromatin, is to stress the fact that the presumptive action of heterochromatin *per se* may be called non-specific only as a first approximation. We should really think of heterochromatin more in the plural than in the singular, and this way of thinking ought to extend to the heterochromatic functions. In the past this has been emphasized in the clear-cut distinction made, for example, in *Drosophila,* between chromocentric heterochromatin, contained in large blocks within chromosomes or even making up almost an entire chromosome (with the densely coiled α- and the looser meshed β-heterochromatins) (182) and the intercalary variety which forms several small blocks within the mitotic chromosomes. It has been suggested that there is justification for restricting the name 'heterochromatin' to the chromocentric type, finding a different name for the intercalary variety. It is to this type that the function was attributed of carrying tight blocks of genes with similar, small, plus and minus, supplementary effects all contributing to the same quantitative character (polygenic blocks) (183). Indeed, some (184) have tended to equate all heterochromatic functions with those thought to be characteristic attributes of polygenic systems. This view had not had great support, but the idea of multiple duplications and thus the presence of several copies of specific genes in some chromosome structures within the genome is very acceptable now. Be this as it may, powerful techniques are providing new facts and information about the heterochromatins in higher organisms, including mammals and man. First, there are the methods of biochemical isolation of DNA and the studies of the kinetics of DNA denaturation-renaturation which permit inferences to be made on repetitiveness or uniqueness of special DNA sequences in the genome and their distribution (185, 186). Second is the related preparative method of cutting up the genomic DNA into segments of different lengths, which allows inferences to be made about the alternation within the organized chromosome of repetitive with unique DNA sequences (187). Third, there is the complementary method of *in situ* hybridization (188, 189), valuable in seeing the distribution and localization in the actual chromosomes of the various 'satellite' DNA fractions (reviewed in 190); and fourth, the various other chromosome procedures from fluorescence to the various types of Giemsa banding. All this gives information about the organization of the genome into chromosomes, their DNA make-up and the types and distribution of heterochromatin. As a result, the constitutive centromeric heterochromatin (reviewed in 191), the 'intercalary' type (192), possibly the telomeric variety and those of the Y-chromosome are joining the ranks of the facultative (and other) heterochromatins of the mammalian X chromosomes.

Undoubtedly as far as human sex chromosomes and their anomalies are concerned, heterochromatin is of particular interest, and the ideas on heterochromatin which I have reviewed, fit these chromosomes well. First the X chromosome that forms the X-chromatin mass of normal females—or those that form additional X-chromatin masses in cases of X chromosome polysomy—is clearly heterochromatic when it forms a distinct chromocentre in the interphase nucleus, though whether this X-chromatin mass represents the whole of the chromosome is unknown. And this chromosome, or, in the case of X polysomy, these chromosomes, synthesize their DNA very late during the synthetic period of the mitotic cycle. Finally, it is (or: they are) alleged to be genically inactive according to the Lyon hypothesis and thus, at least from the viewpoint of the expression of the major gene content, inert (reviewed in 193).

The Y chromosome is also thought to be at least largely heterochromatic. The cytological evidence from fluorescence and banding studies is supported by autoradiography and by the fact that hardly any major alleles have been shown to be transmitted in a holoandric manner, at least in humans.

Genetic role of heterochromatin

We have seen that heterochromatin is thought to be genically inert, but there are many data that deny the idea of total inertness. It seems that heterochromatin exerts an effect, but the explanation for the findings relating to this effect are not straightforward and we lack a detailed molecular framework on heterochromatin: 'One thing must be said with certainty: heterochromatin must play a considerable role in the history of the chromosomes and in their function and an important, but unorthodox, genetic role is expected' (194). Present views on repression and de-repression of whole chromosomes or chromosome segments during development and their relationship to heterochromatization are beginning to provide a background for a general hypothesis on one important aspect of heterochromatin function.

Looking particularly, but not exclusively, at the facultative variety, the prime function of heterochromatin (or, more precisely, of its molecular correlate) would be to turn off genes, or some of them, when they are not wanted in a given cell, tissue, sex and developmental stage. The fundamental question is whether or not, once it has done this, heterochromatin has any further function and activity as such, that is, as heterochromatin. If not, then any effect on, say, a quantitative character under study, which seems attributable to heterochromatin *per se*, is in reality the effect of the action of one or more standard genes within it, observed at a distance in time and space and therefore far removed from when the gene was active during earlier development. Alternatively, heterochromatin may act also in its own right, independent of the genes within it that were active earlier on or are active only in some tissues.

It seems clear that the X-chromatin-forming, facultatively heterochromatic X chromosomes are not fully inert, neither the single heterochromatic X in the normal female—which, at the very least, seems required for fertility—nor the plural heterochromatic Xs in subjects with multiple X chromosomes. An increasing number of them, as we have seen, causes various abnormalities of brain function and the evidence points to a quantitative relationship between the number of Xs and the severity of brain dysfunction. In the more extreme examples there are not only severe subnormality but also somatic anomalies, including cardiovascular changes. These facts could be taken to support the idea that the X or Xs present in excess of one, act as heterochromatic elements by their charge of heterochromatin, though other general suggestions are possible.

The heterochromatin of the X and those of the Y differ in several important respects, even apart from the respective sizes of these two chromosomes. If sex is determined by heterochromatin controlling the essential developmental steps that lead to the primary sex differences—an old idea in experimental and theoretical genetics (195) which has been recently discussed (196, 197, 198, 199)—the heterochromatin of the mammalian Y would clearly have a different function from that of the heterochromatic X. Although the sex-determining role of the Y chromosome may well be attributed to the presence in a discrete part of the Y chromosome of structural or other major genes (197), it has been argued that there is no need to postulate the existence of such genes (198), the presence of which is not proved, and that heterochromatin may be the genetic agent that influences the 'generalized processes of early development that decide the growth properties of the cells which after all make up the morphological sex differences' (200).

If we accept, as a working hypothesis, the view that heterochromatin may act in its own right, though keeping in mind the alternative touched upon above, and not forgetting that we may be dealing with an interplay of both effects, the question is: what does heterochromatin do and how does it do it? As for its manifestations, a few can be listed and will be briefly discussed: a general effect on the cell cycle, on the pattern of cell division and particularly its control, especially when it is fast (201); regulation of cell growth and size particularly during development (202); and a quantitative effect on cell metabolism (201, 203).

Additional chromosomes usually increase the length of the mitotic cycle (204). In plants, for example, supernumerary heterochromatic chromosomes may make pollen grains undergo additional divisions (205) and quicken cell division (206), though in other cases heterochromatin seems to lengthen the mitotic cycle (207). Supernumerary chromosomes which, however, are not invariably heterochromatic, have been known to induce precocity of seed germination in some plants (208) and delays in others (209), and other quantitative variations are attributable to these chromosomal elements (209, 210).

Accepting the 'second' X of normal females, and the Y, as examples of heterochromatic chromosomes, we have some knowledge as to what happens when they are absent in man, in the 45,X condition. Angell (211), by subculturing fibroblasts from mosaics with a 45,X line, showed the proliferative advantage of these cells, and a considerably shorter mitotic cycle of 45,X cells was demonstrated by Barlow (212). It was attributed to a shortening of the G^1, pre-DNA synthesis (or S) phase. This, *in vivo*, could have a powerful influence on cell division during early development when the process is already fast (see, for example, 213). If tissues, as seems to be the case for total body size in developing mammals, or at least some organs, are subject to control of size rather than cell numbers, this rapid cell cycle might result in an excessive number of cells at the time of differentiation and may possibly account for the high prenatal mortality of 45,Xs and for the other effects (214). In the haploid axolotl, in which we can assume that the cell cycle is fast, there are twice as many neural crest-derived cells as in the diploid larvae (215). Extrapolating to the 45,X condition, it may be hypothesized that a similar specific cell excess could be the reason for the significantly increased number of pigmented naevi and for the high frequency of dark hair observed in Turner's syndrome and Ovarian Dysgenesis survivors, compared with age-matched normal controls (216).

We have little information about the effect on the cell cycle of added sex chromosomes but, in view of the low prenatal lethality of embryos with this type of imbalance, it might be argued that the effect is small, or that, at any rate, it does not grossly affect global development, that any effect on the cell cycle should be a lengthening of the G^1 phase and that there should result an overall limitation of cell numbers during development, but that there could be some complementary increase in cell size (see below). In a few animals, and in many plants (particularly rye, maize and some lilies), variable numbers (more usually even) of additional chromosomes, called B chromosomes, are often found. They are generally heterochromatic, in the cytological sense, and are not essential to normal growth and development, yet seemingly they are not devoid of adaptive meaning. Each extra B chromosome lengthens the G^1 phase and thus retards the mitotic cycle by almost 10% (207) or a little less

(217), depending on the plant. Whether or not heterochromatic elements act on the cell cycle merely by the extra DNA which they add (218)—about one twentieth of the total DNA is added with each B chromosome (219)—or by their late DNA synthesizing property is unknown. It has been found, for example, that plants with extra B chromosomes have a higher nuclear histone content and histone/DNA ratio, which increases with the number, from 0 to 8, of these chromosomes and is especially marked in the odd-numbered chromosome classes (220, 221, 222). With the increment of nuclear histone there is a corresponding fall of nuclear RNA (222). It is of interest that histone f1, the very lysine-rich histone, is produced, albeit in small amounts, during the G^1 phase of the mammalian cell cycle (223). While one should stress that the role of histones generally is by no means settled, and that various substances would seem to interact with them (224, 225), they probably play an important part in regulating gene expression. Histone f1 in particular inhibits transcription of repetitive DNA into RNA, and DNA 'packing' and condensation are highly dependent on it. It should be noted that one model of heterochromatin is based on repeated gene sequences which specifically are required to function genically only at special developmental stages but are otherwise partly or wholly inactivated (224), and, clearly, could be excessively masked by a surplus of histone produced, with consequent untoward developmental effects. While an excess of masking histones is thought to be capable of completely switching-off genic chromosomal segments, one has to consider the alternative possibility that it may instead shorten the time during which a given stretch of DNA, previously tightly packed, becomes uncoiled, opens up and is thus available for copying into RNA and hence for delivering its genetic message. This curtailment of time could result in impaired gene transcription and translation, a well known quantitative effect on the products of genes located within heterochromatin. But there is another way in which we can visualize that biochemical effects could stem from changes in the cell cycles. We have seen that f1 histone seems to be produced, in small amounts, during the G^1 phase of the cycle, while the bulk is produced during S. Also the manufacture, or release, of other proteins and enzymes seems to be geared to phases of the cell cycle, both in the case of substances continuously produced (and thus influenced by total duration of the cycle) and those periodically synthesized. For each substance there may be a characteristic 'step' or 'peak' production- (or expression-) profile which depends on its stability, on type of cell and, presumably, on developmental stage (226, 227). So, to the influence of surplus (or deficient) heterochromatin on the cell cycle, on cell division and thus on the number of cells at differentiation, and on other derived cellular properties (such as migratory ability), we must add the correlated biochemical effect, which at times may be serious enough to upset cellular viability and interfere with development in a gross way. Thus there are at least two interrelated ways by which heterochromatin imbalance may affect development. In addition, there is the problem of how sex chromosome imbalance can affect cells in differentiated tissues, *after* the division cycle is over. We are considering cells, like the neurons, that are not going to re-enter the mitotic cycle, though naturally, within the nervous system, they are in equilibrium with cells which are capable of division and which therefore are influenced in a direct way by alterations of the mitotic cycle.

A first assumption we can make is that the neurons may be numerically inadequate and morphologically deviant having emerged as 'resting cells' from cells with an abnormal cycle due to chromosome imbalance. Clearly these cells could be also functionally impaired, subject to greater wear and tear than normal cells and prone to abiotrophic involution. In addition, it is possible that heterochromatin might continue to disturb gene-mediated effects in a more direct manner. For example, it has been thought that heterochromatin influences general cell size and nuclear volume (202, 228). Changes in nuclear volume are known to be related to heterochromatization, for example sex chromatin formation (229), and it is possible that dispersion and condensation of chromatin may determine volume changes, perhaps by influencing permeability of nuclear membranes (230). The spatial relationship of heterochromatin, and of chromosomes generally, to the nuclear membrane is of interest in this context. Therefore it is entirely possible that persistent effects in differentiated tissues of heterochromatin *per se,* may rest on alterations of cell volume and membrane permeability. Other suggestions have been put forward (203), but have not been found convincing, for biochemical reasons also (231).

Quantitative effects

Leaving aside hypotheses concerning mechanisms of action, it is clear that heterochromatic chromosomes can influence quantitative characters. In plants, for example, B chromosomes depress height, tiller number, straw weight and degree of fertility in a manner which strictly depends on the number of additional chromosomes (222). In man, too, there are marked quantitative effects: on stature (33), on IQ and on birth weight (for example, 72). The quantitative effect on height is rather complex, but each extra heterochromatic X chromosome was found to depress the IQ by sixteen points

TABLE 8   Total digital ridge count (TRC) in sex chromosome anomalies and in normal males and females

Chromosome complement	Number of subjects	Mean TRC
45,X	126	168.14
46,XY	825	144.98
46,XX	825	127.23
47,XYY	226	128.21
47,XXY	210	117.55
⎰ 47,XXX	32	103.94
⎱ 48,XYYY	1	83.00
48,XXYY	46	97.34
48,XXXY	15	89.85
48,XXXX	19	73.93
49,XXXYY	1	71.43
49,XXXXY	10	55.36
49,XXXXX	2	17.00

Refs. 130, 239-56, and unpublished work by myself and N. Polani.

and the birth weight by 305 g (see also 214). In each case the Y chromosome seems to exercise a similar, but smaller quantitative influence. By contrast the IgM level, which is greater in normal females than males, rises with each X chromosome added (72, 232, 233). The quantity control of this immunoglobulin has been attributed to genes on the X chromosome (234, 235), and the effect could be related to synthesis geared to cell cycle stage (72). However, the most striking effect of sex chromosome imbalance in man is on number of dermal ridges on finger tips, the so-called total ridge count. This is an almost perfect metrical characteristic which follows the rules for the correlation between relatives in respect to quantitative traits on the supposition of Mendelian inheritance (56). The total ridge count is, with very little environmental interference, thought to be genetically determined by a few autosomal genes with strictly additive effect (236). There is no indication (57) of an effect of X-linked genes (58, 237), but the effect of numerical anomalies of sex chromosomes is turning out to be most interesting from the viewpoint of the heterochromatin hypothesis. Sex chromosome increments depress the total ridge count, as Alter pointed out (238), and Penrose (237, 239) has shown a quantitative and inverse relationship between the number of sex chromosomes in the set and the total ridge count.

It is estimated that each X chromosome depresses the total ridge count by about thirty ridges, and that each Y chromosome has about two-thirds this effect. If this quantitative effect were an effect of the heterochromatins of these two chromosomes, it might be possible to show, in normal circumstances, and if proportionally important, an influence of sex heterochromatin added to any effects of the autosomes. In this situation family studies should show

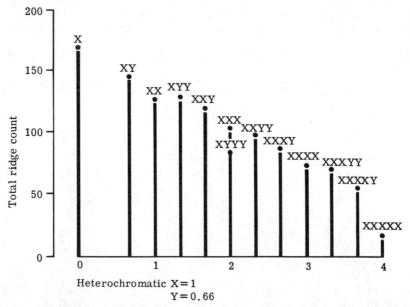

Figure 1 Relationship between number of sex chromosomes and total ridge count on fingers (from Table 8, modified from ref. 239).

daughters to be more highly correlated with their mothers—they possess one Barr-body-forming, heterochromatic X, the same as their mothers. Sons should be more strongly correlated with their fathers, whose Y chromosome they inherit. On the other hand, fathers and daughters, and mothers and sons, should be less strongly correlated, expectations that differ from those of X-linked inheritance. For a character completely controlled by an X-linked gene, disregarding the details of the inter-sibling correlations, the father/son correlation should be zero and the father/daughter and mother/son correlations should be high, in keeping with X chromosome transmission. Completely holoandrically transmitted characters due to Y-linked genes would cause the correlation coefficients between father and son and that between brothers to be near unity (57).

TABLE 9   Correlation coefficient for the 'total ridge count' between parents and offspring according to sex

	No. of pairs	r		Standard error of r
Mother/daughter	155	0.60	±	0.05
Father/son	159	0.55	±	0.06
Father/daughter	145	0.45	±	0.07
Mother/son	165	0.41	±	0.06

Ref. 97

Unfortunately, data are scanty and correlations, though showing a trend in the right direction, are not significant, at least if the four correlation coefficients are considered against the theoretical value of 0.5 (Table 9). A comparison of the two correlation coefficients, mother/daughter and mother/son, however, shows them to be significantly different; also, the difference between the values for mother/daughter and father/daughter almost reaches the conventional level of statistical significance. The father/son correlation, while stronger than that between father and daughter, does not differ significantly from it. The sib/sib correlations have not been instructive (237). A more recent study (58) based on a sample of Polish rural family isolates has given somewhat similar results, but with lower correlation coefficient in all pairwise comparisons, and the trend indicated in Table 9 and discussed above has not been maintained.

All these observations on quantitative effects of sex chromosome imbalance are important in relation to heterochromatic effects. For the ridge-count effect, Penrose (237) proposed a mechanism involving imbibition of tissues with fluid, based on the cystic hygroma findings in 45,X abortuses. A lymphoedema state in 45,X survivors is also well known, and there may be some evidence, though not supported by other findings, of a relationship between this state and the ridge count on finger tips (discussed in 33). There is no evidence that tissues of subjects with an excessive number of sex chromosomes are dehydrated, to account for an opposite effect on the ridge count. So it is possible that the effect of numerical sex chromosome anomalies is mediated instead by an influence on number *and* size of cells, in accordance with the views expressed above; and when cells are mixed, in mosaics, the resulting patterns will also be mixed, as indeed they are (258). It is clear that these two cell features could profoundly influence the formation and size of the characteristic ridges of the skin during early embryonic life, and exercise their influence in other tissues and organs as hypothesized above.

Summary

With few exceptions, errors of the sex chromosomes allow near-normality of bodily appearance, though they may cause a variety of behavioural disorders, ranging from minor deviations of brain function, through subnormality, to psychopathic disorders that may pave the way to various forms of social maladaptation and may bring the afflicted person into conflict with the law. There are trends that link some of these disorders to specific sex chromosome anomalies. The absence of a sex chromosome has little overall effect on cognition, but may specifically affect brain function. The presence of an extra X chromosome in females and in males may cause moderate mental subnormality and may introduce a risk of psychotic illness, at times schizophrenia. Further additions of sex chromosomes cause more serious mental subnormality. An additional Y chromosome in males may produce a greater than usual risk of involvement with the law.

It is possible that the effect of numerical sex chromosome anomalies on brain function be related rather to whole specific chromosomes than to their content of specific genes, an effect attributable to their 'heterochromatin'. There is evidence that measured intelligence (IQ) and other characteristics are affected by sex chromosome anomalies in a manner which is quantitatively correlated with the number of these 'heterochromatic' chromosomes in the set. The way this heterochromatin imbalance acts is unknown, but it could affect cell cycles during development and thus upset the number of cells at differentiation. It could, in addition, or in parallel, exercise other quantitative effects on cells and, by a combination of developmental and other influences, affect not only cell morphology but also directly cell function and hence integrity.

References

(1)   Polani, P.E. (1967) Occurrence and effect of human chromosome abnormalities. In *Social and Genetic Influences on Life and Death*, Eds. R. Platt and A.S. Parkes, pp. 3-19. Edinburgh and London, Oliver and Boyd.

(2)   Polani, P.E. (1969) Autosomal imbalance and its syndromes, excluding Down's. *Br. med. Bull.*, *25*, 81-93.

(3)   Alberman, E. and Creasy, M.R. (1975) Factors affecting chromosome abnormalities in human conceptions. In *Chromosome Variations in Human Evolution* (Symposium of the Society for the Study of Human Biology), *14*, pp. 83-95. London, Taylor and Francis.

(4)   Dhadial, R.K., Machin, A.M. and Tait, S.M. (1970) Chromosome anomalies in spontaneously aborted human fetuses. *Lancet*, *2*, 20-1.

(5)   Boué, J. and Boué, A. (1973) Anomalies chromosomiques dans les avortements spontanes. In *Les accidents chromosomiques de la reproduction*, Eds. A. Boué and C. Thibault, pp. 29-55. Paris: Institute National de la Santé et de la Recherche Médicale.

(6) Machin, G.A. (1974) Chromosome abnormality and perinatal death. *Lancet, 1*, 549-51.
(7) Sutherland, G.R., Bauld, R. and Bain, A.D. (1974) Chromosome abnormality and perinatal death. *Lancet, 1*, 752 (letter).
(8) Robinson, A. (1974) Neonatal deaths and sex-chromosome anomalies. *Lancet, 1*, 1223 (letter).
(9) Kajii, T., Ohama, K., Niikawa, N., Ferrier, A. and Avirachan, S. (1973) Banding analysis of abnormal karyotypes in spontaneous abortion. *Am. J. hum. Genet., 25*, 539-47.
(10) Creasy, M.R. and Crolla, J.A. (1974) Prenatal mortality of trisomy 21 (Down's syndrome). *Lancet, 1*, 473-4.
(11) Hamerton, J.L., Ray, M., Abbott, J., Williamson, C. and Ducasse, G.C. (1972) Chromosome studies in a neonatal population. *Canadian Medical Association Journal, 106*, 776-9.
(12) Friedrich, U. and Nielsen, J. (1973) Chromosome studies in 5,049 consecutive newborn children. *Clin. Genet., 4*, 333-43.
(13) Lubs, H.A. and Ruddle, F.H. (1970) Application of quantitative karyotype to chromosome variation in 4,400 consecutive newborns. In *Human Population Cytogenetics*, Eds. P.A. Jacobs, W.H. Price and P. Law, pp. 119-42. Edinburgh, Edinburgh University Press.
(14) Caspersson, T., Lomakka, G. and Zech, L. (1971) The 24 fluorescence patterns of the human metaphase chromosomes—distinguishing characters and variability. *Hereditas (Lund), 67*, 89-102.
(15) Arrighi, F.E. and Hsu, T.C. (1971) Localization of heterochromatin in human chromosomes. *Cytogenetics, 10*, 81-6.
(16) Gagné, R., Tanguay, R. and Laberge, C. (1971) Differential staining patterns of heterochromatin in man. *Nature New Biology, 232*, 29-30.
(17) Bobrow, M., Madan, K. and Pearson, P.L. (1972) Staining of some specific regions of human chromosomes, particularly the secondary constriction of No. 9. *Nature New Biology, 238*, 122-4 (letter).
(18) Gagné, R. and Laberge, C. (1972) Specific cytological recognition of the heterochromatic segments of No. 9 chromosome in man. *Exp. cell Res., 73*, 239-42.
(19) Pearson, P.L., Geraedts, J.P.M. and van der Linden, A.G.J.M. (1972) Human chromosome polymorphism. In *Modern Aspects of Cytogenetics: Constitutive Heterochromatin in Man*, Ed. R.A. Pfeiffer, pp. 201-13. Symposia Medica Hoechst No. 6. Stuttgart and New York, Schattauer.
(20) Craig-Holmes, A.P., Moore, F.B. and Shaw, M.W. (1973) Polymorphism of human C-band heterochromatin. I. Frequency of variants. *Am. J. hum. Genet., 25*, 181-92.
(21) Mutton, D.E. and Daker, M.G. (1973) Pericentric inversion of chromosome 9. *Nature New Biology, 241*, 80 (letter).
(22) Jacobs, P.A. (1974) Correlation between euploid structural chromosome rearrangements and mental subnormality in humans. *Nature (London), 249*, 164-5.
(23) Polani, P.E., Hamerton, J.L., Giannelli, F. and Carter, C.O. (1965) Cytogenetics of Down's syndrome (Mongolism) III. Frequency of interchange trisomics and mutation rate of chromosome interchanges. *Cytogenetics, 4*, 193-206.
(24) Lubs, H. (1972) Neonatal cytogenetic surveys. In *Perspectives in Cytogenetics*, Eds. S.W. Wright, B.F. Crandall and L. Boyer, pp. 297-304. Springfield, Ill., C.C. Thomas.
(25) Court Brown, W.M. (1969) Sex chromosome aneuploidy in man and its frequency, with special reference to mental subnormality and criminal behaviour. In *International Review of Experimental Pathology*, Eds. G.W. Richter and M.A. Epstein, 7, pp. 31-97. London and New York, Academic Press.
(26) Jacobs, P.A. (1972) Chromosome mutations: frequency at birth in humans. *Hum. Genet., 16*, 137-40.
(27) Ratcliffe, S.G. and Keay, A.J. (1973) Chromosome studies on 11,000 newborn infants. *Archives of Disease in Childhood, 48*, 407.
(28) Bochkov, N.P., Kuleshov, N.P., Chebotarev, A.N., Alekhin, V.I. and Midian, S.A. (1974) Population cytogenetic investigation of newborns in Moscow. *Hum. Genet., 22*, 139-52.
(29) Eller, E., Frankenburg, W., Puck, M. and Robinson, A. (1971) Prognosis in newborn infants with X-chromosomal abnormalities. *Pediatrics, 47*, 681-8.
(30) Polani, P.E. (1967) Chromosome anomalies and the brain. *Guy's Hospital Reports, 116*, 365-96.
(31) Maclachlan, T.K. (1969) Criminological implications of sex chromosome abnormalities: a review. In *Criminal Implications of Chromosome Abnormalities*, Ed. D.J. West, pp. 9-31. University of Cambridge, Institute of Criminology.

(32) Fujita, H., Yoshida, Y., Tanigawa, Y., Yamamoto, K. and Sakamoto, Y. (1972) A survey of sex chromosome anomalies among normal children and mental defectives. *Japanese Journal of Human Genetics, 16,* 198-211.

(33) Polani, P.E. (1970) Chromosome phenotypes—sex chromosomes. In *Congenital Malformations,* Eds. F.C. Fraser and V.A. McKusick, pp. 233-50, (Proceedings of the third international conference on congenital malformations, The Hague, 7-13 September 1969.) Excerpta Medica International Congress Series No. 204. Amsterdam and New York, Excerpta Medica.

(34) Haddad, H.M. and Wilkins, L. (1959) Congenital anomalies associated with gonadal aplasia. Review of 55 cases. *Pediatrics, 23,* 885-902.

(35) Bishop, P.M.F., Lessof, M.H. and Polani, P.E. (1960) Turner's syndrome and allied conditions. In *Sex Differentiation and Development.* Memoirs of the Society for Endocrinology, No. 7, Ed. C.R. Austin, pp. 162-72. London, Cambridge University Press.

(36) Polani, P.E. (1960) Chromosomal factors in certain types of educational subnormality. In *Mental Retardation,* Eds. P.W. Bowman and H.V. Mautner, pp. 421-38. New York, Grune and Stratton.

(37) Polani, P.E. (1962) Chromosomes in mental deficiency. In *Proceedings of the London Conference on Scientific Study of Mental Deficiency,* Eds. B.W. Richards, A.D.B. Clarke and A. Shapiro, *1,* 19-37. England: May and Baker.

(38) Money, J. and Granoff, D. (1965) IQ and the somatic stigmata of Turner's syndrome. *Am. J. ment. Defic., 70,* 69-77.

(39) Garron, D.C. and Vander Stoep, L.R. (1969) Personality and intelligence in Turner's syndrome. A critical review. *Archs gen. Psychiat., 21,* 339-46.

(40) Bekker, F.J. and van Gemund, J.J. (1968) Mental retardation and cognitive defects in XO-Turner's syndrome. *Maandschrift Kindergeneesk, 36,* 148-56.

(41) Cohen, H. (1962) Physiological test findings in adolescents having ovarian dysgenesis. *Psychosom. Med., 24,* 249-56.

(42) Shaffer, J.W. (1962) A specific cognitive deficit observed in gonadal aplasia (Turner's syndrome). *J. clin. Psychol., 18,* 403-6.

(43) Money, J. (1964) Two cytogenetic syndromes: psychologic comparisons. I. Intelligence and specific factor quotients. *J. psychiat. Res., 2,* 223-31.

(44) Buckley, F. (1971) Preliminary report on intelligence quotient scores of patients with Turner's syndrome: a replication study. *Br. J. Psychiat., 119,* 513-14 (abstract).

(45) Theilgaard, A. (1972) Cognitive style and gender role in persons with sex chromosome aberrations. *Danish Medical Bulletin, 19,* 276-82.

(46) Cohen, J. (1959) The factorial structure of the WISC at ages 7-6, 10-6 and 13-6. *J. consult. Psychol., 23,* 285-99.

(47) Money, J. (1963) Cytogenetic and psychosexual incongruities with a note on space-form blindness. *Am. J. Psychiat., 119,* 820-7.

(48) Alexander, D., Walker, jun. H.T. and Money, J. (1964) Studies in direction sense. I. Turner's syndrome. *Archs gen. Psychiat., 10,* 337-9.

(49) Alexander, D., Ehrhardt, A.A. and Money, J. (1966) Defective figure drawing, geometric and human in Turner's syndrome. *J. nerv. ment. Dis., 142,* 161-7.

(50) Alexander, D. and Money, J. (1965) Reading ability, object constancy and Turner's syndrome. *Percept. mot. Skills, 20,* 981-4.

(51) Alexander, D. and Money, J. (1966) Turner's syndrome and Gerstmann's syndrome: neuropsychologic comparisons. *Neuropsychologia, 4,* 265-73.

(52) Stafford, R.E. (1961) Sex differences in spatial visualization as evidence of sex-linked inheritance. *Percept. mot. Skills, 13,* 428.

(53) Hartlage, L.C. (1970) Sex-linked inheritance of spatial ability. *Percept. mot. Skills, 31,* 610.

(54) Bock, R.D. (1973) Word and image: sources of the verbal and spatial factors in mental test scores. *Psychometrika, 38,* 437-57.

(55) Bock, R.D. and Kolakowski, D. (1973) Further evidence of sex-linked major-gene influence on human spatial visualizing ability. *Am. J. hum. Genet., 25,* 1-14.

(56) Fisher, R.A. (1918) The correlation between relatives on the supposition of Mendelian inheritance. In *Transactions of the Royal Society of Edinburgh, Series B, 52,* 399-433. (Commentary by Moran, P.A.P. and Smith, C.A.B., 1966, Eugenics Laboratory Memoirs *41,* London, Cambridge University Press.)

(57) Hogben, L. (1932) Filial and fraternal correlations in sex-linked inheritance. *Proceedings of the Royal Society of Edinburgh, Series B, 52,* 331-6.
(58) Loesch, D. (1971) Genetics of dermatoglyphic patterns on palms. *Ann. hum. Genet., 34,* 277-93 (with appendix by Penrose, L.S.).
(59) Garron, D.C. (1970) Sex-linked, recessive inheritance of spatial and numerical abilities, and Turner's syndrome. *Psychol. Rev., 77,* 147-52.
(60) Petersen, A.C. (1973) Quoted by Bock, R.D. (1973) Word and image: sources of the verbal and spatial factors in mental test scores. *Psychometrika, 38,* 437-57.
(61) Henkin, R.I. (1967) Abnormalities of taste and olfaction in patients with chromatin negative gonadal dysgenesis. *J. clin. Endocr., 27,* 1436-40.
(62) Sabbath, J.C., Morris, jun., T.A., Menzer-Benaron, D. and Sturgis, S.H. (1961) Psychiatric observations in adolescent girls lacking ovarian function. *Psychosom. Med., 23,* 224-31.
(63) Shaffer, J.W. (1963) Masculinity-femininity and other personality traits in gonadal aplasia (Turner's syndrome). In *Advances in Sex Research,* Ed. H.G. Beigel, pp. 219-32. New York, Hoeber.
(64) Ehrhardt, A.A., Greenberg, N. and Money, J. (1970) Female gender identity and absence of fetal gonadal hormones: Turner's syndrome. *Johns Hopkins Medical Journal, 126,* 237-48.
(65) Money, J. and Mittenthal, S. (1970) Lack of personality pathology in Turner's syndrome: relation to cytogenetics, hormones and physique. *Behav. Genet., 1,* 43-56.
(66) Nielsen, J. (1970) Turner's syndrome in medical, neurological and psychiatric wards. A psychiatric, cytogenetic and clinical study. *Acta psychiat. Scand., 46,* 286-310.
(67) Kessler, S. and Moos, R.H. (1973) Behavioural aspects of chromosomal disorders. In *Annual Review of Medicine,* Eds. W.P. Creger, C.H. Coggins and E.W. Hancock, *24,* 89-102. Palo Alto, California, Annual Reviews.
(68) Childs, B. (1972) Genetic analysis of human behaviour. In *Annual Review of Medicine,* Eds. A.C. De Graff, and W.P. Creger, *23,* 373-406. Palo Alto, California, Annual Reviews.
(69) Garvey, M. and Mutton, D.E. (1973) Sex chromosome aberrations and speech development. *Archives of Disease in Childhood, 48,* 937-41.
(70) Van Denberg, S.G. (1971) What do we know today about the inheritance of intelligence and how do we know it? In *Intelligence: Genetic and Environmental Influences,* Ed. R. Cancro, pp. 182-218. New York, Grune and Stratton.
(71) Moor, L. (1967) (The intelligence level and polygonosomia: a comparative study of the karyotype and of the mental level in 374 patients with excessive numbers of X or Y chromosomes in the karyotype.) *Revue de Neuropsychiatrie infantile, 15,* 325-48 (in French).
(72) Barlow, P. (1973) The influence of inactive chromosomes on human development. Anomalous sex chromosome complements and the phenotype. *Hum. Genet., 17,* 105-36.
(73) Züblin, W. (1953) Zur psychologie des Klinefelter-syndroms. *Acta endocr., 14,* 137-44.
(74) Pasqualini, R.Q., Vidal, G. and Bur, G.E. (1957) Psychopathology of Klinefelter's syndrome. A review of 31 cases. *Lancet, 2,* 164-7.
(75) Nowakowski, II., Lenz, W., Bergmann, S. and Reitalu, J. (1960) Chromosomenbefunde beim echten Klinefelter-syndrom. *Acta endocr., 34,* 483-95.
(76) Hunter, H. (1967) Some clinical observations on Klinefelter's syndrome in a subnormal population in England. A survey of all hospitals for the subnormal in Sheffield Regional Hospital Board. M.D. Thesis. University of London.
(77) Breg, W.R., Castilla, E.E., Miller, O.J., and Cornwell, J.G. (1963) Sex chromatin and chromosome studies in 1,562 institutionalized mental defectives. *J. Pediat., 63,* 738 (abstract).
(78) De la Chapelle, A. (1963) Sex chromosome abnormalities among the mentally defective in Finland. *J. ment. Defic. Res., 7,* 129-46.
(79) Breakey, W.R. (1961) Sex chromatin analyses in a mentally defective population. *J. Anat., 95,* 618 (abstract.)
(80) Carr, D.H., Barr, M.L. and Plunkett, E.R. (1961) A probable XXYY sex-determining mechanism in a mentally defective male with Klinefelter's syndrome. *Canadian Medical Association Journal, 84,* 873-8.
(81) Gustavson, K-H. and Åkesson, H.O. (1961) Mental deficiency and aberrant sex chromatin. *Lancet, 2,* 724 (letter).
(82) Anderson, I.F., Goeller, E.A. and Wallace, C. (1964) Sex chromosome abnormalities in a population of 1,622 mental defectives. *South African Medical Journal, 38.* 346-9.

(83) Benirschke, K., Brownhill, L., Efron, M.L. and Hoefnagel, D. (1962) Phenylketonuria associated Klinefelter's syndrome. *J. ment. Defic. Res., 6,* 44-55.

(84) Maclean, N., Court Brown, W.M., Jacobs, P.A., Mantle, D.J. and Strong, J.A. (1968) A survey of sex chromatin abnormalities in mental hospitals. *J. med. Genet., 5,* 165-72.

(85) Close, H.G., Goonetilleke, A.S.R., Jacobs, P.A. and Price, W.H. (1968) The incidence of sex chromosome abnormalities in mentally subnormal males. *Cytogenetics, 7,* 277-85.

(86) Court Brown, W.M. (1968) Males with an XYY sex chromosome complement. *J. med. Genet., 5,* 341-59.

(87) Márquez-Monter, H., Santiago-Payán, H. and Kofman-Alfaro, S. (1968) Sex chromatin survey in mentally handicapped children in Mexico. *J. med. Genet., 5,* 40-4.

(88) Robinson, A., Puck, M. and Tennes, K. (1974) The 47,XXY karyotype. *Lancet, 1,* 1343 (letter).

(89) Court Brown, W.M. (1962) Sex chromosomes and the law. *Lancet, 2,* 508-9 (letter).

(90) Mosier, H.D., Scott, L.W. and Dingman, H.F. (1960) Sexually deviant behaviour in Klinefelter's syndrome. *J. Pediat., 57,* 479-83.

(91) Nielsen, J. (1969) Klinefelter's syndrome and the XYY syndrome. A genetical, endocrinological and psychiatric-psychological study of thirty-three severely hypogonadal male patients and two patients with karyotype 47,XYY. *Acta psychiat. Scand., 45,* Supplement No. 209.

(92) Nielsen, J., Sørensen, A., Theilgaard, A., Frøland, A. and Johnsen, S.G. (1969) A psychiatric-psychological study of fifty severely hypogonadal male patients, including thirty-four with Klinefelter's syndrome, 47,XXY. *Acta Jutlandica, 41,* 3.

(93) Theilgaard, A., Nielsen, J., Sørensen, A., Frøland, A. and Johnsen, S.G. (1971) A psychological-psychiatric study of patients with Klinefelter's syndrome, 47,XXY. *Acta Jutlandica, 43,* 1.

(94) Nielsen, J. (1972) Gender role identity and sexual behaviour in persons with sex chromosome aberrations. *Danish Medical Bulletin, 19,* 269-75.

(95) Money, J. and Pollitt, E. (1964) Cytogenetic and psychosexual ambiguity. Klinefelter's syndrome and transvestism compared. *Archs gen. Psychiat., 11,* 589-95.

(96) Hoenig, J. and Torr, J.B.D. (1964) Karyotyping of transexualists. *J. psychosom. Res., 8,* 157-9.

(97) Harms, S. (1967) Anomalien der Geschlechtschromosomenzahl (XXX- und XO-Zustand) bei Hamburger Hilfsschülerinnen. *Pädiatrie und Pädologie, 3,* 34-52.

(98) Nielsen, J. and Fischer, M. (1965) Sex chromatin and sex chromosome abnormalities in male hypogonadal mental patients. *Br. J. Psychiat., 111,* 641-7.

(99) Jancar, J. (1964) 11 mentally defective males with XXXXY chromosomes. In *Proceedings of the International Copenhagen Congress on the Scientific Study of Mental Retardation,* Eds J. Øster and H.V. Sletved, pp. 179-95. Denmark: Det. Berlingske Bogtrykkeri.

(100) Carr, D.H., Barr, M.L. and Plunkett, E.R. (1961) An XXXX sex chromosome complex in two mentally defective females. *Canadian Medical Association Journal, 84,* 131-7.

(101) Kesaree, N. and Woolley, Jun., P.V. (1963) A phenotypic female with 49 chromosomes, presumably XXXXX. *J. Pediat., 63,* 1099-103.

(102) Brody, J., Fitzgerald, M.G. and Spiers, A.S.D. (1967) A female child with five X chromosomes. *J. Pediat., 70,* 105-9.

(103) Anders, J.M., Jagiello, G., Polani, P.E., Giannelli, F. Hamerton, J.L. and Leiberman, D.M. (1968) Chromosome findings in chronic psychotic patients. *Br. J. Psychiat., 114,* 1167-74.

(104) Tsuboi, T., Asaka, A., Hamada, S. and Nagumo, Y. (1966) Frequency of sex chromosome anomaly among schizophrenic patients. *Japanese Journal of Human Genetics, 11,* 39-40.

(105) Judd, L.L. and Brandkamp, W.W. (1967) Chromosome analyses of adult schizophrenics. *Archs. gen. Psychiat., 16,* 316-24.

(106) Nielsen, J. (1968) Prevalence of sex-chromatin abnormalities among female patients in a mental hospital (sex-chromatin percentage in relation to age, diagnosis and menstrual cycle). *Acta psychiat. Scand., 44,* 124-40.

(107) Vartanyan, M.E. and Gindilis, V.M. (1972) The role of chromosomal aberrations in the clinical polymorphism of schizophrenia. *Int. J. ment. Health, 1,* 93-106.

(108) Schulz, F.W. (1965) quoted by Hessing, J., Kabarity, A. and Schade, H. (1969) Über X-chromosomale Zahlabweichungen, in besondere Mosaike, bei Anstalespatienten. *Deutsche Medizinische Wochenschrift, 94,* 2675-8.

(109) Casteel, B. (1967) quoted by Hessing, J., Kabarity, A. and Schade, H. (1969) Über X-

chromosomale Zahlabweichungen, in besondere Mosaike, bei Anstalespatienten. *Deutsche Medizinische Wochenschrift, 94,* 2675-8.

(110) Dasgupta, J., Dasgupta, D. and Balasubrahmanyan, M. (1973) XXY syndrome XY/XO mosaicism and acentric chromosomal fragments in male schizophrenics. *Indian Journal of Medical Research, 61,* 62-70.

(111) Hambert, G. (1966) *Males with Positive Sex Chromatin. An Epidemiologic Investigation followed by Psychiatric Study of Seventy-five Cases.* Reports from the Psychiatric Research Centre, St Jörgen's Hospital, University of Goteborg, Sweden. Goteborg: Scandinavian University Books.

(112) Forssman, H. and Hambert, G. (1963) Incidence of Klinefelter's syndrome among mental patients. *Lancet, 1,* 1327 (letter).

(113) Swanson, D.W. and Stipes, A.H. (1969) Psychiatric aspects of Klinefelter's syndrome. *Am. J. Psychiat., 126,* 814-22.

(114) Thomsen, O. (1962) Klinefelter's syndrom hos 5 patienter med psykiatriske lidelser. *Ugeskrift for Laeger, 124,* 1276-85.

(115) Dumermuth, G. (1961) Untersuchungen beim jugendlichen Klinefelter-syndrom. *Helvetica paediatrica Acta, 16,* 702-10.

(116) Hambert, G. and Frey, T.S. (1964) The electroencephalogram in the Klinefelter syndrome. *Acta psychiat. Scand., 40,* 28-36.

(117) Sperber, M.A., Salomon, L., Collins, M.H. and Stambler, M. (1972) Childhood schizophrenia and 47,XXY Klinefelter's syndrome. *Am. J. Psychiat., 128,* 1400-8.

(118) Kaplan, A.R. and Cotton, J.E. (1968) Chromosomal abnormalities in female schizophrenics. *J. nerv. ment. Dis., 147,* 402-17.

(119) Kaplan, A.R. (1967) Sex-chromatin variation in institutionalized females. 1. Sex chromosome anomalies in hospitalized schizophrenics, adult prisoners, confined juvenile offenders and non-institutionalized volunteers. In *Recent Advances in Biological Psychiatry,* Ed. J. Wortis, *9,* 21-7. New York, Plenum Press.

(120) Kaplan, A.R. (1970) Chromosomal mosaicisms and occasional acentric chromosomal fragments in schizophrenic patients. *Biol. Psychiat., 2,* 89-94.

(121) Olanders, S. (1967) Double Barr bodies in women in mental hospitals. *Br. J. Psychiat., 113,* 1097-9.

(122) Kidd, C.B., Knox, R.S. and Mantle, D.J. (1963) A psychiatric investigation of triple-X chromosome females. *Br. J. Psychiat., 109,* 90-4.

(123) Mellbin, G. (1966) Neuropsychiatric disorders in sex chromatin negative women. *Br. J. Psychiat., 112,* 145-8.

(124) Ferguson-Smith, M.A. (1958) Chromatin-positive Klinefelter's syndrome (primary microrchidism) in a mental-deficiency hospital. *Lancet, 1,* 928-31.

(125) Wegmann, T.G. and Smith, D.W. (1963) Incidence of Klinefelter's syndrome among juvenile delinquents and felons. *Lancet, 1,* 274 (letter).

(126) Casey, M.D., Segall, L.J., Street, D.R.K. and Blank, C.E. (1966) Sex chromosome abnormalities in two state hospitals for patients requiring special security. *Nature, 209,* 641-2.

(127) Court Brown, W.M. (1967) *Human Population Cytogenetics.* Amsterdam, North Holland Publishing Company.

(128) Jacobs, P.A., Brunton, M., Melville, M.M., Brittain, R.P. and McClemont, W.F. (1965) Aggressive behaviour, mental subnormality and XYY male. *Nature, 208,* 1351-2.

(129) Casey, M.D., Blank, C.E., Street, D.R.K., Segall, L.J., McDougall, J.H., McGrath, P.J. and Skinner, J.L. (1966) YY chromosomes and antisocial behaviour. *Lancet, 2,* 859-60 (letter).

(130) Noel, B., Quack, B., Durand, Y. and Rethoré, M-O. (1969) Les hommes 47,XYY. *Annales de Génétique, 12,* 223-36.

(131) Hunter, H. (1968) Klinefelter's syndrome and delinquency. *Br. J. Crim., 8,* 203-7.

(132) Wiener, S., Sutherland, G., Bartholomew, A.A., and Hudson, B. (1968) XYY males in Melbourne Prison. *Lancet, 1,* 150 (letter).

(133) Nielsen, J. (1968) The XYY syndrome in a mental hospital. Genetically determined criminality. *Br. J. Crim., 8,* 186-203.

(134) Åkesson, H.O., Forssman, H. and Wallin, L. (1968) Chromosomes of tall men in mental hospitals. *Lancet, 2,* 1040 (letter).

(135) Price, W.H., Strong, J.A., Whatmore, P.B. and McClemont, W.F. (1966) Criminal patients with XYY sex chromosome complement. *Lancet, 1,* 565-6.

(136) Jacobs, P.A., Price, W.H., Court Brown, W.M., Brittain, R.P. and Whatmore, P.B. (1968)

Chromosome studies on men in a maximum security hospital. *Ann. hum. Genet., 31*, 339-58.

(137) Goodman, R.M., Smith, W.S. and Migeon, C.J. (1967) Sex chromosome abnormalities. *Nature, 216*, 942-3 (letter).

(138) Welch, J.P., Borgaonkar, D.S. and Herr, H.M. (1967) Psychopathy, mental deficiency, aggressiveness and the XYY syndrome. *Nature, 214*, 500-1 (letter).

(139) Telfer, M.A., Baker, D., Clark, G.R. and Richardson, C.E. (1968) Incidence of gross chromosomal errors among tall criminal American males. *Science, 159*, 1249-50.

(140) Nielsen, J., Tsuboi, T., Stürup, G. and Romano, D. (1968) XYY chromosomal constitution in criminal psychopaths. *Lancet, 2*, 576 (letter).

(141) Griffiths, A.W. and Zaremba, J. (1967) Crime and sex chromosome anomalies. *Br. med. J., 4*, 622 (letter).

(142) Hunter, H. (1968) Chromatin-positive and XYY boys in approved schools. *Lancet, 1*, 816 (letter).

(143) Nielsen, J. (1971) Prevalence and a 2½ years incidence of chromosome abnormalities among all males in a forensic psychiatric clinic. *Br. J. Psychiat., 119*, 503-12.

(144) Kahn, J., Carter, W.I., Dernley, N. and Slater, E.T.O. (1969) Chromosome studies in remand home and prison populations. In *Criminological Implications of Chromosome Abnormalities*, Ed. D.J. West, pp. 44-8. Cambridge, Institute of Criminology, University of Cambridge.

(145) Shah, S.A. (1970) *Report on the XYY chromosomal abnormality*. The National Institute of Mental Health. National Clearing House for Mental Health Information. U.S.P.H.S. Publication. No. 2103. Washington, US Government Printing Office.

(146) Hunter, H. (1966) YY chromosomes and Klinefelter's syndrome..*Lancet, 1*, 984 (letter).

(147) Goodman, R.M., Miller, F. and North, C. (1968) Chromosomes of tall men. *Lancet, 1*, 1318 (letter).

(148) Zeuthen, E., Nielsen, J. and Yde, H. (1973) XYY males found in a general male population. Cytogenetic and physical examination. *Hereditas (Lund), 74*, 283-90.

(149) Nielsen, J. (1970) Criminality among patients with Klinefelter's syndrome and the XYY syndrome. *Br. J. Psychiat., 117*, 365-9.

(150) Price, W.H. and Whatmore, P.B. (1967) Criminal behaviour and the XYY male. *Nature, 213*, 815.

(151) Clark, G.R., Telfer, M.A., Baker, D. and Rosen, M. (1970) Sex chromosomes, crime and psychosis. *Am. J. Psychiat., 126*, 1659-63.

(152) Cowie, J. and Kahn, J. (1968) XYY constitution in prepubertal child. *Br. med. J., 1*, 748-9.

(153) Gustavson, K-H. and Verneholt, J. (1968) The XYY syndrome in a prepubertal boy. *Hereditas (Lund), 60*, 264-6.

(154) Price, W.H. and Whatmore, P.B. (1967b) Behaviour disorders and pattern of crime among XYY males identified at a maximum security hospital. *Br. med. J., 1*, 533-6.

(155) Gibbens, T.C. (1968) Genetics and ethics. *New Scientist, 40*, 236.

(156) Daly, R.F. (1969) Neurological abnormalities in XYY males. *Nature, 221*, 472-3 (letter).

(157) Bartlett, D.J., Hurley, W.P., Brand, C.R. and Poole, E.W. (1968) Chromosomes of male patients in a security prison. *Nature, 219*, 351-4.

(158) Price, W.H. (1968) The electrocardiogram in males with extra Y chromosomes. *Lancet, 1*, 1106-8.

(159) Hope, K., Philip, A.E. and Loughran, J.M. (1967) Psychological characteristics associated with XYY sex-chromosome complement in a state mental hospital. *Br. J. Psychiat., 113*, 495-8.

(160) Jacobs, P.A., Price, W.H., Richmond, S. and Ratcliff, R.A.W. (1971) Chromosome surveys in penal institutions and approved schools. *J. med. Genet., 8*, 49-58.

(161) Jacobs, P., Lubs, H., Sergovich, F. and Walzer, S. (1972) Table: Individuals with XYY karyotype ascertained among consecutively examined males. In *Perspectives in Cytogenetics. The next decade*, Eds. S.W. Wright, B.F. Crandall and L. Boyer, pp. 305-7. Springfield, Ill., C.C. Thomas.

(162) Townes, P.L., Ziegler, N.A. and Lenhard, L.W. (1965) A patient with 48 chromosomes (XYYY). *Lancet, 1*, 1041-3.

(163) Gracey, M. and Fitzgerald, M.G. (1967) The XXYYY sex chromosome complement in a mentally retarded child. A case report. *Australasian Paediatric Journal, 3*, 119-21.

(164) Berg, J.M., Ridler, M.A.C. and McQuaid, A. (1969) Sex chromatin survey of women in a special psychiatric hospital. *Nature, 222*, 896-7.

(165) Barr, M.L., Sergovich, F.R., Carr, D.H. and Shaver, E.L. (1969) The triplo-X female: an appraisal based on a study of 12 cases and a review of the literature. *Canadian Medical Association Journal, 101,* 247-58.

(166) Polani, P.E. (1968) Congenital malformations. A clinico-pathological conference held at the Royal Alexandra Hospital for Sick Children, Brighton, on Friday, 14 January 1966. *Postgraduate Medical Journal, 44,* 156-66.

(167) Marimo, B. (1974) Personal communication.

(168) Sadler, J.R. and Novick, A.J. (1965) The properties of repressor and the kinetics of its action. *J. mol. Biol., 12,* 305-27.

(169) Yielding, K.L. (1967) Chromosome redundancy and gene expression: an explanation for trisomy abnormalities. *Nature, 214,* 613-14.

(170) McDaniel, R.G. and Ramage, R.T. (1970) Genetics of a primary trisomic series in barley: identification by protein electrophoresis. *Canadian Journal of Genetics and Cytology, 12,* 490-5.

(171) Henderson, A.S., Warburton, D. and Atwood, K.C. (1972) Location of ribosomal DNA in the human chromosome complement. *Proceedings of the National Academy of Sciences (Washington), 69,* 3394-8.

(172) Bross, K. and Krone, W. (1973) Ribosomal cistrons and acrocentric chromosomes in man. *Hum. Genet., 18,* 71-5.

(173) Heitz, E. (1956) Die Chromosomenstruktur im Kern während der Kernteilung und der Entwicklung. In *Chromosomes, Lectures held at the Conference on Chromosomes, Wageningen, April 1956.* pp. 5-26. Zwolle, Netherlands, W.E.J. Tjeenk Willink.

(174) Brown, S.W. (1966) Heterochromatin. *Science, 151,* 417-25.

(175) Hsu, T.C. (1962) Differential rate in RNA synthesis between euchromatin and heterochromatin. *Exp. cell Res., 27,* 332-4.

(176) Littau, V.C., Burdick, C.J., Allfrey, V.G. and Mirsky, A.E. (1965) The role of histones in the maintenance of chromatin structure. *Proceedings of the National Academy of Sciences (Washington), 54,* 1204-12.

(177) Comings, D.E. (1966) Uridine-5-H^{3}radioautography of the human sex chromatin body. *J. cell. Biol., 28,* 437-41.

(178) Lewis, E.B. (1950) The phenomenon of position effect. In *Advances in Genetics,* Ed. M. Demerec, 3, 73-115. New York, Academic Press.

(179) Baker, W.K. (1968) Position-effect variegation. In *Advances in Genetics.* Ed. E.W. Caspari, 14, 133-69. New York, Academic Press.

(180) Prokofyeva-Belgovskaya, A.A. (1947) Heterochromatization as a change of chromosome cycle. *J. Genet., 48,* 80-98.

(181) Cooper, K.W. (1959) Cytogenetic analysis of major heterochromatic elements (especially Xh and y) in *Drosophila melanogaster* and the theory of 'heterochromatin'. *Chromosoma (Berlin), 10,* 535-88.

(182) Heitz, E. (1934) Über α- und β-Heterochromatin sowie Konstanz und Bau der Chromomeren bei *Drosophila. Biologisches Zentralblatt, 54,* 588-609.

(183) Mather, K. (1944) The genetical activity of heterochromatin. *Proceedings of the Royal Society, Series B, 132,* 308-32.

(184) Pontecorvo, G. (1943) Meiosis in the striped hamster (*Cricetulus griseus* Milne-Edw.) and the problem of heterochromatin in mammalian sex-chromosomes. *Proceedings of the Royal Society of Edinburgh Series B, 62,* 32-42.

(185) Britten, R.J. and Kohne, D.E. (1968) Repeated sequences in DNA. Hundreds of thousands of copies of DNA sequences have been incorporated into the genomes of higher organisms. *Science, 161,* 529-40.

(186) Britten, R.J., Hough, B.R., Amenson, C.S., Neufeld, B.R., Graham, D.E. and Davidson, E.H. (1974) Studies of the molecular organization of the genetic material. In *Birth Defects.* Proceedings of the fourth International Conference, Vienna, Austria, 2-8 September 1973. Eds. A.G. Motulsky, W. Lenz and F.J.G. Ebling, pp. 21-31. Amsterdam, Excerpta Medica.

(187) Davidson, E.H. (1973) Sequence organization in the genome of *Xenopus laevis.* In *Genetic Mechanisms of Development,* Ed. F.H. Ruddle, pp. 251-68. New York and London, Academic Press.

(188) Pardue, M.L. and Gall, J.G. (1972) Molecular cytogenetics. In *Molecular Genetics and Developmental Biology,* Ed. M. Sussman, pp. 65-99. Englewood Cliffs, New Jersey: Prentice Hall.

(189) Pardue, M.L. (1974) Repeated DNA sequences in the chromosomes of higher organisms.

In *Birth Defects*. Proceedings of the fourth International Conference, Vienna, Austria, 2-8 September 1973, Eds. A.G. Motulsky, W. Lenz and F.J.G. Ebling, pp. 32-43. Amsterdam: Excerpta Medica.

(190)   Jones, K.W. (1973) Satellite DNA. *J. med. Genet., 10*, 273-81.

(191)   Hsu, T.C. (1973) Longitudinal differentiation of chromosomes. In *Annual Review of Genetics*, Eds. H.L. Roman, L.M. Sandler and A. Campbell, *7*, 153-76. Palo Alto, California, Annual Reviews.

(192)   Comings, D.E. (1974) The role of heterochromatin. In *Birth Defects*. Proceedings of the fourth International Conference, Vienna, Austria, 2-8 September 1973, Eds. A.G. Motulsky, W. Lenz and F.J.G. Ebling, pp. 44-52. Amsterdam, Excerpta Medica.

(193)   Lyon, M.F. (1972) X-chromosome inactivation and developmental patterns in mammals. *Biol. Rev., 47*, 1-35.

(194)   Goldschmidt, R.B. (1955) *Theoretical Genetics, 57*. Berkeley and Los Angeles, University of California Press.

(195)   Goldschmidt, R.B. (1955) *Theoretical Genetics, 90*. Berkeley and Los Angeles, University of California Press.

(196)   Mittwoch, U. (1967) *Sex Chromosomes*. London and New York, Academic Press.

(197)   Hamerton, J.L. (1968) Significance of sex chromosome derived heterochromatin in mammals. *Nature, 219*, 910-14.

(198)   Mittwoch, U. (1969) Do genes determine sex? *Nature, 221*, 446-8.

(199)   Mittwoch, U. (1973) *Genetics of Sex Differentiation*. New York and London, Academic Press.

(200)   Goldschmidt, R.B. (1955) *Theoretical Genetics, 91*. Berkeley and Los Angeles, University of California Press.

(201)   Goldschmidt, R.B. (1955) *Theoretical Genetics, 83*. Berkeley and Los Angeles, University of California Press.

(202)   Barigozzi, C., (1951) The influence of the Y-chromosome on quantitative characters of *D. melanogaster. Heredity, 5*, 415-32.

(203)   Commoner, B. (1964) Deoxyribonucleic acid and the molecular basis of self-duplication. *Nature, 202*, 960-8.

(204)   Lennartz, K.J., Schümmelfeder, N. and Maurer, W. (1966) Dauer der DNA-Synthesephase bei Ascitestumoren der Maus unterschiedlicher Ploidie. *Naturwissenschaften, 53*, 21-2.

(205)   Darlington, C.D. and Thomas, P.T. (1941) Morbid mitosis and the activity of inert chromosomes in *Sorghum, Proceedings of the Royal Society, Series B, 130*, 127-51.

(206)   Rutishauser, A. and Röthlisberger, E. (1966) Boosting mechanisms of B chromosomes in *Crepis capillaris*. In *Chromosomes Today*, Eds. C.D. Darlington and K.R. Lewis, *1*, 28-30. Edinburgh and London, Oliver and Boyd.

(207)   Ayonoadu, U.W. and Rees, H. (1968) The regulation of mitosis by B-chromosomes in rye. *Exp. cell Res., 52*, 284-90.

(208)   Vosa, C.G. (1966) Seed germination and B chromosomes in the leek *(Allium porram)*. In *Chromosomes Today*, Eds. C.D. Darlington and K.R. Lewis, *1*, 24-7. Edinburgh and London, Oliver and Boyd.

(209)   Moss, J.P. (1966) The adaptive significance of B chromosomes in rye. In *Chromosomes Today*, Eds. C.D. Darlington and K.R. Lewis, *1*, 15-23. Edinburgh and London, Oliver and Boyd.

(210)   Müntzing, A. (1967) Some main results from investigations of accessory chromosomes. *Hereditas (Lund), 57*, 432-8.

(211)   Angell, R.R. (1969) *Cytogenetic and genetic studies in Turner's syndrome and allied conditions in man*. Ph.D. Thesis. University of London.

(212)   Barlow, P.W. (1972) Differential cell division in human X-chromosome mosaics. *Hum. Genet., 14*, 122-7.

(213)   Graham, C.F. (1973) The cell cycle during mammalian development. In *The Cell Cycle in Development and Differentiation*. Eds. M. Balls and F.S. Billett, pp. 293-310 (British Society for Developmental Biology Symposium, July 1972). London, Cambridge University Press.

(214)   Polani, P.E. (1974) Chromosomal and other genetic influences on birth weight variation. In *Size at Birth*. CIBA Foundation Symposium, 12-14 March 1974. Eds. K.E. Elliott and J. Knight. Amsterdam: Associated Scientific Publishers.

(215)   Fankhauser, G. and Schott, B.W. (1952) Inverse relation of number of melanophores to

chromosome number in embryos of the newt *Triturus viridescens. J. exp. Zool., 121*, 105-19.

(216) Polani, P.E., Polani, N. and Zampa, G. (1974) Unpublished observations.
(217) Barlow, P.W. (1973) Mitotic cycles in root meristems. In *The Cell Cycle in Development and Differentiation*, Eds. M. Balls and F.S. Billett, pp. 133-65. (British Society for Developmental Biology, Symposium, July 1972.) London, Cambridge University Press.
(218) Van't Hof. J. (1966) Comparative cell population kinetics of tritiated thymidine labeled diploid and colchicine-induced tetraploid cells in the same tissue of *Pisum. Exp. cell Res., 41*, 274-88.
(219) Jones, R.N. and Rees, H. (1968) The influence of B-chromosomes upon the nuclear phenotype in rye. *Chromosoma (Berlin), 24*, 158-76.
(220) Kirk, D. and Jones, R.N. (1970) Nuclear genetic activity in B-chromosome rye, in terms of the quantitative interrelationships between nuclear protein, nuclear RNA and histone. *Chromosoma (Berlin), 31*, 241-54.
(221) Ayonoadu, U.W. and Rees, H. (1971) The effects of B chromosomes on the nuclear phenotype in root meristems of maize. *Heredity, 27*, 365-83.
(222) Rees, H. and Jones, R.N. (1971) Chromosome gain in higher plants. In *Cellular Organelles and Membranes in Mental Retardation*, Ed. P.F. Benson, pp. 185-208. Institute for Research into Mental Retardation. Study Group No. 2. Edinburgh and London: Churchill Livingstone.
(223) Gurley, L.R., Walters, R.A. and Tobey, R.A. (1972) The metabolism of histone fractions. IV. Synthesis of histones during the G^1-phase of the mammalian life cycle. *Archs. Biochem., 148*, 633-41.
(224) Georgiev, G.P. (1969) Histones and the control of gene action. In *Annual Review of Genetics*, Eds. H.L. Roman, L.M. Sandler and A. Campbell, *3*, 155-80. Palo Alto, California, Annual Reviews.
(225) Allfrey, V.G. (1971) Functional and metabolic aspects of DNA-associated proteins. In *Histones*, Ed. D.M.P. Phillips, pp. 241-94. London and New York, Plenum Press.
(226) Mitchison, J.M. (1971) *The Biology of the Cell Cycle*. London, Cambridge University Press.
(227) Mitchison, J.M. (1973) Differentiation in the cell cycle. In *The Cell Cycle in Development and Differentiation*, Eds. M. Balls and F.S. Billett, pp. 1-11. (British Society for Developmental Biology, Symposium, July 1972.) London, Cambridge University Press.
(228) Barigozzi, C. and di Pasquale, A. (1953) Heterochromatic and euchromatic genes acting on quantitative characters, in *D. melanogaster. Heredity, 7*, 389-99.
(229) Mittwoch, U., Lele, K.P. and Webster, W.S. (1965) Relationship of Barr bodies, nuclear size and deoxyribonucleic acid value in cultured human cells. *Nature, 205*, 477-9.
(230) Harris, H. (1967) The reactivation of the red cell nucleus. *J. cell Sci., 2*, 23-32.
(231) Davidson, J.N. (1967) A sceptical chemist in a biological wonderland. *Proceedings of the Royal Society of Edinburgh, Series B, 70*, 169-91.
(232) Rhodes, K., Markham, R.L., Maxwell, P.M. and Monk-Jones, M.E. (1969) Immunoglobulins and the X-chromosome. *Br. med. J., 3*, 439-41.
(233) Wood, C.B.S., Martin, W., Adinolfi, M. and Polani, P.E. (1970) Levels of γM and γG globulins in women with XO chromosomes. *Atti della Associazione Genetica Italiana, 15*, 228-39.
(234) Grundbacher, F.J. (1972) Human X chromosome carries quantitative genes for immunoglobulin M. *Science, 176*, 311-12.
(235) Grundbacher, F.J. (1974) Heritability estimates and genetic and environmental correlations for the human immunoglobulins G,M and A. *Am. J. hum. Genet., 26*, 1-12.
(236) Holt, S.B., (1968) *The Genetics of Dermal Ridges*, p. 64. Springfield, Ill., C.C. Thomas.
(237) Penrose, L.S. (1967) Finger-print pattern and the sex chromosomes. *Lancet, 1*, 298-300.
(238) Alter, M. (1965) Is hyperploidy of sex chromosomes associated with reduced total finger ridge count? *Am. J. hum. Genet., 17*, 473-5.
(239) Penrose, L.S. (1968) Medical significance of finger prints and related phenomena. *Br. med. J., 2*, 321-5.
(240) Holt, S.B. and Lindsten, J. (1964) Dermatoglyphic anomalies in Turner's syndrome. *Ann. hum. Genet., 28*, 87-100.
(241) Hunter, H. and Quaife, R. (1973) Case Report. A 48,XYYY Male: A somatic and psychiatric description. *J. med. Genet., 10*, 80-3.

(242) Borgaonkar, D.S., Mules, E. and Char, F. (1970) Do the 48,XXYY males have a characteristic phenotype? A review. *Clin. Genet., 1,* 272-93.
(243) Saldaña-Garcia, P. (1973) A dermatoglyphic study of sixty-four XYY males. *Ann. hum. Genet., 37,* 107-16.
(244) Shiono, H. (1969) Dermatoglyphics of XXYY Klinefelter's syndrome. *Tohoku Journal of Experimental Medicine, 98,* 1-6.
(245) Rerrick, E.G. (1972) A female with XXXX sex chromosome complement. *J. ment. Defic. Res., 16,* 84-9.
(246) Berkeley, M.I.K. and Faed, M.J.W. (1970) A female with the 48,XXXX karyotype. *J. med. Genet., 7,* 83-5.
(247) Telfer, M.A., Richardson, C.E., Helmken, J. and Smith, G.F. (1970) Divergent phenotypes among 48,XXXX and 47,XXX females. *Am. J. hum. Genet., 22,* 326-35.
(248) Sokolowski, J., Knaus, A. and Kleczkowska, A. (1969) Dermatogylphics in cases of X-tetrasomy. *Genetica Polonica, 10,* 332-3.
(249) Hunter, H. (1968) Finger and palm prints in chromatin-positive males. *J. med. Genet., 5,* 112-17.
(250) Cushman, C.J. and Soltan, H.C. (1969) Dermatoglyphics in Klinefelter's syndrome (47,XXY). *Human Heredity, 19,* 641-53.
(251) Tsuboi, T. and Nielsen, J. (1969) Dermatoglyphic study of six patients with the XYY syndrome. *Human Heredity, 19,* 299-306.
(252) Málková, J. (1972) (The use of dermatoglyphics in the diagnosis of Klinefelter's syndrome.) *Sbornik lékařsky, 74,* 276-81 (in Czech).
(253) Parker, C.E., Mavalwala, J., Weise, P., Koch, R., Hatashita, A. and Cibilich, S. (1970) The 47,XYY syndrome in a boy with behaviour problems and mental retardation. *Am. J. ment. Defic., 74,* 660-5.
(254) Mavalwala, J., Parker, C.E. and Melnyk, J. (1969) Dermatoglyphics of the XYY syndrome. *Am. J. phys. Anthrop., 30,* 209-13.
(255) Málková, J. (1970) (Dermatoglyphics in cases of ovarian dysgenesis of the masculine and feminine fenotype.) *Ceskoslovenska pediatrie, 25,* 176-9(in Czech).
(256) Hubbell, H.R., Borgaonkar, D.S. and Bolling, D.R. (1973) Dermatoglyphic studies of the 47,XYY male. *Clin. Genet., 4,* 145-57.
(257) Holt, S.B. (1968) *The Genetics of Dermal Ridges,* 61. Springfield, Ill., C.C. Thomas.
(258) Polani, P.E. and Polani, N. (1974) Unpublished observations.

8. Neurological findings in newborn infants after prenatal and perinatal complications

Heinz F.R. Prechtl

In the past years, several attempts have been made to assess the hazards of prenatal and perinatal obstetric complications. There is little doubt that such complications carry an increased risk of mortality (1-3). Moreover, where several complications are present in combination, it would be expected, *a priori,* that the risks will be additive. While the exact causes of mortality in any case may be complex, a major factor is damage to the central nervous system. Post-mortem examination of the brains of babies who have died after obstetric complications or unfavourable events during the neonatal period have clearly shown that these factors may produce lesions in the nervous system (4-10). Studies in monkeys (11-17) have provided evidence of harmful consequences of experimentally induced perinatal complications.

It is supposed that the same conditions which cause perinatal mortality because of severe brain lesions may also be responsible for the neurological morbidity of the infant. However, while mortality-rate studies have a strict criterion available—death of the fetus within a given period of time—the assessment of damage to the surviving infant is much more difficult. Signs have to be found which indicate the condition of the baby's nervous system. These signs must have high inter-observer reliability and must indicate long-term effects. Apgar's technique has merits but is restricted to the first few minutes after birth and deliberately covers only general aspects of physiological status (18, 19). A quite different approach has been used by Graham (20, 21) and in revised form by Rosenblith (22) who measured a small number of behaviour patterns of babies a few days old in order to assess the neonatal condition. This can never be more than an indirect indicator of the condition of the infant's nervous system.

A comprehensive assessment of the structural and functional integrity of the nervous system of the newborn infant can only be obtained by a neurological examination. The specific properties of the baby's brain makes techniques based on concepts derived from adult neurology unsuitable. The assessment of the nervous system in infants must take into account the dynamic aspects of development. Neural maturation brings different sub-systems of the nervous system into play at different times. It is against this background that I have designed an examination technique for the full-term newborn (23). The following principles have been observed in order to develop an optimal strategy of the examination:

A revised form of the Sir Geoffrey Vickers Lecture of 22 February 1967, an abridged version of which was published in the *British Medical Journal,* 1967, *4*, 763-7.

1. The design has to take into account the age-specific properties of the nervous system.

2. Tests must deal with sufficiently complex functions of the nervous system, not merely with artificially fragmented performances or signs.

3. The examination method must indicate not only defects in structure and function, but also deviant maturation. However, it is essential to keep these two aspects separate, since they are completely different kinds of deviation from the optimum.

4. It is necessary to standardize the examination technique in respect of the behavioural state, because of the wide but systematic fluctuations in the readiness of particular nervous functions to act. Particular functions should only be assessed in particular states.

5. Since the evaluation procedure often influences the behavioural state of the infant, it is essential to design and strictly adhere to a rigid sequence of test procedure which take this effect into consideration.

6. Because of the complex nature of the nervous system, a meaningful and reliable assessment must be an elaborate technique.

With this technique more than 2700 newborn infants have been examined in our department since 1954. Certain constellations of neonatal abnormal signs have been designated as hyperexcitability, apathy syndrome and hemi-syndrome in addition to hypo- and hypertonia, neonatal convulsions, etc. Beintema (24) has studied the consistency of abnormal signs and the normal developmental course of the items from the first to the ninth day in fifty infants and found a high reliability and consistency.

The present paper studies some inter-relationships between obstetric complications and the results of the examination. Our hypothesis is that obstetric complications carry a high risk of neurological damage to the surviving infant. The data upon which the present study is based, have been collected over a period of twelve years. The paper will be restricted to presentation of a number of global findings.

Method

The sample

A neurological examination was carried out on 1515 infants born between 1954 and 1966 in the Department of Obstetrics of the University Hospital. At that time, in the Netherlands about 70% of all infants were born at home. The 30% of mothers delivered in hospital are therefore primarily cases with a risk of obstetric complication, although a minority goes to hospital for social reasons, such as poor housing.

From this total, the following were eliminated:

1. Babies of women who did not regularly attend the out-patient unit of the obstetric department during pregnancy;

2. Babies whose birthweight was less than 2500 g and whose gestational age was less than 38 weeks;

3. Babies with gross malformations;

4. Babies whose mother was in a poor nutritional state, suffered from

psychiatric disease, epilepsy, diabetes or heart disease, or whose basal metabolism was low;

5. Babies whose mothers had suffered prolonged infertility.

Both categories 4 and 5 occurred rarely (fewer than fifteen cases) in our material. Babies whose condition was poor or dangerous in the first week were not subjected to full neurological examination. The sample remaining, after exclusion of the above cases, consisted of 1378 babies.

The neurological examination

All infants were examined once with our standard neurological examination technique two or three hours after a feed. All examinations were carried out between the second and fourteenth day, 91% of them being between the third and tenth day. The babies were picked at random from the obstetric department and were examined without knowledge of the obstetric history.

Data processing

The obstetric and neurological data were entered on precoded forms and later transferred to punch cards. Seventy-six items were related to the mother, the course of pregnancy and delivery and the general aspects of the infant, and 142 items to the neurological examination. All computations were carried out on a general-purpose computer (TR 4) at the Computer Centre of the University.

Results

Incidence of obstetric complications and the optimality concept

An obstetric complication may be defined as any factor or group of factors in the pre- and perinatal environment which increases the risk of fetal mortality. These will be symptoms of maternal disease during pregnancy, signs of fetal distress and mechanical intervention in the delivery. Few of these factors are independent of each other and many are causally related. For example, maternal toxaemia may lead to fetal distress which in turn will lead to instrumental extraction.

In order, therefore, to give a more precise meaning to the rather loosely used term 'complications', the following procedure was adopted. For every case, forty-two variables of the obstetric history were analysed and a count was made of the number of variables which did not deviate from optimal conditions (the 'Obstetric Score'), according to generally accepted criteria. Optimality has a more precise connotation than 'normal' (25). Table 1 gives the criteria. In 6.2% of our sample, all forty-two variables were in the optimal condition (Figure 1). The largest number of *non*-optimal conditions was fifteen.

Table 2 shows some of the most frequently occurring obstetrical complications in the traditional sense.

The data were next divided into six sub-groups: those with 0; 1-2; 3-4; 5-6; 7-9; 10 or more non-optimal conditions. The percentage of cases in each subgroup is given for boys and girls separately in Figure 2.

There were no statistically significant sex differences with respect to

TABLE 1   Criteria of optimal obstetric conditions

Maternal factors

1.	Maternal age primipara	18-30 years
	Maternal age multipara	20-30 years
2.	Marital state	married
3.	Parity	1-4
4.	Abortions in history	0-1
5.	Pelvis	no disproportion
6.	Luetic infection	absent
7.	Rh incompatibility	absent
8.	Blood group incompatibility	absent
9.	Nutritional state	well nourished
10.	Haemoglobin level	70% or more
11.	Bleeding during pregnancy	absent
12.	Infection during pregnancy	absent
13.	X-ray abdomen during pregnancy	no
14.	Toxaemia	absent or mild
15.	Blood pressure	not exceeding 90/135
16.	Albuminuria and oedema	absent
17.	Hyperemesis	absent
18.	Psychological stress	absent
19.	Prolonged unwanted sterility (2 years)	absent
20.	Maternal chronic diseases	absent

Parturition

21.	Twins or multiple birth	no
22.	Delivery	spontaneous
23.	Duration 1st stage	6-24 hours
24.	Duration 2nd stage	10 min—2 hours
25.	Contractions	moderate or strong
26.	Drugs given to mother	O^2, local anaesthetic
27.	Amniotic fluid	clear
28.	Membranes broken	not longer than 6 hours

Fetal factors

29.	Intrauterine position	vertex
30.	Gestational age	38-41 weeks
31.	Fetal presentation	vertex
32.	Cardiac regularity	regular
33.	Fetal heart rate (2nd stage)	100-160
34.	Cord around the neck	no or loose
35.	Cord prolapse	no
36.	Knot in the cord	no
37.	Placental infarction	no or small
38.	Onset respiration	within first minute
39.	Treatment, resuscitation	no
40.	Drugs given	nil
41.	Body temperature	normal
42.	Birth weight	2500-4990 g

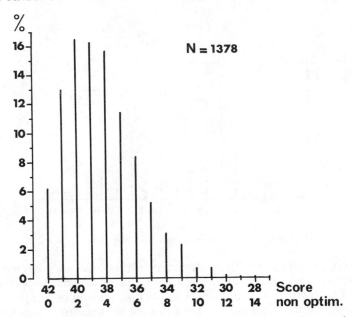

Figure 1   Percentage distribution of the obstetric scores. Below each score is given the corresponding number of non-optimal conditions.

TABLE 2   Frequency of occurrence of obstetrical complications

Condition	N	%
Maternal age above 30 years	342	25.0
Moderate toxaemia	250	18.1
Severe toxaemia	108	8.5
Other than vertex presentations	235	17.2
Non spontaneous delivery	427	31.0
Caesarean sections	81	6.0
Middle forceps	75	5.4
Low forceps	133	9.7
Prolonged labour ≥24 hours	170	12.3
Second stage longer than two hours	96	7.0
Tight cord around the neck	101	7.3
Fetal bradycardia <100/min.	188	13.6
Postpartum apnoea >1 min.	224	16.3

occurrence of non-optimal obstetric conditions. In the subsequent analysis the data for boys and girls are combined.

Interrelationships between non-optimal obstetric conditions

It is of interest to examine which conditions occur in combination with others and which do not. This summary will be confined to three examples only, illustrating respectively: complications of pregnancy, delivery and fetal state.

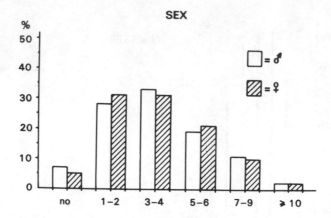

Figure 2   Incidence of non-optimal conditions in boys and girls.

Toxaemia. If all cases with moderate or severe toxaemia (characterized by blood pressure ⩾ 140/95, and proteinuria and/or oedema respectively) are compared with the rest, with respect to the distribution of complications, it will be seen that there is a marked tendency for the toxaemia cases to occur in association with a large number of other non-optimal conditions (Figure 3).

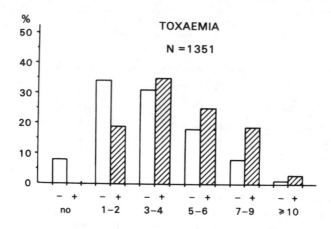

Figure 3   Percentage of non-toxaemic (-), and moderate and severe toxaemic cases (+) (*N* = 370) in each sub-group of non-optimal conditions. The difference is significant.

Delivery. A similar picture emerges, as might be expected, for instrumental, as compared with spontaneous, deliveries (Figure 4). Since the introduction of the vacuum extractor, the use of forceps has dramatically decreased in recent years.

Fetal heart-rate and apnoea. Signs of fetal distress, such as tachycardia or bradycardia during the second stage (Figure 5) and postpartum apnoea lasting longer than one minute (Figure 6), show a similar picture to the complications above.

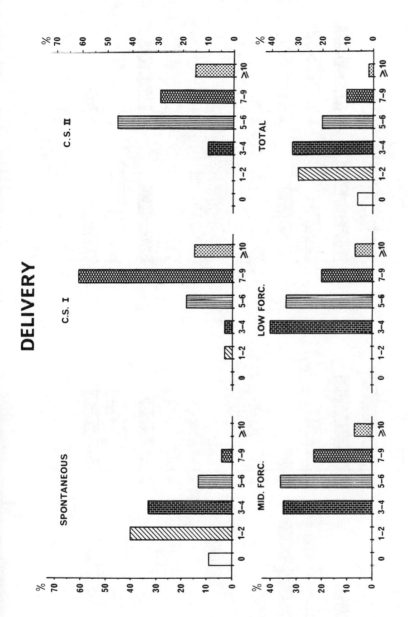

Figure 4 Type of delivery and obstetric sub-group. Spontaneous delivery, elective caesarean sections C.S.I. (*N* = 33), non-elective C.S. 11 (*N* = 48), middle forceps (*N* = 85), and low forceps (*N* = 133) are presented separately.

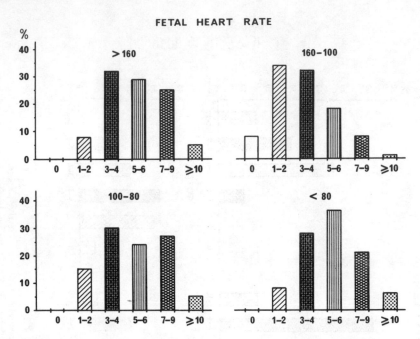

Figure 5   Fetal heart rate and non-optimal conditions. The tachycardia group with a heart rate >160/min(N=59) and the two groups of bradycardia 100—80/min (N=101) and ≤80/min (N = 89) are all significantly different from the group with normal heart rate (100—160).

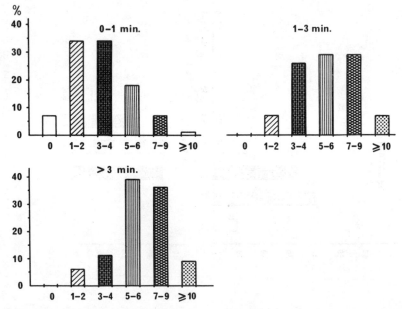

Figure 6   Onset of respiration and incidence of non-optimal conditions. The longer the apnoea, the more non-optimal conditions are present. The difference is highly significant: 1-3 min, N = 187; >3 min, N = 37.

Non-optimal obstetric conditions and neurological symptoms

Most of the items of the neurological examination are assessed on an ordinal scale with three or four points. For instance, the palmar grasp reflex is recorded as being absent (-), being weak or just discernable (+), giving a good sustained response for ten seconds (++), or giving an exaggerated forceful grasp (+++). The rooting response is recorded as being absent (-), showing only a weak turn toward the stimulated side (+), giving a full turn and a grasp with the lips (++), and consisting of a very vigorous turn with grasping (+++). The intensity of the Moro reflex is recorded as low, middle or high. In the case of the palmar grasp reflex and rooting response, the (++) category may be regarded as the optimal response, whereas for the Moro reflex, the optimal response would be that of intermediate intensity and threshold.

If we assume that for each item of the neurological examination there is an optimal response, we may examine the frequency with which cases with varying numbers of obstetric complications, fall into the optimal and non-optimal categories.

For the purpose of this analysis the data were divided on the basis of the obstetric optimality into three sub-groups:

1. A 'low risk' group (*N* = 264; 19.2%) with no or only one non-optimal condition;
2. A 'middle risk' group (*N* = 943; 68.4%) with two to six non-optimal conditions;
3. A 'high risk' group (*N* = 171; 12.4%) with seven or more non-optimal conditions.

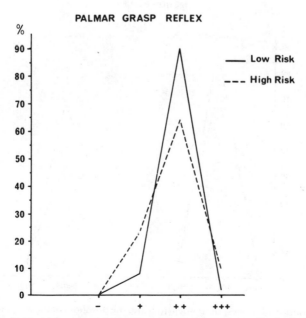

Figure 7 Distribution of response intensities of the palmar grasp reflex in the low and high risk groups. The difference is significant (X^2 = 22.2, *p* = 0.001).

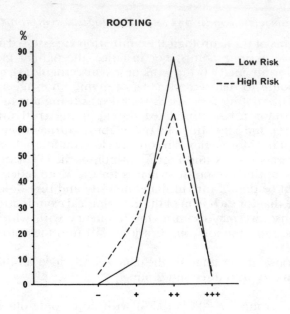

Figure 8 Distribution of response intensities of the rooting response in the low and high risk group. The difference is significant ($X^2 = 22.2$, $p = 0.001$).

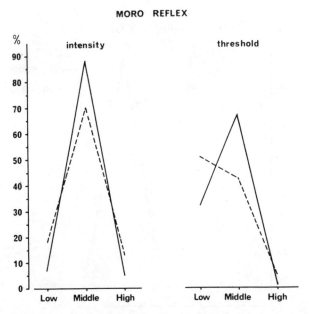

Figure 9 Distribution of the response intensities and the threshold of the Moro response in the low (solid line) and the high risk (broken line) group ($X^2 = 19.8$, $p < 0.01$; and $X^2 = 19.9$, $p < 0.01$ respectively).

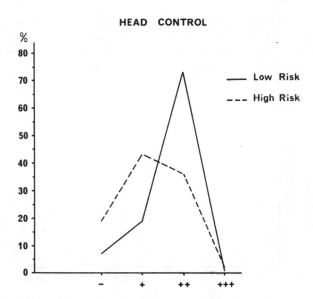

Figure 10 Distribution of the scores of head control in the sitting posture in the low and the high risk group (χ^2 = 20.1, p<M 0.01).

The word 'risk' is used to denote a raised probability of mortality during delivery and the first two weeks of life. It involves no assumptions about the possible outcome of the neurological examination.

For illustration the distributions of response intensities of the palmar grasp reflex (Figure 7), the rooting response (Figure 8), the Moro-response (Figure 9), and the head control in sitting posture (Figure 10) are shown for the low and high risk group.

Fifty-eight neurological items were selected which, like those above, could be assigned a position on a four-point ordinal scale. Contingency tables were constructed showing the frequency with which patients from the three 'risk' groups fell into different positions on each scale. In forty-two of the tests, the differences between expected and observed frequencies as measured by χ^2 tests were significant at least at the 1% level of confidence. The 'low-risk' group predominantly showed those responses described as 'optimal', whereas the 'high-risk' group showed relatively few optimal responses. In all forty-two of these items, the 'middle-risk' group was intermediate between the other two with respect to the number of optimal responses. In other words, there is a highly significant association between the number of non-optimal obstetric conditions and neurological abnormalities in the newborn.

The relationship between non-optimal obstetric conditions and neurological abnormality is seen even more clearly, if we carry out the following transformation. For each ordinal item of the neurological examination, a score of 1 was given if the baby's response was in the 'optimal' category. It was thus possible to obtain a 'neurological optimality score', the number of items of the neurological examination upon which the baby gave an optimal response. For all babies on whom the full neurological examination had been carried out   ($N = 1000$) the neurological scores were plotted against the corresponding number of non-optimal conditions.

It was found that the mean neurological score decreased as the number of obstetric non-optimal conditions increased (Figure 11).

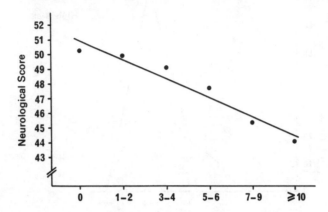

Figure 11   Mean neurological scores plotted against the corresponding number of non-optimal conditions.

The neurological scores were next separated into three main groups, taking the following cut-off points: scores equal to less than 47 (abnormal); scores between 48 and 52 (suspected abnormal) and scores between 53 and 58 (normal). The babies in each of these three groups were then allocated, on the basis of their obstetric scores, to the high, middle and low risk groups. The relationship between the neurological and obstetric findings is shown in Table 3. There was a highly significant difference between the observed and expected frequencies with which the three neurological sub-groups were represented in the three risk groups ($x^2 = 38.5$, d.f. $= 4$, $p < 0.001$). It is clear therefore that there is a high association between obstetric conditions as measured by the obstetric scores and the occurrence of neonatal neurological optimal conditions.

It is of interest to examine the relationship between the obstetric and neurological findings and birthweight. Babies with a relatively low birthweight of 2500 to 3000 g were compared with those whose birthweight was

TABLE 3   Relation between neurological score and obstetric risk group

Neurological	Risk Group			
Scores	Low	Middle	High	Totals
$\leqslant 47$	73 (101.7)	375 (363.4)	83 (65.9)	531
48-52	84 (87.9)	316 (314.1)	59 (57)	459
53-58	107 (74.3)	252 (265.5)	29 (48.1)	388
Totals	264	943	171	1378

Figures in parentheses are expected frequencies.

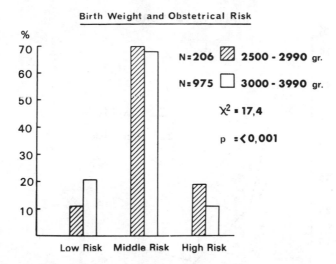

Figure 12 Comparison of percentages of lower and higher birthweight babies in low, middle and high risk groups.

3000 to 4000 g. The percentages of babies in each range who fell into the three obstetric groups, low, middle and high risk, are shown in Figure 12. Babies with the lower birthweight are significantly over-represented in the high risk and under-represented in the low risk groups respectively. Similarly, the lower birthweight babies are significantly under-represented in the neurologically normal and over-represented in the suspect abnormal and abnormal groups respectively (Figure 13).

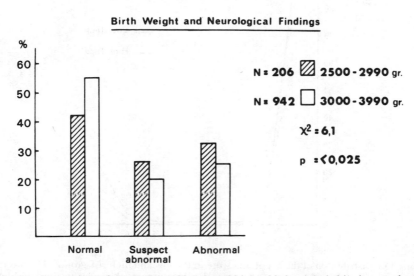

Figure 13 Comparison of percentages of lower and higher birthweight babies in neurological normal, suspected abnormal and abnormal groups.

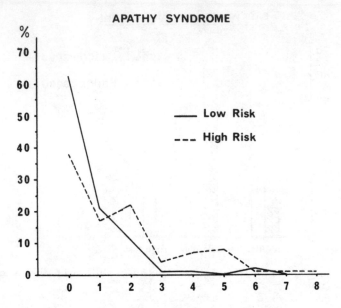

Figure 14   Distributions of apathy scores in low and high risk groups.

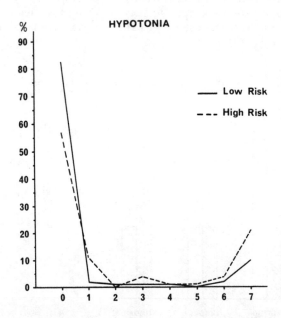

Figure 15   Distribution of the hypotonia score in the low and high risk groups. The rise at the right-hand end of the curves is due to the generalized hypotonic babies who obtained the highest scores.

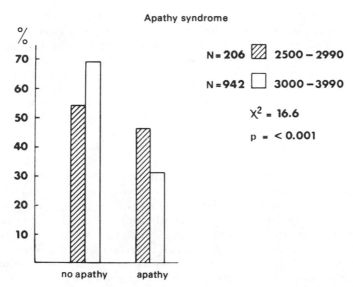

Figure 16 Comparison of percentages of lower and higher birthweight babies with respect to the presence or absence of the apathy syndrome.

Obstetric risks and neurological syndromes

If a group of symptoms occurs repeatedly in combination, they may be said to constitute a syndrome. We have previously described as the *apathy syndrome* (26), a combination of low intensity of general motor activity and of sucking, rooting, hand- and foot-grasping, head-lifting in prone position, recoil of forearms and the labyrinthine reflex. Similarly, babies showing lowered resistance to passive movements of the neck, trunk, shoulder, elbow, hand, hip, knee and ankle joints, have been described as hypotonic. Significantly more babies showing both the apathy syndrome and hypotonia were found in the high risk group than in either the middle or low risk groups (Figures 14 and 15). The apathy syndrome was also found significantly more often among the babies whose birthweight was relatively lower (2500 to 3000g) (Figure 16). Babies with asymmetries of posture, tendon reflexes and skin reflexes (which we have previously described as the *hemisyndrome*) were equally distributed among the three risk groups. Interestingly, however, babies with the hemisyndrome and those with facial palsies, occurred significantly more frequently after forceps delivery and version-extraction. Babies who are what we have called *hyperexcitable* (26) were significantly over-represented in the middle risk group. Hyperexcitability occurred significantly more frequently among the boys.

Neurological scores and classical neurological signs

We have so far argued that there is a high positive correlation between non-optimal conditions and neurological abnormality as measured by our standardized procedure. Because neonatal abnormalities using this technique are predictive of continuing abnormality and future behavioural disturbance, we believe it is essential for full neurological examination to be carried out on all babies who are obstetrically at higher risk. It might be argued however, that since the full examination is a time-consuming and expensive procedure, it is sufficient to record the presence of obvious neurological signs which any well trained obstetrician or paediatrician could not fail to see. In fact, twenty-five of our babies showed one or more obvious neurological signs: facial palsies; bulging fontanelles; deviation of eye position; absence of sucking; Moro or palmar grasp reflexes; severe floppiness or marked asymmetry. It is of interest to examine the distribution of the neurological scores of these babies relative to that of the remainder. No baby with an obvious neurologically abnormal condition, ever obtains fewer than four non-optimal sub-test items, i.e. it is never misclassified as normal by our examination. On the other hand, a very large number of babies with no classical neurological signs, obtain the same neurological scores as those with such classical signs. It is clear therefore that examination merely for gross signs of pathology will result in the omission of a considerable amount of neurological abnormality which is prognostically ominous. Thus, the presence of 'classical neurological signs' is not exclusive evidence of neurological abnormality. Moreover, we have shown that neurological abnormality, as measured by the full standardized procedure, increases in relation to the number of non-optimal obstetric conditions. It therefore follows that the urgency for full neurological examination of the newborn increases also as a function of the number of non-optimal conditions present (27).

Discussion

The identification of what constitute obstetric hazards remains an urgent clinical problem. An approach to this question through mortality rate studies has great merits, but the answers must remain incomplete, since the majority of infants survive obstetric complications. Among these babies, however, may be many who suffer major or minor impairment of brain function. The early recognition of nervous dysfunction is of great importance both with respect to the possibility of early treatment, and in relation to handling difficulties arising during the development of the mother-infant relationship. Many studies seem to indicate that besides handicaps such as cerebral palsy, due to pre- and perinatal brain damage, minor brain dysfunctions, undramatic from the clinical neurological point of view, may lead to severe problems in the life of children and their parents. Although well controlled studies are still scarce, the available data are alarming.

In the context of these aspects the need for early indicators of risks is evident. The attempt to design risk registers which would select those babies from the population who are at special risk of brain damage is a major task. If only for the purpose of practical management, criteria are needed which do not select for special attention half or even more of all newborn babies. In the light of our study, one possible approach is through the obstetric score. It will be remembered that obstetric scores were highly correlated with neurological findings which were themselves predictive of continuing abnormality. In practice, this would mean filling in a checklist of optimal conditions which results in a risk score. This is obviously a more reliable strategy than to look only for the presence of particular dangerous obstetric complications in the baby's history.

As a further result of our study new criteria are suggested for the interpretation of the quantitative results of our neurological test items. Although it was possible previously to indicate the optimal intensity of responses, it was still questionable for many responses, at what points of the scale one should speak of an abnormal response, a fact we have indicated in our Manual for the neurological examination of the full-term newborn infant. Differences found between the neurological item scores of the obstetrically high risk group and those of the low risk group are very suggestive of a more valid demarcation of neurological abnormality. For example, with respect to the rooting response, the differences between the two risk groups are apparent in the scores (-) and (+), but the incidence of (+++) is no higher in the high risk group than in the low risk group. This offers a possible operational definition of 'abnormal' as being the (-) and (+) responses only, in contrast to the normal responses (++) and (+++). In the case of the palmar grasp response, on the other hand, the (+++) response would still be considered as abnormal.

This new information is valid for many test items of the neurological examination. There remain certain neurological signs which are undoubtedly abnormal, such as the absence of sucking or of the Moro response, and persistent deviation of the eyes. Our study has shown, however, that application of these generally accepted criteria of abnormality alone would leave many neurologically abnormal babies unrecognized. The French technique as advocated by St Anne Dargassies (28) uses only such qualitative signs. The quantitative assessment of neurological signs is not however a mere academic refinement of neurological examinations but a clinical necessity.

Summary

A group of 1378 full-term newborn infants, born in the Obstetric Department of the University of Groningen were subjected to a standardized quantitative neurological examination in their first ten days of life. Data on pregnancy, delivery, and condition of the infant at birth were available.

Since previous correlation analysis of neurological results with obstetric complications failed to give instructive results a new approach was carried out. Forty-two variables of the pre- and perinatal history were analysed and counted if they deviated from optimal conditions, giving an obstetric risk score for each baby. The distributions of response intensities of many neurological items were shown to be different in the low, middle and high risk groups. This held true also for some syndromes. The number of optimal neurological responses was negatively correlated with the number of non-optimal obstetric conditions.

Non-optimal conditions tended to occur in association with each other. The more a condition deviated from the norm, the greater was the number of other non-optimal conditions associated with it. A simple count of the number of such non-optimal conditions present, offers promise as a means of identifying those babies at risk of neurological damage. Though the presence of 'classical' neurological signs is diagnostic, absence of such signs by no means excludes a high non-optimal score on our scale.

It is suggested that the criteria for assessing what is an abnormal neurological response may be refined to the responses of our low and high risk groups.

References

(1) De Haas-Posthuma, J.H. (1962) *Perinatale sterfte in Nederland*. Assen, Van Gorcum.
(2) Butler, N.R. and Bonham, D. (1963) *Perinatal Mortality*. Edinburgh and London, Livingstone.
(3) Butler, N.R. and Alberman, E.D. (1969) *Perinatal Problems*. Edinburgh and London, Livingstone.
(4) Debre, R., Bargeton, E., Mozziconacci, P. and Habib, R. (1955) Lésions cérébrales par anoxie neo-natale. *Archives francaises de Pediatric, 12*, 673-84.
(5) Norman, A.P. (1956) Birth trauma. *Br. med. J., 1*, 37-40.
(6) Malamud, N. (1959) Sequelae of perinatal trauma. *Journal of Neuropathology and Experimental Neurology, 18*, 141-55.
(7) Towbin, A. (1969) Mental retardation due to germinal matrix infarction. *Science, 164*, 156-61.
(8) Towbin, A. (1969) Cerebral hypoxic damage in foetus and newborn. *Archs Neurol., 20*, 35-43.
(9) Towbin, A. (1970) Central nervous system damage in the human foetus and newborn infant. *Am. J. Dis. Child, 119*, 529-42.
(10) Towbin, A. (1971) Organic causes of minimal brain dysfunction. *'J. Am. med. Ass., 217*, 1207-14.
(11) Ranck B. Jr. and Windle, W.F. (1959) Brain damage in the monkey, *Macaca mulatta*, by asphyxia neonatorum. *Exp. Neurol., 1*, 130-54.
(12) Windle, W.F. (1957) Neurological and psychological deficits from asphyxia neonatorum. *Public Health Reports, 72*, 646-50.
(13) Windle, W.F. (1960) Effects of asphyxiation of the foetus and the newborn infant. *Pediatrics, 25*, 565-9.
(14) Windle, W.F., De Ramirez De Arellano, M.I.R., Ramirez De Arellano, M. and Hibbard, E. (1961) Rôle de l'asphyxie pendant la naissance dans le genèse des troubles du jeune singe. *Revue Neurologique, 105*, 142-52.
(15) Windle, W.F. (1970) Cerebral hemorrhage in relation to birth asphyxia. *Science, 167*, 1000-1.
(16) Myers, R.E. (1970) Brain damage induced by umbilical cord compression at different gestational ages in monkeys. Proc. 2nd. Conf. exp. Med. Surg. Primates, New York. *Medical Primatology*, 394-425.
(17) Myers, R.E. (1972) Two patterns of perinatal brain damage and their conditions of occurrence. *American Journal of Obstetrics and Gynecology, 112*, 246-76.
(18) Apgar, V. (1966) The newborn (Apgar) scoring system: Reflections and advice. *Pediatric Clinics of North America*, Symposium on the Newborn, *1*, 13/3, 645-50.
(19) Drage, J.S. and Berendes, H. (1966) Apgar scores and outcome of the newborn. *Pediatric Clinics of North America*, Symposium on the Newborn, *1*, 13/3, 635-44.
(20) Graham, F.K. (1956) Behavioral differences between normal and traumatized newborns. I. Test Procedures. II. Standardization, reliability and validity. *Psychol. Monogr., 70*, nos. 20 and 21.
(21) Graham, F.K., Pennoyer, M., Caldwell, B., Greenman, M. and Hartmann, A.F. (1957) Relationship between clinical status and behaviour test performance in a newborn group with histories suggesting anoxia. *J. Pediat., 50*, 177-89.
(22) Rosenblith, J.F. (1961) The modified Graham behavior test for neonates: test-retest reliability, normative data, and hypotheses for future work. *Biologia Neonatorum, 3*, 174-92.
(23) Prechtl, H.F.R. and Beintema, D. (1964) *The Neurological Examination of the Full-Term Newborn Infant. Clinics in Developmental Medicine, 12*. London, Spastics International and Heinemann Medical.
(24) Beintema, D.J. (1968) *A Neurological Study of Newborn Infants. Clinics in Developmental Medicine, 28*. London, Spastics International and Heinemann Medical.

(25) Prechtl, H.F.R. (1972) Strategy and Validity of Early Detection of Neurological Dysfunction. In *Mental Retardation: Prenatal Diagnosis and Infant Assessment,* Eds. C.P. Douglas and K.S. Holt. London, Butterworths.

(26) Prechtl, H.F.R. (1960) Die neurologische Untersuchung des Neugeborenes: Voraussetzungen, Methode und Prognose. *Wiener medizinische Wochenschrift, 110,* 1035-9.

(27) Prechtl, H.F.R, (1970) Hazards of oversimplification. *Developmental Medicine and Child Neurology, 12,* 522-4.

(28) St Anne Dargassies, (1962) Le nouveau-né à terme: Aspect neurologique. *Biologie Neonatale, 4,* 174-200.

9. Parent-child separation: psychological effects on the children

Michael Rutter

The importance of the family as a formative influence on a child's personality growth needs no arguing. Particularly in early childhood, it is the matrix within which the child develops, the area where his strongest emotional ties are formed and the background against which his most intense personal life is enacted (1). The family is the most intimate, one of the most important and most studied of all human groups and yet our knowledge of it remains rudimentary (2).

Misconceptions, myths and false knowledge on the effects of different patterns of child-rearing are rife. Generations of doctors, psychologists, nurses and educators have pontificated on what parents need to do in order to bring up their children to be healthy and well adjusted adults. Over the last fifty years we have been exhorted in the name of mental health to suppress masturbation, to feed children by the clock, and then to let them gratify their impulses in whatever way they wish (3, 4). However, the claims that these policies were necessary for normal emotional development were made in the absence of supporting evidence. Research findings have failed to show any significant effects stemming from patterns of feeding, time of weaning, type of toilet-training and the like (5) and the consequences of different patterns of discipline appear surprisingly slight (6).

Uninterrupted mother-child contact has also been the subject of firm claims. Bowlby (7) suggested that 'prolonged separation of a child from his mother (or mother substitute) during the first five years of his life stands foremost among the causes of delinquent character development and persistent misbehaviour.' More recently, he reiterated that because of its long-term consequences a child should be separated from his parents only in exceptional circumstances (8, 9). These statements are arguable (10), but are cautious compared with those of some other writers. For example, Baers (11) claimed that the normal growth of children is dependent on the mother's full-time occupation in the role of child-rearing and that 'anything that hinders women in the fulfilment of this mission must be regarded as contrary to human progress.' Similarly, a WHO Expert Committee (12) concluded that the use of day nurseries and creches inevitably caused 'permanent damage to the emotional health of a future generation.' It is, perhaps, noteworthy that assertions of this kind have mostly been made by men and from the tenor of their comments we might well agree with Margaret Mead (13) when she suggests that the campaign on the evils of mother-child separation is just

A revised form of the Sir Geoffrey Vickers Lecture of 24 February 1971, the original version of which was published in the *Journal of Child Psychology and Psychiatry*, 1971, *12*, 233-60.

another attempt by men to shackle women to the home. Nevertheless, it would be wrong to dismiss the argument on these grounds. If mother-child separation actually does lead to delinquent character formations and if care by fathers cannot compensate, then, however much the Women's Liberation Movement may protest, it is necessary for women to be tied to their children during the growing years.

But first we must know the facts. We are still not sufficiently in the habit of critically examining the facts before arriving at our conclusions (14). Many of the statements quoted above imply that we understand exactly what sort of upbringing a child needs, and precisely which factors cause psychiatric disorder in children. But we do not, and it is our failure to *recognize* our ignorance which has led to these confident but contradictory claims. It is not the ignorance as such which is harmful but rather our 'knowing' so many things that are not true. Our theories on the importance of the family have multiplied and become increasingly certain long before we know what are the facts the theories have to explain.

Of course, it would be quite futile to collect facts without a purpose. As Medawar (15, 16) has described so well, science consists of both discovery and proof, hypothesis and then careful testing to discriminate between alternative hypotheses.

My purpose here is to illustrate this process with respect to family studies. In order to emphasize that research is the *act* of scientific enquiry, the *search* for truth and not the *statement* of knowledge, I am going to describe how my colleagues and I set out to answer one simple question on the psychological effects of a child's separation from his mother. The question chosen was one which has aroused great interest, which carries with it wide-ranging implications for community policies and which has been the subject of very strong claims concerning its consequences.

The research method used is that of epidemiology, which is simply the study of the distribution of disorders in a community together with an examination of how the distribution varies with particular environmental circumstances. Originally this was a technique used with great success in the study of the cause of infectious diseases and other medical conditions (17, 18). It can also be used to study the social causes of psychiatric disorder (19, 20) and the psychological effects of family influences (21), which is how I shall be using it here.

In order to give some 'feel' of the successive steps of research I shall confine more detailed descriptions to the work carried out over the last ten years by my collaborators and myself. In doing this I serve as the representative of a research team, or more accurately several research teams, and many of the ideas I express stem as much from them as from me. However, the validity of any observation is upheld only when it is repeated in other independent investigations. There are now many family studies using a variety of methods (2, 22, 23) and I shall try to point out which of our findings have been supported by other research.

Measurement of family characteristics

The first task was to measure the family characteristics in which we were interested and to assess children's psychological development. We wanted to determine what actually happened in the home with regard to different aspects of family life, and interview methods were developed for this purpose (24, 25).

The interview served two quite distinct functions: (*a*) to obtain an accurate account of various events and happenings in the family (who put the children to bed, how often the parents played or talked with the children, how often they quarrelled and so forth), and (*b*) to provide a standard stimulus for eliciting emotions and attitudes (warmth, criticism, hostility, dissatisfaction and the like). Different techniques were necessary for these two aspects of the interview, and these have been outlined previously (24, 25). Some three years were spent in devising methods which could differentiate successfully between different aspects of family life. In particular it was found essential to distinguish between what people did in the home and what they felt about it— between the acts and the emotions accompanying the acts. It was also necessary to measure emotions separately in relation to different members of the family, since parents may be very warm towards one child and yet reject another. Finally, it was important to consider negative and positive feelings separately. Frequently, people have 'mixed' feelings, both loving and hating someone at the same time. By making these distinctions it proved possible to devise reasonably accurate measures of the central features of family life. Systematic investigation showed that the ratings had a satisfactory level of reliability and validity.

Measurement of psychiatric state

Similar care had to be taken in the measurement of the children's emotional and behavioural state. For this purpose we used both questionnaire and interview measures of behaviour in different situations. As with the family measures, the reliability and, as far as possible, the validity of the ratings were tested and found adequate (26, 27, 28, 29).

Samples

The effects of different family influences on children's psychological development have been examined in several populations. Here I shall refer to only two—both of which, as it happens, were being studied primarily for other reasons. This has the advantage that we have a lot of information on additional aspects of children's circumstances and development which help to put the family findings into perspective.

The first group studied consisted of the families of nine- to twelve-year-old children living in a community of small towns on the Isle of Wight. This study* investigated the educational, physical, and psychiatric handicaps in school-age children (29, 30). The second sample was a representative group of London families, in which one or both parents had been under psychiatric care (31). The study† was designed to investigate the difficulties faced by

*This study was carried out in collaboration with Professor J. Tizard, Dr K. Whitmore, Professor P. Graham, Mr W. Yule and Mr L. Rigley.
†This study was undertaken together with Mrs S. George, Professor P. Graham, Mrs B. Yule, Mr D. Quinton, Miss O. Rowlands, Miss C. Tupling and Mr P. Ziffo.

families when one parent became sick, and to determine to what extent their needs were being met by the current provision of services. In both cases we have been extremely fortunate in the cooperation we have received and we are most grateful to the many families who have helped us in this work.

Parent-child separation

If separation is such a serious hazard to mental health as claimed, there are vital implications for public health policy and important opportunities for the prevention of psychiatric disorder.

All children must separate from their parents at some time if they are to develop independent personalities. Furthermore, most youngsters experience some form of temporary separation from their parents during childhood. For example, Douglas *et al.* (32) found that one in three children was separated from its parents for at least one week before the age of four and a half years. Obviously most of these turn out to be quite normal boys and girls, so the question to be asked is not whether separation should be allowed but rather what sort of separation, at what age, for how long, and for what reason leads to psychological disturbance. Also, we need to specify separation from which parent? Most emphasis has been placed on *mother*-child separation, the father being regarded as a relatively insignificant figure with respect to a child's personality development. Is this so? Finally, it has been suggested that it is necessary for children to have a relationship with a *single* mother-figure and that harm will come if mothering is divided among several people. So the apparently simple question whether separation from their parents is bad for children turns out to be quite complicated.

Short-term effects

In attempting to provide a solution to the problem it may be appropriate to begin with the short-term effects of parent-child separation. This has been most studied in children admitted to hospital. Bowlby and his colleagues noted the frequency with which children were upset after admission and described three phases to the disturbance (33, 34, 35, 36). First, the child cries and shows acute distress, the period of *protest*; he then appears miserable and withdrawn, the phase of *despair*; and finally there is a time when he seems to lose interest in his parents, the stage of *detachment*. When the child returns to his parents he often ignores them at first and then becomes clinging and demanding.

Some investigators have failed to confirm these findings (37), but on the whole the observations have received support from other studies (38, 39). Nevertheless, a number of important qualifications have had to be introduced. The response described is most marked in children aged six months to four years, but even at this age it occurs in only some children (40, 41, 42). Moreover, it is misleading to regard the separation as being only from mother. While children at this age are often most attached to their mother they are also attached to their father and to their brothers and sisters (43, 44). In the past the strength of these other attachments has often been underestimated. Their importance is shown by the finding that when children are admitted to hospital with their brother or sister they show less distress (45). Although the separation is probably the principal factor even in hospital admission, the care during the separation is also relevant (41, 46, 47).

Some of the reasons why children differ in their response to separation can be found in their temperamental characteristics prior to separation (48). Similar findings have been reported in sub-human primates (49). Finally, with regard to the short-term effects of separation it appears that children used to brief separations of a happy kind are less distressed by *unhappy* separations such as hospital admission (48). This last point suggests that in some circumstances separation experiences may actually be beneficial to the child.

In summary, children are not inevitably distressed by separation from their parents and we are beginning to learn what factors determine whether they are upset, and how we may take steps to diminish the emotional disturbance associated with separation. Even so, despite these qualifications the main point that a child's separation from his family is a potential cause of short-term distress and emotional disturbance has received substantial support from research findings.

Long-term effects

It is the long-term effects that my colleagues and I have been concerned to investigate. In order to discuss our findings it will be necessary to divide separation experiences into several categories.

Working mothers

This is a situation which exemplifies both recurrent very brief separations and maternal care provided by several or even many mother-figures. In the past it has been claimed that the children of working mothers are particularly likely to become delinquent or develop some form of psychiatric disorder, but there is abundant evidence from numerous studies, including our own, that this is not so (29, 50, 51). Indeed, in some circumstances, children of working mothers may be *less* likely to become delinquent (52). There is no evidence that children suffer from having several mother-figures so long as stable relationships and good care are provided by each (53). This is an important proviso, but one which applies equally to mothers who are not working. A situation in which mother-figures keep changing so that the child does not have the opportunity of forming a relationship with any of them may well be harmful, but such unstable arrangements usually occur in association with poor quality maternal care, so that up to now it has not been possible to examine the effects of each independently.

Day nurseries and creches have come in for particularly heavy criticism and, as already noted, the World Health Organization actually asserted that their use inevitably caused permanent psychological damage. There is *no* evidence in support of this view. Of course, day nurseries vary greatly in quality and some are quite poor. Bad child-care whether in day nurseries or at home is to be deplored, but there is no reason to suppose that day nurseries, as such, have a deleterious influence. Indeed, day care need not interfere with normal mother-child attachment (54) and to date there is no reason to suppose that the use of good day nurseries has any long-term ill-effects (50). Although the evidence is still incomplete, the same conclusions probably apply also to communities such as the Israeli kibbutzim where children are, in effect, raised in residential nurseries although retaining strong links with their parents (55, 56).

The claim that working mothers and day nurseries cause delinquency and psychiatric disorder was made in good faith but without substantiating evidence, and subsequent research has shown the charge to be wrong. It is important that we listen carefully to the advice and testimony of individuals who have studied a problem, but it is equally important that we demand that they present the evidence relevant to their recommendations. Science does not consist of experts' answers, but rather of the process by which questions may be investigated and the means of determining the relative merits and demerits of different explanations and answers.

Transient separations

Transient parent-child separation can lead to acute short-term distress as already discussed. Can it also lead to long-term psychological disturbance? Several independent investigations have shown that children can be separated from their parents for quite long periods in early childhood with surprisingly

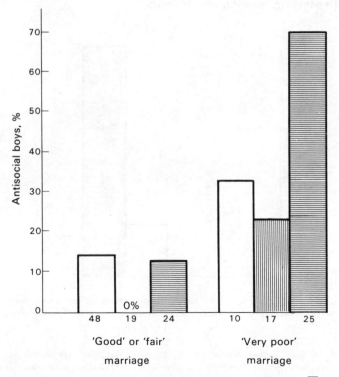

Figure 1   Discord or separation as causes of anti-social behaviour in boys. ☐ No separation; ▥ Separation from one parent at a time; ▤ Separation from both parents or institutional care.

On this and all subsequent Figures, the numbers at the base of the histogram refer to the number of cases for that column.

little in the way of long-term ill-effects (51, 57, 58, 59).* Yet, most studies have shown that children subjected to separation experiences in early childhood do have a slightly increased risk of later psychological disturbance (61) and it is necessary to explore the possible explanations for this association. To do this we must examine more closely the nature of the separation experiences.

In our study of patients' families we divided separation experiences into those involving separation from one parent only and those involving separations from both parents at the same time. In each case separations were counted only if they had lasted at least four consecutive weeks.

It was immediately apparent that children separated from both parents came from more disturbed homes than did children who had never experienced separation. Many of the children were separated because they had been taken into care following some family crisis and often this occurs against a background of more long-standing difficulties (62, 63).

As a measure of family disturbance we used one of our most reliable summary ratings on the quality of the parental marriage. This is based on a wide range of information concerning such items as affectional relationships between the parents, marital dissatisfaction, shared leisure activities, communication between husband and wife, mutual enjoyment of each other's company, quarrelling, tension and hostility.

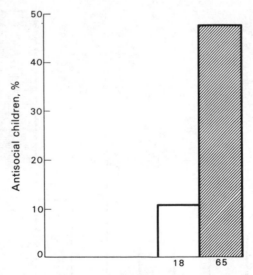

Figure 2   Reasons for total parent-child separation and anti-social behaviour in children. □ Separation due to physical illness or holiday; ▨ Separation due to family discord or psychiatric illness.

*A further study by Naess (60) confirmed that prolonged separation experiences were no more frequent in delinquents than in controls, but also suggested that separations might be more frequent in a small group of serious delinquents. As this study is sometimes quoted in support of Bowlby's 1946 paper, it may be appropriate to give Naess' conclusions in full: 'Our conclusion is that mother-child separation as such is a minor criminogenic factor; it does not stand "foremost among the causes of a delinquent character development", but may be conceived as part of the picture of an unstable family life.'

Figure 1 (total N = 151) shows the association between parent-child separation and anti-social behaviour in boys, after controlling for the quality of the parental marriage. In this and in subsequent figures the measure of children's behaviour used is the score on a behavioural questionnaire completed by teachers (28). This has been shown to be a reliable and valid instrument, and it can be scored to differentiate between neurotic and anti-social disturbance (28, 29). We chose to use this measure because it is the one most independent of our family measures and because it concerns the child's behaviour outside the home. However, the comparisons have also been made using more detailed clinical assessments and the findings are closely similar regardless of which behavioural measure is employed.

The largest differences in anti-social behaviour are associated with the marriage rating and not with separation experiences. In each type of separation circumstance the proportion of anti-social boys was higher when there was a 'very poor' marriage than when there was a 'good' or 'fair' marriage.* Furthermore, regardless of the parental marriage relationship, separations from one parent only carried *no* increase in the rate of anti-social disorder. Indeed, although the differences are well short of statistical significance rather *fewer* of the separated children showed anti-social behaviour.

This comparison took into account neither *which* parent had been separated from the child nor the *age* of the child at the time of separation. Accordingly the comparisons were repeated making these differentiations. Again we found *no* difference. Comparisons were repeated for neurotic disorders and still no differences were found. It may be concluded that in the sample studied there was *no* association between separation from one parent only and any type of psychiatric or behavioural disorder in children.

But there was an association between separation from *both* parents and anti-social disorder in the children. On the face of it this might seem to indicate that this type of separation experience is a factor leading to psychological disturbance in later childhood. But it can be seen that this difference applied *only* in homes where there was a very poor marriage relationship between the parents ($p<0.05$). No such difference was found in cases where there was a 'fair' or 'good' marriage. This difference according to the marriage rating suggests that the association may not be due to the fact of separation from both parents, but rather to the discord and disturbance which surrounded the separation.

To investigate this possibility we divided separations from both parents into those due to some event *not* associated with discord (namely the child's admission to hospital for some physical illness or his going on a prolonged, usually convalescent, holiday), and those in which the separation was due to some deviance or discord. In the majority of cases this followed family break-up due to quarrels but in some instances separation was due to one parent having a mental disorder and the other parent being unable to keep the family together, the child staying with relatives or going into care.

As shown in Figure 2 (total N = 83), it is the *reason* for the separation that

---

*The marital rating scale has three main subdivisions, each being split into two parts making a six-point scale in all. There are instructions for raters defining each point.

mattered, not the separation itself. When the children were separated from both their parents because of physical illness or a holiday, the rate of anti-social disorder was quite low. When the separation was due to some type of family discord or deviance, on the other hand, nearly half the children exhibited anti-social behaviour, a rate over four times as high as in the other children ($p < 0.05$).

It seems that transient parent-child separation as such is unrelated to the development of anti-social behaviour. It only appears to be associated with anti-social disorder because separation often occurs as a result of family discord and disturbance. I should add that this conclusion still holds after taking into account the child's age at the time of separation. As other studies have produced contradictory and statistically insignificant associations with age of separation (64, 65), we may conclude that this is not a crucial variable with respect to long-term effects, although it is with respect to short-term effects.

Permanent separations

If we accept that transient separations are of little long-term importance, can we also conclude that prolonged or permanent separations are equally innocuous? To answer that question let us examine what happens when there is an irreversible break-up of the family due to parental death, divorce, or separation. In our several family studies we found that children who were in some type of anomalous family situation showed a higher rate of anti-social disorder than did children living with their two natural parents. This finding agrees with the large literature linking broken homes with delinquency (25, 29, 30, 38, 66, 67) and it may be accepted as a fact that, overall, children from a broken home have an increased risk of delinquency. This association does not apply to neurosis, but it may apply to some types of depression as well as to delinquency (68, 69).

But is this association due to parent-child separation, and if not, how is it to be explained? Bowlby (70) has laid most emphasis on loss of the maternal figure and has suggested that disorder in the child arises from a disruption of the affectional bond with his mother or other parent substitute (34, 35). Thus, he suggests that it is the separation or loss which is important and that the disorder in the child has some of the elements of grief and mourning (71). This explanation may well be correct with respect to the short-term effects of mother-child separation (45), but there are good reasons for doubting the hypothesis with respect to long-term effects and it is these with which we are concerned here.

One important issue concerning the mechanisms involved in the association between broken homes and delinquency is whether the harm comes from disruption of bonds or distortion of relationships. This question may first be examined by comparing homes broken by death (where relationships are likely to have been fairly normal prior to the break), and homes broken by divorce or separation (where the break is likely to have been preceded by discord and quarrelling—or at least by a lack of warmth and affection). Figure 3 shows this comparison as made in three independent investigations.

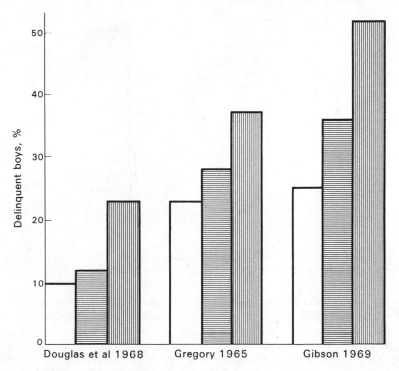

Figure 3   Cause of family disruption and delinquency.   ☐ Unbroken family; 📊 Broken by death; ⦀ Broken by divorce/separation.

In all three studies the delinquency rates are nearly *double* for boys whose parents had divorced or separated (64, 72, 73), but for boys who had lost a parent by death the delinquency rate was only slightly (and non-significantly) raised. In other studies, too, delinquency and conduct disorders have been found to be associated with parental divorce or separation but *not* with parental death (74, 75).

This suggests that it may be the discord and disharmony, rather than the break-up of the family as such, which lead to anti-social behaviour. To test that hypothesis it is first necessary to show directly that parental discord is associated with anti-social disorder in the children even when the home is unbroken. There is good evidence from several studies that this is the case (76, 77, 78) and Figure 4 (total N = 124) shows our own findings in this connection from the study of patients' families.*

*These findings still apply after controlling for social class. In our sample, parental occupation was not related to either the marriage rating or to anti-social behaviour. It is frequently assumed that delinquency is commoner in the lower social classes (66), but the evidence is contradictory (29). Furthermore, even in communities where social class is associated with behavioural disorder or delinquency in the children, this association often disappears once the effects of IQ are partialled out (29) or family discord and disruption are taken into account (79, 80, 81, 82). The association between social class and marital discord or family disorganization is also inconsistent; it applies in some communities but not in others (83, 22).

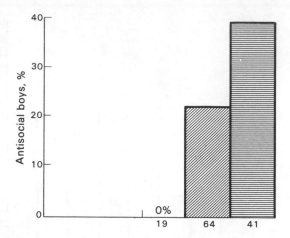

Figure 4 Marital relationship and anti-social behaviour in boys living with both natural parents. ☐ Good marriage; ▨ Fair marriage; ☰ Very poor marriage.

The rate of disorder in boys rises steadily from 0% in homes where there is a 'good' marriage to 22% when the marriage is 'fair' to 39% when there is a 'very poor' marriage (linear trend significant: $p < 0.001$). Parental discord is associated with anti-social disorder in the children. However, we can take the matter one stage further. If parental discord is more important than break-up of the home as a cause of deviant behaviour, the rate of anti-social disorder should be higher for children living with their two natural, but unhappily married, parents than for children living in harmonious but broken homes. In our study we had too few cases of the latter variety for the comparison to be meaningful, but information is available from several other investigations which have shown that delinquency tends to be commoner in unhappy unbroken homes than in harmonious but broken ones (77, 84). For example, the McCords (77) in a well-controlled study showed that broken homes resulted in significantly less juvenile delinquency than did unbroken but quarrelsome and neglecting homes.

The conclusions on broken homes are surprisingly straightforward. Although parental death may play a part in the pathogenesis of some disorders (25, 85), delinquency and anti-social disorder are mainly associated with breaks which follow parental discord rather than with the loss of a parent as such. Even within the group of homes broken by divorce or separation, it appears that it is the discord prior to separation rather than the break itself which was the main adverse influence.

The present findings suggest that separation as such is of negligible importance in the causation of anti-social disorder. It is important not to generalize too readily from the results of one study and it could be said that the sample studied was one with a rather high rate of family discord. Perhaps in families with happier relationships, separation experiences could be more influential in the causation of anti-social behaviour but our evidence suggests not. In this study separation from both parents had some association with anti-social disorders when there was a very poor marriage, but none at all when there was a good marriage. As Gibson's (64) findings were somewhat different it would be unwise to be dogmatic. I cannot state that a single separation experience has no adverse effects on a child's psychological development; we can conclude that, at most, they can only be a minor factor in the development of delinquent behaviour.*

Could it be, though, that we have been looking at the wrong index of psychological development and that separations lead to neurosis rather than delinquency? The evidence is firmly against this proposition. Separation experiences of any kind have never been shown to be associated with child neurosis (29, 30). Indeed, we know surprisingly little about the causes of child neurosis. Disturbed family relationships are associated with anti-social behaviour but not neurosis. Family disruption has been associated also with depression (69) and with enuresis (65), but in neither case has it been shown that the disorders are due to separation as such rather than with the family disturbance surrounding separation.

Lastly, in defence of the proposition that separation *per se* is an adverse factor it might be suggested that there is a delayed effect, that the ill-effects are to be found in adult life and not in childhood. This remains a possibility and some studies have suggested that bereavement in childhood is followed by depressive disorders in adult life (86, 87, 88). However, others have found this association only in severe depression (89, 90, 91) or not at all (92, 93, 94, 95). It remains uncertain whether or not this is a valid finding. Even if it is, it is probably of little relevance to the present discussion in that most studies indicate that the association is particularly with deaths during *adolescence*, not early childhood. We may still conclude that parent-child separation in early childhood, in itself, is probably of little consequence as a cause of serious long-term psychological disturbance.†

This is not to say that separation experiences in early childhood are without long-term effect. Unhappy separations in a *few* children may lead to clinging behaviour lasting many months or even a year or so. These experiences may also render the child more likely to be distressed by separations when older. However, many children show *no* such long-term effects and even in those that do the effects are generally relatively minor. Serious sequelae are so rare that taken overall they are of very little pathogenic importance.

Parental death and delinquency

Before discussing the effects of parental discord we need to consider why parental death is followed by *any* increase in disorder. Although in the delinquency studies quoted in Figure 3 the differences were small and statistically not significant, there was an apparent trend for parental death to be associated with a slight increase in delinquency. If it is, and the evidence is only weakly suggestive, it could mean that, after all, parent-child separation is

---

*It should be noted that *multiple* acute stresses, such as repeated hospital admissions, may have long-term sequelae in the form of antisocial behaviour (133, 134). However, even in these cases it remains uncertain whether separation as such is the crucial variable.

†Studies have demonstrated important links between family break-up in childhood and subsequent poor functioning as a parent, but the links apply to homes broken by divorce or separation rather than death so that again separation as such is not the key influence (135).

of some importance in its own right, even if it is a minor influence compared with parental discord, but there are other equally plausible explanations (96). In the first place, death often follows a long illness and it has been shown that chronic physical illness (probably by virtue of the accompanying emotional distress and tension) may be associated with an increased risk of disorder in the children (97). A second factor is the grief of the surviving parent, which often lasts as long as two years (98). Children may well be more affected by the distress and emotional disorder of the bereaved parent than they are by the death of the other. Thirdly, families in which a father dies tend to be characterized by other adverse factors and the death is frequently followed by economic and social deterioration (51, 99). Again, these may be more important than the death itself. At the moment, we do not know which of these influences is the greater. It is clear that when a parent dies the situation is much more complex than just a disruption of parent-child relationship. The association between parental death and delinquency is quite weak and even this weak association may not be attributable to parent-child separation.

Parental discord and disharmony

We should now consider in more detail the effects of parental discord and disharmony. So far we have said little more than that bad homes lead to bad children, which does not take us very far. We need to know in more detail how long disharmony has to last before the child is affected, how permanent are its effects, what sorts of disharmony are particularly associated with anti-social behaviour, what factors in the home may mitigate the effects of discord and tension, and what factors in the child determine why only some children are affected by quarrelsome homes. At present we have only partial answers to some of these questions.

We have no direct measure of the duration of discord and tension in the home but we do have some indirect measures in the study of patients' families, all of which suggest that the longer the tension lasts the more likely the children are to develop anti-social problems. First, we can look at children going through their second experience of a home with unhappily married parents. When children have experienced parental discord followed by divorce and then, after the parents remarry, a second very poor marriage, the rate of disorder is double that for children going through the first experience of parents who cannot get on together ($p < 0.05$). Secondly, where children were separated from their parents in early childhood because of family discord and were *still* in a quarrelsome home at the time we interviewed the parents, the rate of anti-social disorder was again unusually high (see Fig. 5). Thirdly, within homes with a very poor marriage the children were more likely to be deviant if one or both parents had shown impaired personal relationships throughout the whole of their adult life (see Fig. 11). In each case the differences were large and statistically significant. The evidence is circumstantial but it strongly suggests that the longer the family disharmony lasts the greater the risk to the children, but we have no findings which enable us to estimate how long there must be disharmony before there is any effect on the children.

However, we can look at what happens when disharmony *stops*, in order to

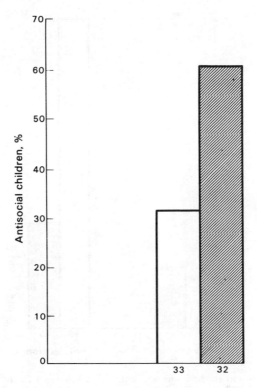

Figure 5   Anti-social behaviour in children previously separated through family discord/devi-ance in relation to current family situation. ☐ Current family situation fair or good; ▨ Current family situation very poor.

determine whether the ill-effects of bad family relationships in early childhood are transient or permanent. Figure 5 (total $N = 65$) shows the findings on children all of whom were separated from their parents through family discord or deviance and compares them with those whose present family situation is still very poor and with those whose present situation is fair or good. In most cases the family situation remained rather unsatisfactory and there were only a few children living in happy and harmonious homes. Accordingly, the comparison more accurately concerns children with very poor homes and children with less poor homes. Nevertheless, there is a large and significant difference ($p < 0.05$); the rate of anti-social disorder was double in children currently in a very poor family situation. The effects are *not* permanent and given a change for the better in the family situation the outlook for the child's psychological development correspondingly improves. How readily, how completely and how often the adverse effects of disturbed relationships in early childhood may be reversed, we cannot answer. That remains one of the many important questions requiring further research.

The next issue is what *type* of family disharmony leads to anti-social disorder in the children. Broadly speaking, unhappy families can be divided

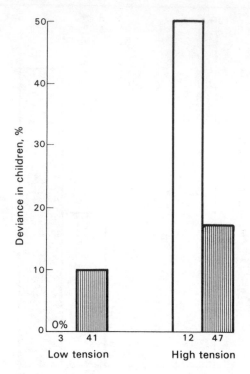

Figure 6   Warmth/tension in the home and anti-social behaviour in the children. □ Low warmth; ▥ High warmth.

into those where there is active disturbance (quarrelling, hostility, fighting and the like) and those which merely lack positive feelings (where relationships are cold and formal and the home is characterized by emotional uninvolvement and lack of concern).

Figure 6 (total N = 103) compares these two situations. As a measure of active disturbance I have taken 'tension', a rating which reflects the extent to which discord leads to a persistent atmosphere in the home so that visitors sense the disharmony and feel ill at ease. The warmth rating assesses positive feelings. It is based on feelings expressed by the parents at interview in terms of tone of voice, facial expression and words used. It has been shown to be a reliable measure which accurately predicts emotional expression in other situations. A rating of 'low' warmth means that *both* the parent-child *and* the husband-wife relationship lacked warmth. This is a rather infrequent situation, so that the numbers are small. In particular, there needs to be study of more families where there is low warmth but also low tension. However, it seems that there is an interaction effect. There is little disorder in the children when there is low tension but when there is high tension the rate of disorder is significantly higher ($p < 0.05$) if there is also low warmth. In short, both a lack of feeling and active discord are associated with deviant behaviour in the children.

This last comparison did not differentiate between the marital relationship

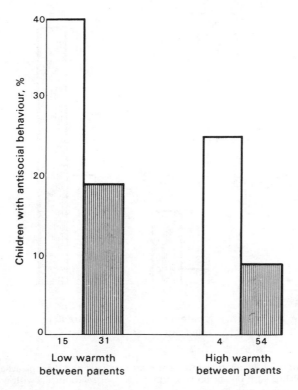

Figure 7 Warmth in family relationships and anti-social behaviour in the children. ☐ Low warmth to children; ▥ High warmth to children.

and the parent-child relationship. So Figure 7 makes this comparison with regard to warmth (total N = 104). On the whole, adults who are warm towards their spouse are also warm towards their children, so that the number of cases when the two are discrepant is small. Nevertheless (although the differences fall just short of statistical significance), it does seem that the rate of anti-social behaviour in the children is raised if *either* relationship lacks warmth; the rate is particularly high if both relationships are cold.

Quite often in clinical practice one is faced with the problem of a very disturbed home situation with one parent behaving in a very deviant fashion, but with the child still having a good relationship with the other parent. The question then is to what extent a good relationship with one parent can 'make up' for a family life which is grossly disturbed in all other respects. Figure 8 (total N = 60) shows a comparison which provides some answer to this question. Families were first divided according to the quality of the marriage relationship and then within each marriage rating a comparison was made between children who had a good relationship with one parent and children who had a good relationship with neither parent. For this purpose, a good relationship was defined in terms of the parent expressing both positive warmth *and* very little negative feeling. No account was taken of the child's behaviour toward the parent in making the rating.

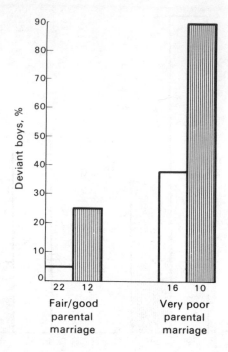

Figure 8   Parent/child relationships, parental marriage and deviant behaviour in boys. □ Good relationship with one or both parents; ▥ Poor relationship with both parents.

There was again an interaction effect. Whatever the parent-child relationship the rate of disorder in the sons was significantly higher ($p < 0.05$ for good parent-child relationship and $p < 0.01$ for poor parent-child relationship) if the marital relationship was bad. Conversely, whatever the marital relationship the child was better off if he had a good relationship with at least one parent ($p < 0.05$ for difference within 'very poor' marriage). A good relationship with one parent was *not* sufficient to remove the adverse effect of marital discord but it could go quite a long way in mitigating its effects.

Father-child and mother-child relationships

So far, not much attention has been paid to whether good or bad relationships have been with the father or with the mother, because, for the most part, in our current studies this has not proved to be a relevant variable. It has not made much difference which parent the child got on well with so long as he did so with one. Yet, it would be wrong to assume that it never matters, as other studies have suggested its importance.

For example, in an earlier study of mine (97) examining the effects of parental death and of parental mental illness in children attending a psychiatric clinic there was a sex-linked association. Boys were more likely to show psychiatric disorder if it was the father who had died ($p < 0.05$) or who

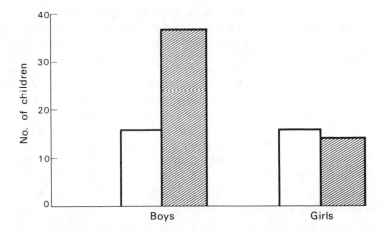

Figure 9 Association between sex of dead parent and sex of child attending psychiatric clinic. ☐ Mother dead; ▨ Father dead.

was ill ($p < 0.05$). Figure 9 shows the findings for parental death but the association for parental mental illness was similar.

Or, again, in a study of delinquent children (Figure 10) Gregory (72) found that delinquency rates were higher in boys if the father was absent from home, but in girls the rate was higher if the mother was missing.

We did not find this association in the present study and it has not always been found in other investigations (64), so the matter must remain open for the moment. It may be that the importance of the same-sexed parent is marked only at certain ages, perhaps in adolescence. The issue requires further study.

I have touched on the subject here, in spite of the inconclusive findings, because, however the problem is finally resolved, it is evident that the father-

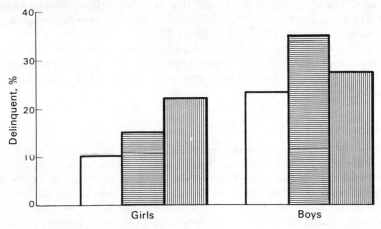

Figure 10 Family composition and delinquency. ☐ Child with both parents; ▤ Father absent; ▥ Mother absent.

child relationship is an important one, and in some circumstances it may even be more influential than the mother-child relationship (100, 101, 102). Of course, it is also true that mothers generally have more contact with very young children and her influence on them often predominates (103). The point, quite simply, is that both parents are important with respect to their children's development and which parent is more important varies with the situation and with the child. It should be added that the influence of each parent cannot be regarded as independent factors. The mental health of one parent may influence that of the other (104) and may also affect the marriage relationship (83). It is useful to try to separate the effects of different dyads in the family but it is also important to remember that the family is a social group in its own right (23).

The direction of the relationship

So far the effects of parental discord have been discussed with the implicit assumption that it was the discord that led to the anti-social behaviour, not that the anti-social children caused their parents' marriage to be disturbed. This assumption must be tested, for it is important not to forget that children can influence parents just as parents can influence children (105), as has been shown, for example, by studies of foster parents (106), nursing mothers (105, 106) and of parents of children with congenital handicaps (107, 108).

Accordingly, we must ask whether the anti-social behaviour is a cause or a consequence of family discord (109). Our own study provides only circumstantial evidence on this point. However, we found that when children were separated from their parents in the first few years of life because of family discord, anti-social disorders often developed later. In some of these cases the marital difficulties must have preceded the child's birth because older children had already been taken into care following some family crisis.

Other investigations have measured parental behaviour when the children were young and then have followed the development of the children into early adolescence. These studies have shown that it is possible, on the basis of the early family assessment, to predict the development of later delinquency at a considerably better than chance level (52, 76, 78).

The effects are not entirely unidirectional and a circular process is probable (110), but we may conclude that parental discord can start off a maladaptive process which leads to anti-social disorder in the children. This may fairly be regarded as a causal relationship.

Parental personality

Genuine and spurious relationships have still to be distinguished (111). Because parental discord leads to later anti-social behaviour it does not necessarily follow that it is the discord itself which is the cause of the anti-social disorder. It could be that the discord is only important because it is associated with some other factor of a more basic kind, such as parental personality. In many of the very bad marriages one or both parents has a gross personality disorder. The question is whether the children were anti-social because their parents were abnormal rather than because the home was

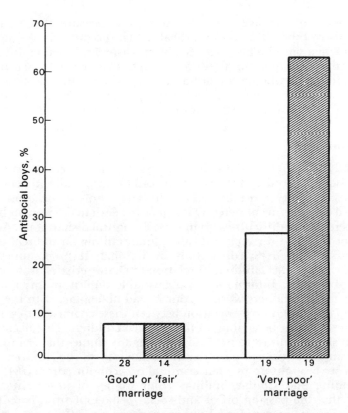

Figure 11 Personality of parents, parental marriage and anti-social behaviour in boys. □ Neither parent has personality disorder; ▨ One or both parents have personality disorder.

unhappy. Figure 11 (total N = 70) shows findings relevant to that question.

Families have been sub-divided both according to the quality of the marriage, as before, and also on the basis of whether either parent showed a handicapping personality disorder. Much the most important factor in relation to anti-social disorder in the sons was the parental marriage rating. Regardless of whether one parent had a personality disorder, anti-social behaviour was many times more common when the marriage was 'very poor' than when it was 'good' or 'fair'. Furthermore, within the group of families with a satisfactory marriage there was *no* effect attributable to parental personality disorder. These findings make it most unlikely that the association between parental discord and anti-social disorder is due to the presence of abnormalities of personality in the parent.

Even so, the difference associated with parental personality within the families with a 'very poor' marriage requires explanation although the difference falls just short of statistical significance at the 5% level (X^2 = 3.832). By definition, the parents with a personality disorder had shown disordered behaviour or relationships throughout their adult life and in most cases this was associated with prolonged marital discord (in some cases occurring throughout two marriages). We do not have a measure of the duration of marital discord, but it is highly probable that discord was of much longer duration when one parent had a personality disorder. Whether this is so, and if so, whether it accounts for the difference is not known. All that can be said is that regardless of whether or not a parental personality disorder acts as a contributory factor in the causation of anti-social disorder, its influence is not such as to account for the effects of parental discord.

Genetic influences

This result makes it less likely that the association between parental discord and anti-social disorder in the children could be explicable in genetic terms, but this possibility must be examined. The whole association could be accounted for in terms of heredity if a gene led both to delinquent behaviour and to personality difficulties giving rise to marital disharmony. Again, this could not be tested directly, but other studies allow an indirect test of the hypothesis. A recent Swedish study by Bohman (112) examined deviant behaviour in *adopted* children in relation to characteristics of the children's biological parents. Information was available on criminality and alcohol abuse in the true fathers who, of course, had no contact with the children. Bohman (112) found *no* association between these characteristics of the true fathers and deviant behaviour in the adopted children. This negative result stands in sharp contrast to the findings of many studies that criminality and alcoholism *are* associated with deviant behaviour in the children when the children are brought up by their criminal or alcoholic parents (84, 102, 113). This finding and similar findings from studies of foster children (114) suggests that the passing on of anti-social behaviour from parent to child largely involves environmental rather than genetic influences.

Twin studies also suggest that genetic factors play but a relatively small part in the pathogenesis of juvenile delinquency (115, 116, 117). The concordance of monozygotic pairs with regard to anti-social disorders is only slightly greater than that of dizygotic pairs, showing that genetic factors have only a minor influence. That concordance rates are high in both types of twins suggests the importance of familial influences of an environmental type.

In short, the evidence shows that delinquent behaviour is not inherited as such and that personality disorders in the parents probably lead to anti-social difficulties in the children in considerable part through their association with family discord and disturbance rather than through any direct genetic influence. Of course, that is not to say that genetic factors play no part. They probably are of importance with respect to the temperamental features which render children more susceptible to psychological stress (see below), and also more directly with respect to the psychopathy (118) which is the end result in some cases of persistent anti-social disorder (102).

Factors in the child

Although I have concentrated on the effects associated with family discord, it should not be thought that this is the only factor involved in the causation of anti-social behaviour. Other studies have shown that a variety of social, cultural, psychological and biological factors all play a part in the genesis of delinquency (119). The Tower Hamlets studies by Power and his colleagues (120) suggest that factors in the school as well as in the home may be important. In addition, there are a number of factors in the child himself which may make him more likely to develop some type of behavioural disorder. For example, our own studies on the Isle of Wight showed that children with organic brain disorders were more likely to develop deviant behaviour (30) and that children with severe reading difficulties were especially prone to exhibit anti-social tendencies (29).

However, at the moment we can only be concerned with the factors which aggravate or ameliorate the adverse influence of family discord. Two factors in the child which have to be discussed are sex and temperament.

Sex

Nearly all the findings mentioned so far have referred to boys. This is not accidental, since in our studies the effects of parental discord have been found to be much more marked in boys than in girls. The size of this difference is illustrated in Figures 12 and 13. Figure 12 (total N = 151) shows the association between marital disharmony and deviant behaviour in boys. As noted previously, the rate of deviant behaviour rises steeply the worse the parental marriage, and there is an association with parental personality disorder.

In girls this association was not found (Figure 13; total N = 139). The rate of deviant behaviour was much the same in girls regardless of whether a parent had an abnormal personality and regardless of the state of the parental marriage. This implies that boys may be more susceptible to the effects of

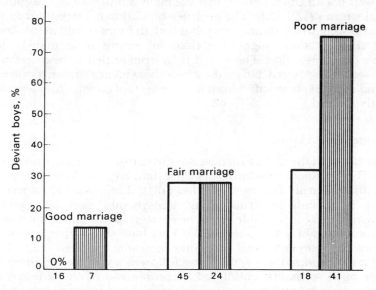

Figure 12 Personality of patient, parental marriage and deviant behaviour in boys. ☐ Parent/patient has normal personality; ▥ Parent/patient has personality disorder. Unlike Fig. 11, Figs. 12 and 13 refer to personality disorder in the patient alone (not both parents). This information was available on a larger sample.

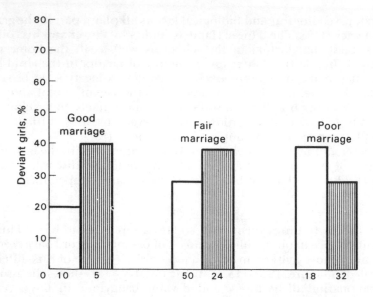

Figure 13 Personality of patient, parental marriage and deviant behaviour in girls. □ Parent/patient has normal personality; ▥ Parent/patient has personality disorder.

family discord than are girls. The evidence from other studies is incomplete and rather unsatisfactory, but there does seem to be a tendency for the male to succumb more readily to psychological stresses (121), in parallel perhaps with the very well-documented finding that the male is much more susceptible to biological stresses (121, 122). The evidence on children's responses to acute separation is somewhat contradictory, but both in humans and in sub-human primates there is some suggestion that the young male may be more vulnerable (39, 48, 49, 123). The matter is far from settled at the moment and further research is required, but on the whole the evidence tends to point to the male being more likely to suffer from the ill-effects of parent-child separation and family discord.

Temperamental make-up

The other factor in the child which we have to consider is his temperamental make-up. There is now substantial evidence that, even in the infancy period, children differ sharply one from another (124). The young child responds selectively to stimuli in terms of his idiosyncratic and developmental characteristics; to a considerable extent he *elicits* responses from other people (110). Thomas and his colleagues in New York have shown that it is possible to measure the temperamental attributes of young children (125). In the course of a longitudinal study, they have followed a group of children from soon after birth to middle childhood. A proportion of the children have developed emotional and behavioural difficulties and it has been found that the children's temperamental attributes as measured at the age of 1 to 3 years were associated with the development of behavioural difficulties a few years later (126). Children who were irregular in their eating and sleeping habits, who were very intense in their emotional responses, who adapted slowly to new situations and who showed much negative mood were those most likely to develop behavioural problems. This study showed that a child's own characteristics influenced the development of emotional and behavioural disorders and it seemed that it did so through effects on parent-child interaction (127).

In our study of patients' families (128) we investigated children's temperamental attributes in a somewhat similar way. These were assessed when the children were four to eight years old and the influence of temperament was measured against behavioural deviance in the school (i.e. in a different situation) one year later. Figure 14 shows the findings.

Children who lacked fastidiousness (that is, they did not mind messiness and disorder) were significantly more likely ($p \cdot < 0.05$) to show deviant behaviour one year later. The same was true of children who lacked malleability ($p < 0.05$), whose behaviour was difficult to change (a measure quite similar to the New York group's category of non-adaptability). As in the New York study, children who were markedly irregular in their eating and sleeping patterns were also more likely to develop behavioural problems ($p < 0.01$). There was a similar, but statistically insignificant ($p < 0.2$), tendency for highly active children to be at greater risk.

The findings demonstrated that children differed in their susceptibility to family stress and they showed which temperamental attributes were important in this respect. The attributes were not ones concerned with deviance, but rather were features which determined *how* a child interacted with his environment. That we were measuring more than just aspects of

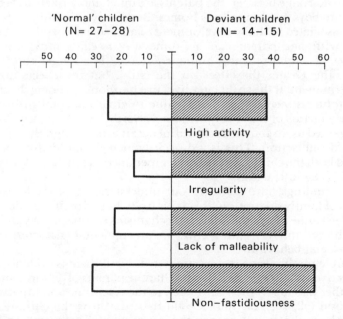

Figure 14 Temperamental characteristics and deviant behaviour (one year later) in children of mentally ill parents.

deviant behaviour is suggested by the finding that the attributes tended to have a stronger association with deviance one year later than with deviance at the time. Furthermore, the association was as strong with respect to the child's deviance at school as at home in spite of the fact that temperament was assessed only in relation to the child's mode of behaviour when with his family.

It is no new observation that children differ in their responses to stress situations but until recent years surprisingly little attention has been paid to this side of parent-child interaction. It warrants further study and the dividends of such study should be great.

Theoretical explanations

It has been found that a child's separation from his family constitutes a potential cause of short-term distress, but that separation is of little direct importance as a cause of long-term disorder. Moreover, even the short-term effects cannot be regarded solely as a response to maternal separation. Other family members are also very important in this context. Although separation experiences have an association with the later development of anti-social behaviour, this is due not to the fact of separation itself, but rather to the family discord which accompanies the separation. The same applies to the more permanent separations due to family disruption consequent upon parental death or divorce. For the most part, the child is adversely affected by the tension and disharmony; the break-up of the family is only a minor influence. Studies of unbroken families show that boys in homes where there is an unhappy marriage between the parents are much more likely to become deviant than are boys in harmonious homes. Both active discord and lack of affection are associated with the development of anti-social disorders. A good relationship with one parent can go some way towards mitigating the harmful effect of a quarrelsome, unhappy home. The longer the family discord lasts, the greater the effect on the child, but the effects are not necessarily permanent. If the child later lives in a harmonious home the risk of anti-social problems seems to be largely due to environmental influences, with hereditary factors of lesser importance. Nevertheless, the family discord cannot be regarded as an independent influence; it acts through the medium of parent-child interaction. This is a dyad in which the child also plays an active role and both the child's sex and his temperamental attributes have been shown to affect the interaction.

While these findings have added to our understanding of the long-term consequences of family disruption, this is far from the end of the problem. We have still to determine the psychological mechanisms involved. *Why* and *how* does family discord interact with a child's temperamental characteristics to produce anti-social behaviour?

Three possible mechanisms can be suggested. First, there is evidence from both retrospective and prospective studies that the parents of delinquent boys differ from other parents in their approach to the discipline and supervision of their children (52, 76, 129, 130). Could it be that it is the child-rearing practices which are the main factor in the causation of delinquency and that the discord is important only in so far as it is associated with erratic and deviant methods of bringing up children? Secondly, experimental studies have shown how readily children imitate other people's behaviour and how a model of aggressive or deviant behaviour may influence the children to behave similarly (131). Perhaps the family discord is important only because it provides the child with a model of aggression, inconsistency, hostility and anti-social behaviour which he copies. The third possibility is that the child learns social behaviour through having a warm stable relationship with his parents, that this relationship provides a means of learning how to get on with other people and that difficulties in interpersonal relationships constitute the basis of anti-social conduct (132). It is not difficult to think of situations in which these three hypotheses might lead to different predictions, but the relevant comparisons have yet to be made.

We have come a long way from the simple question whether separation from their parents is bad for children. The conclusions from research suggest a more complex interaction than that implied in the original question, but one which is still susceptible to critical analysis. There is some distance yet to go before we understand the mechanisms and processes by which family life helps shape children's psychological development. However, the problems are soluble and the solutions should be of practical importance in knowing how best to help children and families who are going through a period of psychological difficulties.

Acknowledgment

The studies were financed in part by a grant from the Foundation for Child Development.

References

(1) Lewis, A.J. (1956) Social Psychiatry, In *Lectures on the Scientific Basis of Medicine VI*. London, British Postgraduate Medical Federation.
(2) Anthony, E.J. and Koupernik, C. (Eds.) (1970) *The Child in His Family*. New York, Wiley-Interscience.
(3) Stendler, C.B. (1950) Sixty years of child training practices. *J. Pediat., 36*, 122-34.
(4) Wolfenstein, M. (1953) Trends in infant care. *Am. J. Orthopsychiat., 23*, 120-30.
(5) Caldwell, B.M. (1964) The effects of infant care. In *Review of Child Development Research*, Vol. 1. Eds. M.L. Hoffman, L.W. Hoffman. New York, Russell Sage Foundation.
(6) Becker, W.C. (1964) Consequences of different kinds of parental discipline. In *Review of Child Development Research*, Vol.1. Eds. M.L. Hoffman, and L.W. Hoffman. New York, Russell Sage Foundation.
(7) Bowlby, J. (1946) *Forty-four Juvenile Thieves: Their Characters and Home-life*. London, Bailliere, Tindall and Cox.
(8) Bowlby, J. (1958) Separation of mother and child. *Lancet, 1*, 480.
(9) Bowlby, J. (1958) Separation of mother and child. *Lancet, 1*, 1070.
(10) O'Connor, N. (1956) The evidence for the permanently disturbing effects of mother-child separation. *Acta Psychol., 12*, 171-91.
(11) Baers, M. (1954) Women workers and home responsibilities. *International Labour Review, 69*, 338-55.
(12) WHO (1951) Expert Committee on Mental Health, Report on the Second Session 1951. Technical Report Series No. 31. Geneva, WHO.
(13) Mead, M. (1954) Some theoretical considerations of the problem of mother-child separation. *Am. J. Orthopsychiat., 24*, 471-83.
(14) Fletcher, R. (1966) *The Family and Marriage in Britain*. Harmondsworth, Penguin.
(15) Medawar, P.B. (1967) *The Art of the Soluble*. London, Methuen.

(16) Medawar, P.B. (1969) *Induction and Intuition in Scientific Thought*. London, Methuen.
(17) Morris, J.N. (1957) *Uses of Epidemiology*. Edinburgh, Livingstone.
(18) Terris, M. (Ed.) (1964) *Goldberger on Pellagra*. Baton Rouge, Louisiana State University Press.
(19) Lin, T. and Standley, C.C. (1962) *The Scope of Epidemiology in Psychiatry*. Geneva, WHO.
(20) Shepherd, M. and Cooper, B. (1964) Epidemiology and mental disorder: A review. *J. Neurol. Neuros. Psychiat., 27*, 277-90.
(21) Christensen, H.T. (1969) Normative theory derived from cross-cultural family research. *Journal of Marriage and the Family, 31*, 209-22.
(22) Christensen, H.T. (1964) *Handbook of Marriage and the Family*, Chicago, Rand McNally.
(23) Handel, G. (Ed.) (1967) *The Psychosocial Interior of the Family: a sourcebook for the study of whole families*. London, Allen and Unwin.
(24) Brown, G.W. and Rutter, M. (1966) The measurement of family activities and relationships—a methodological study. *Hum. Relat., 19*, 241-63.
(25) Rutter, M. and Brown, G.W. (1966) The reliability and validity of measures of family life and relationships in families containing a psychiatric patient. *Soc, Psychiat., 1*, 38-53.
(26) Rutter, M. and Graham, P. (1968) The reliability and validity of the psychiatric assessment of the child—I: Interview with the child. *Br. J. Psychiat., 114*, 563-79.
(27) Graham, P. and Rutter, M. (1968) The reliability and validity of the psychiatric assessment of the child—II: Interview with the parent. *Br. J. Psychiat., 114*, 581-92.
(28) Rutter, M. (1967) A children's behaviour questionnaire for completion by teachers: Preliminary findings. *J. child Psychol. Psychiat., 8*, 1-11.
(29) Rutter, M., Tizard, J. and Whitmore, K. (Eds.) (1970) *Education, Health and Behaviour*. London, Longman.
(30) Rutter, M., Graham, P. and Yule, W. (1970) *A Neuropsychiatric Study in Childhood. Clinics in Developmental Medicine 35/36*. London, Spastics International and Heinemann Medical.
(31) Rutter, M. (1970) Sex differences in children's responses to family stress. In *The Child in His Family*, Eds. E.J. Anthony and C. Koupernik, New York, Wiley-Interscience.
(32) Douglas, J.W.B., Ross, J.M., Hammond, W.A. and Mulligan, D.G. (1966) Delinquency and social class. *Br. J. Crim., 6*, 294-302.
(33) Bowlby, J. (1958) The nature of the child's tie to his mother. *Int. J. Psychoanal., 39*, 350-73.
(34) Bowlby, J. (1968) Effects on behaviour of disruption of an affectional bond. In *Genetic and Environmental Influences on Behaviour*, Eds. J.M. Thoday and A.S. Parker. Edinburgh, Oliver and Boyd.
(35) Bowlby, J. (1969) *Attachment and Loss. Vol. 1: Attachment*. London, Hogarth Press.
(36) Robertson, J. and Bowlby, J. (1952) Responses of young children to separation from their mother—II: Observations of the sequences of response of children aged 18-24 months during the course of separation. *Courrier, 2*, 131-41.
(37) Davenport, H.T. and Werry, J.S. (1970) The effect of general anesthesia, surgery and hospitalization upon the behaviour of children. *Am. J. Orthopsychiat., 40*, 806-24.
(38) Yarrow, L.J. (1964) Separation from parents during early childhood. In *Review of Child Development Research*, Vol. 1. Eds. M.L. Hoffman and L.W. Hoffman. New York, Russell Sage Foundation.
(39) Vernon, D.T.A., Foley, J.M., Sipowicz, R.R. and Schulman, J.L. (1965) *The Psychological Responses of Children to Hospitalization and Illness*. Springfield, Ill., C.C. Thomas.
(40) Illingworth, R.S. and Holt, K.S. (1955) Children in hospital: some observations on their reactions with special reference to daily visiting. *Lancet, 2*, 1257-62.
(41) Prugh, D.G., Staub, E.M., Sands, H.H., Kirschbaum, R.M. and Lenihan, E.A. (1953) A study of the emotional reactions of children and families to hospitalization and illness. *Am. J. Orthopsychiat., 23*, 70-106.
(42) Schaffer, H.R. and Callender, W.M. (1959) Psychological effects of hospitalization in infancy. *Paediatrics, 24*, 528-39.
(43) Ainsworth, M.D. (1967) *Infancy in Uganda: Infant Care and the Growth of Love*. Baltimore, Johns Hopkins University Press.
(44) Schaffer, H.R. and Emerson, P.E. (1964) The development of social attachments in infancy. *Monographs of the Society for Research in Child Development, 29, 3*, 1-77.
(45) Heinicke, C.M. and Westheimer, I.J. (1965) *Brief Separations*. London, Longman.

(46) Faust, O.A., Jackson, K., Cermak, E.G., Burtt, M.M. and Winkley, R. (1952) *Reducing Emotional Trauma in Hospitalized Children.* Albany Res. Proj., Albany, New York. Cited in (38).
(47) Robertson, J. and Robertson, J. (1971) Young children in brief separation: a fresh look. *Psychoanal. Study Child, 26,* 264-315.
(48) Stacey, M., Dearden, R., Pill, R. and Robinson, D. (1970) *Hospitals, Children and their Families: The report of a pilot study.* London, Routledge.
(49) Hinde, R.A. and Spencer-Booth,Y.(1970) Individual differences in the responses of rhesus monkeys to a period of separation from their mothers.*J.childPsychol.Psychiat.,11,*159-76.
(50) Yudkin, S. and Holme, A. (1963) *Working Mothers and their Children.* London, Michael Joseph.
(51) Douglas, J.W.B., Ross, J.M. and Simpson, H.R. (1968) *All Our Future.* London, Peter Davies.
(52) West, D.J. (1969) *Present Conduct and Future Delinquency.* London, Heinemann.
(53) Moore, T.W. (1963) Effects on the children. In *Working Mothers and their Children,* Eds. S. Judkin, and A. Holme. London, Michael Joseph.
(54) Caldwell,B.M.,Wright, C.M., Honig, A.S., and Tannenbaum, J. (1970) Infant day care and attachment. *Am. J. Orthopsychiat., 40,* 397-412.
(55) Miller, L. (1969) Child rearing in the kibbutz. In *Modern Perspectives in International Child Psychiatry,* Ed. J.G. Howells, Edinburgh, Oliver and Boyd.
(56) Irvine, E.E. (1966) Children in Kibbutzim: thirteen years after. *J. child Psychol. Psychiat., 7,* 167-78.
(57) Bowlby, J., Ainsworth, M., Boston, M. and Rosenbluth, D. (1956) The effects of mother-child separation: a follow-up study. *Br. J. med. Psychol., 29,* 211-47.
(58) Naess, S. (1959) Mother-child separation and delinquency. *Br. J. Delinq., 10,* 22-35.
(59) Andry, R.G. (1960) *Delinquency and Parental Pathology.* London, Methuen.
(60) Naess, S. (1962) Mother-child separation and delinquency: further evidence. *Br. J. Crim., 2,* 361-74.
(61) Ainsworth, M.D. (1962) The effects of maternal deprivation: a review of findings and controversy in the context of research strategy. In *Deprivation of Maternal Care: A reassessment of its effects. Public Health Papers No. 14.* Geneva, WHO.
(62) Schaffer, H.R. and Schaffer, E.B. (1968) *Child Care and the Family.* London, Bell.
(63) Wolkind, S. and Rutter, M. (1973) Children who have been 'in care': an epidemiological study. *J. child Psychol. Psychiat., 14,* 97-105.
(64) Gibson, H.B. (1969) Early delinquency in relation to broken homes. *J. child Psychol. Psychiat., 10,* 195-204.
(65) Douglas, J.W.B. (1970) Broken families and child behaviour. *Journal of the Royal College of Physicians of London, 4,* 203-10.
(66) Wootton, B. (1959) *Social Science and Social Pathology.* London, Allen and Unwin.
(67) Yarrow, L.J. (1961) Maternal deprivation: toward an empirical and conceptual re-evaluation. *Psychol. Bull., 58,* 459-90.
(68) Wardle, C.J. (1961) Two generations of broken homes in the genesis of conduct and behaviour disorders in childhood. *Br. med. J., 2,* 349-54.
(69) Caplan, M.G. and Douglas, V.I. (1969) Incidence of parental loss in children with depressed mood. *J. child Psychol. Psychiat., 10,* 225-232.
(70) Bowlby, J. (1952) *Maternal Care and Mental Health.* Geneva, WHO.
(71) Bowlby, J. and Parkes, C.M. (1970) Separation and loss within the family. In *The Child in His Family,* Eds. E.S. Anthony and C.M. Koupernik. New York, Wiley-Interscience.
(72) Gregory, I. (1965) Anterospective data following childhood loss of parent. *Archs gen. Psychiat., 13,* 110-20.
(73) Douglas, J.W.B., Ross, J.M., Hammond, W.A., and Mulligan, D.G. (1966) Delinquency and social class. *Br. J. Crim., 6,* 294-302.
(74) Glueck, S. and Glueck, E. (1950) *Unraveling Juvenile Delinquency.* Cambridge, Mass., Harvard University Press.
(75) Brown, F. (1966) Childhood bereavement and subsequent psychiatric disorder. *Br. J. Psychiat., 112,* 1035-41.
(76) Craig, M.M. and Glick, S.J. (1965) *A Manual of Procedures for Applications of the Glueck Prediction Table.* London, University of London Press.
(77) McCord, W. and McCord, J. (1959) *Origins of Crime: a new evaluation of the Cambridge-Somerville Youth Study.* New York, Columbia University Press.

(78) Tait, C.D. and Hodges, E.F. (1962) *Delinquents, their Families and the Community*. Springfield, Ill., C.C. Thomas.

(79) Conger, J.J. and Miller, L. (1966) *Personality, Social Class and Delinquency*. New York, Wiley.

(80) Langner, T.S., Greene, E.L., Herson, J.H., Jameson, J.D. and Goff, J.A. (1969) Mental disorder in a random sample of Manhattan children. Unpubl. paper, American Orthopsychiatry Association.

(81) Langner, T.S., Greene, E.L., Herson, J.H., Jameson, J.D. and Goff, J.A. (1969) Psychiatric Impairment in Welfare and Non-welfare City Children. Unpubl. paper, American Psychological Association.

(82) Robins, L.N. and Hill, S.Y. (1966) Assessing the contributions of family structure, class and peer groups to juvenile delinquency. *Journal of Criminal Law, Criminology and Police Science, 57*, 325-34.

(83) Barry, W.A. (1970) Marriage research and conflict; an integrative review. *Psychol. Bull., 73*, 41-54.

(84) Jonsson, G. (1967) Delinquent boys, their parents and grandparents. *Acta psychiat. Scand., 43*, Suppl. 195.

(85) Schlesinger, B. (1969) *The One-Parent Family: Perspectives and annotated bibliography*. Toronto, University Press.

(86) Brown, F. (1961) Depression and childhood bereavement. *J. ment. Sci., 107*, 754-77.

(87) Dennehy, C.(1966) Childhood bereavement and psychiatric illness. *Br. J. Psychiat., 112*, 1049-69.

(88) Hill, O. and Price, J. (1967) Childhood bereavement and adult depression. *Br. J. Psychiat., 113*, 743-51.

(89) Munro, A. (1966) Parental deprivation in depressive patients. *Br. J. Psychiat., 112*, 443-57.

(90) Munro, A. and Griffiths, A.B. (1969) Some psychiatric non-sequelae of childhood bereavement. *Br. J. Psychiat., 115*, 305-11.

(91) Birtchenall, J. (1970) Depression in relation to early and recent parent death. *Br. J. Psychiat., 116*, 299-306.

(92) Brill, N.Q. and Liston, E.H. (1966) Parental loss in adults with emotional disorders. *Archs. gen. Psychiat., 14*, 307-14.

(93) Pitts, F.N., Meyer, J., Brooks, M. and Winokur, G. (1965) Adult psychiatric illness assessed for childhood parental loss and psychiatric illness in family members: a study of 748 patients and 250 controls. *Am. J. Psychiat., 121*, Suppl. i-x.

(94) Gregory, I. (1966) Retrospective data concerning childhood loss of a parent. *Archs. gen. Psychiat., 15*, 362-7.

(95) Abrahams, M.J. and Whitlock, F.A. (1969) Childhood experience and depression. *Br. J. Psychiat., 115*, 883-8.

(96) Birtchenall, J. (1969) The possible consequences of early parent death. *Br. J. med. Psychol., 42*, 1-12.

(97) Rutter, M. (1966) *Children of Sick Parents: an environmental and psychiatric study*. Maudlsey Monograph No. 16. London, Oxford University Press.

(98) Marris, P. (1958) *Widows and their Families*. London, Routledge.

(99) Rowntree, G. (1955) Early childhood in broken families. *Population Studies, 8*, 247-63.

(100) Peterson, D.R., Becker, W.C., Hellmer, L.A., Shoemaker, D.J. and Quay, H.C. (1959) Parental attitudes and child adjustment. *Child Dev., 30*, 119-30.

(101) Bronfenbrenner, U. (1961) Some family antecedents of responsibility and leadership in adolescents In *Leadership and Interpersonal Behaviour*, Eds. L. Petrullo and B.M. Bass. New York, Holt.

(102) Robins, L.N. (1966) *Deviant Children Grown Up*. Baltimore, Williams and Wilkins.

(103) Wolff, S. and Acton, W.P. (1968) Characteristics of parents of disturbed children. *Br. J. Psychiat., 114*, 593-601.

(104) Kreitman, N., Collins, J., Nelson, B. and Troop, J. (1970) Neurosis and marital interaction—I: Personality and symptoms. *Br. J. Psychiat., 117*, 33-46.

(105) Bell, R.Q. (1968) A reinterpretation of the direction of effects in studies of socialization. *Psychol. Rev., 75*, 81-95.

(106) Yarrow, L.J. (1963) Research in dimensions of early maternal care. *Merrill-Palmer, Q., 9*, 101-14.

(107) Bell, R.Q. (1964) The effect on the family of a limitation in coping ability in a child: a research approach and a finding. *Merrill-Palmer, Q., 10*, 129-42.

(108) Cummings, S.T., Bayley, H.C. and Rie, H.E. (1966) Effects of the child's deficiency on the mother: a study of mothers of mentally retarded, chronically ill and neurotic children. *Am. J. Orthopsychiat., 36*, 595-608.

(109) Robins, L.N. (1969) Social correlates of psychiatric disorders: can we tell causes from consequences? *J. Hlth Hum. Behav., 10*, 95-104.

(110) Yarrow, L.J. (1968) The crucial nature of early experience In *Environmental Influences*, Ed. D.C. Glass. New York, Rockefeller University Press and Russell Sage Foundation.

(111) Hirschi, T. and Selvin, H.C. (1967) *Delinquency Research: an appraisal of analytic methods.* Glencoe, Ill. The Free Press.

(112) Bohman, M. (1970) *Adopted Children and their Families. A follow-up study of adopted children, their background, environment and adjustment.* Stockholm, Proprius.

(113) Nylander, I. (1960) Children of alcoholic fathers. *Acta paediat., 49*, Suppl. 121.

(114) Roe, A. and Burks, B. (1945) *Adult Adjustment of Foster Children of Alcoholic and Psychotic Parentage and the Influence of Foster Homes.* New Haven, Conn., Yale University Press.

(115) Rosanoff, A.J., Handy, L.M. and Plesset, I.R. (1941) The etiology of child behaviour difficulties, juvenile delinquency and adult criminality, with special reference to their occurrence in twins. *Psychiat. Monogr.*, No. 1. Sacramento, Department of Institutions.

(116) Shields, J. (1954) Personality differences and neurotic traits in normal twin school children. *Eugenics Review, 45*, 213-46.

(117) Shields, J. (1968) Psychiatric genetics In *Studies in Psychiatry*, Eds. M. Shepherd and D.L. Davies. London, Oxford University Press.

(118) Schulsinger, F. (1972) Psychopathy: heredity and environment. *International Journal of Mental Health, 1*, 190-206.

(119) West, D.J. (1967) *The Young Offender.* Harmondsworth, Penguin.

(120) Power, M.J., Alderson, M.R., Philipson, C.M., Shoenberg, E. and Morris, J.N. (1967) Delinquent schools? *New Society, 10*, 542-3.

(121) Rutter, M. (1970) Psychosocial disorders in childhood and their outcome in adult life. *Journal of the Royal College of Physicians of London, 4*, 211-18.

(122) Tanner, J.M. (1962) *Growth at Adolescence*, Springfield, Ill., C.C. Thomas.

(123) Sackett, G.P. (1969) Abnormal behaviour in laboratory-reared rhesus monkeys. In *Abnormal Behaviour in Animals*, Ed. M.W. Fox. New York, Saunders.

(124) Berger, M. and Passingham, R.E. (1973) Early experience and other environmental factors: an overview In *Handbook of Abnormal Psychology*, Ed. H.J. Eysenck, 2nd edn. London, Pitman Medical.

(125) Thomas, A., Chess, S., Birch, H.G., Hertzig, M. and Korn, S. (1963) *Behavioural Individuality in Early Childhood.* New York, New York University Press.

(126) Rutter, M., Birch, H.G., Thomas, A. and Chess, S. (1964) Temperamental characteristics in infancy and the later development of behavioural disorders. *Br. J. Psychiat., 110*, 651-61.

(127) Thomas, A., Chess, S. and Birch, H.C. (1968) *Temperament and Behaviour Disorders in Children.* London, University of London Press.

(128) Graham, P., Rutter, M. and George, S. (1973) Temperamental characteristics as predictors of behavior disorders in children. *Am. J. Orthopsychiat., 43*, 328-39.

(129) Glueck, S. and Glueck, E.T. (1962) *Family Environment and Delinquency.* London, Routledge.

(130) Sprott, W.J.H., Jephcott, A.P. and Carter, M.P. (1955) *The Social Background of Delinquency.* University of Nottingham.

(131) Bandura, A. (1969) Social-learning theory of identificatory processes. *Handbook of Socialization Theory and Research*, Ed. D.A. Goslin. New York, Rand McNally.

(132) Rutter, M. (1972) *Maternal Deprivation Reassessed.* Harmondsworth, Penguin.

(133) Douglas, J.W.B. (1975) Early hospital admissions and later disturbances of behaviour and learning. *Develop. Med. Child Neurol., 17*, 456-80.

(134) Quinton, D. and Rutter, M. (1976) Early hospital admissions and later disturbances of behaviour: An attempted replication of Douglas' findings. *Develop. Med. Child Neurol., 18*, 447-59.

(135) Rutter, M. and Madge, N. (1976) *Cycles of Disadvantage: A review of research.* London: Heinemann Educational.

10. Beyond the layman's madness: the extent of mental disease

Michael Shepherd

I am grateful for the opportunity to add my own tribute to the work of the Mental Health Foundation in fostering research into mental illness in Britain and, in particular, to Sir Geoffrey Vickers, who for many years played a central role in developing policy as chairman of the Foundation's Research Committee. Indeed, one of the dividends of this invitation has been the stimulus which it has provided to look up some of Sir Geoffrey's own writings, and I shall be referring specifically to two of his papers, the first of which will serve as my starting point.

The article in question, 'Mental Disorder in British Culture' (1), appeared in a volume commissioned by the Mental Health Research Fund, *Aspects of Psychiatric Research,* published in 1962. This overview still retains much historical interest, underlining as it does the significance of the relatively recent recognition in Britain of the proposition that mental illness calls not only for compassion and custodial care, but also for preventive measures, active treatment and research. We would do well to remember that the acceptance of the psychological or psychosocial component of medicine in Britain has been a slow process which still encounters pockets of resistance. Only recently, for example, an eminent professor of psychology reluctantly concluded that 'Psychologists are often seen as dangerous manipulators and the image of John Bull still survives in Britain; the British feel they should be able to cope with their own lives without professional help and they resent the intrusion on autonomy and privacy that professional help implies. Many liberal-minded people see clinical psychologists as busybodies who attempt to impose their own sexual code on homosexuals by giving them electric shocks while they examine pictures of little Adonises.'

This verdict, I would submit, can now be brought in more credibly on psychology than on psychiatry. Since the publication of Sir Geoffrey's article the rising status of psychological medicine in the United Kingdom has been acknowledged by the customary trappings of recognition. With a Royal Charter for its College, a crop of new academic departments and a steady flow of research monies, its representatives among deans of medical schools and vice-chancellors of universities and appearing regularly in the Honours lists, the subject has entered a new phase of respectability. And, perhaps understandably, its horizons have expanded so that fifteen years later it is not only psychiatrists who would endorse Sir Geoffrey Vickers' observation that the era of exclusive preoccupation with mental illness in the mental hospital

The Sir Geoffrey Vickers Lecture of 4 February 1976, an abridged version of which appeared in the *Canadian Psychiatric Association Journal,* 1976, *21,* 401-9.

is over and that it is time to recognize, in his own words, that: 'the layman's "madness" is only a small part of mental disorder'.

So far, so good. But if psychiatry no longer qualifies as the Cinderella of medical disciplines it still remains within the household of Baron Hardup, which perhaps explains why it has the unfortunate tendency at times to exhibit the characteristics of an Ugly Sister. These disagreeable ladies, it may be recalled, entertained ideas much above their station and failed to impress Prince Charming because they were flat-footed as well as big-headed. A comparable self-importance and grandiloquence has certainly come to characterize the pronouncements of some contemporary psychiatrists. 'Rising living standards in poor countries', writes one of our indigenous authorities, 'often precede and may lead to revolution; similar conditions in more advanced, Western societies lead to a demand for psychotherapy; the hungry mind replaces the empty belly; the emotional sickness shows' (2). With such empty phrase-making goes an attitude of mind which Peter Marin has well termed the 'new narcissism', exquisitely exemplified in a recent paper by two American psychiatrists on what they call 'The Arab-Israel conflict and the development of Arab Ego Identity'. Its content calls to mind nothing so much as the memorable statement in the current edition of Wisden's Almanac, namely that 'the 1956 war against Egypt gave Israeli cricket a jolt from which it took time to recover'.

Such pretensions, of course, rest on the assumption that psychiatrists are in possession of a store of specialized expertise which could equip them to engage in a form of all-purpose human engineering. On the whole, this view is held by a small minority of the profession, at least in Britain, and carries little persuasive force. Probably its most striking achievement to date has been to stimulate the negative reaction of the mistakenly termed anti-psychiatrists who, it cannot be emphasized too often, are concerned not merely to rebut but to appropriate the claims of the psychiatric branch of the medical profession. What doctors call mental illness does not exist as such, they tell us, but if labelled in a different way it becomes the pabulum for their own activities. This form of chop-logic also has a tendency to drag psychiatric issues into the legal and political arenas. Fortunately, the lawyer and the psychiatrist have long recognized the radical differences characterizing their respective approaches to human conduct and they are unlikely to dispense with a very long spoon at table. As for politics, the clinical psychiatrist may well be justified in casting a professional eye in the direction of several public figures on the contemporary scene. In the light of what we hear of the collective behaviour of psychiatrists in some parts of the world, however, we may surely be thankful that most politicians are still inclined to take a sceptical view of psychiatry's potential in their own field.

Yet, even without these extravaganzas it is apparent that psychiatry is coming to take a catalytic part in extending the concerns of traditional medicine. To exemplify this trend, I would cite the activities of the highly respected London Medical Group, a body explicitly devoted to 'the study of issues raised through the practice of medicine which concern other disciplines'. Its listed lectures and symposia for 1975-76 numbered forty-eight, of which no fewer than twenty-nine involved psychiatrists directly. The topics included 'Nurses working under Stress', 'The Misuse of Psychiatry in the

Soviet Union', 'Exorcism', 'The Clincial and Social Significance of Touch', 'Battered Wives', 'Pornography and Violence', 'Incest', 'Teilhard and Jung', 'The Bereaved Child and its Parents', 'Doctors and Torture', 'Can we do without Aggression?', 'Guilt', 'Is Geriatrics the Answer to Old Age?', 'Deviance and the Ethics of Behaviour Modification', 'The impact of the Institution on the Individual', 'Man in Literature', 'Bereavement', 'Marital Breakdown', 'Sex Therapy', 'Homosexuality: is it an Illness?', and 'Should we talk about Dying?'. In the face of so broad a spectrum of involvement one can only speculate as to why psychiatrists were not asked to participate in the Group's symposia on euthanasia, battered children and rape.

It may be that the psychiatrist will eventually make a useful contribution in helping explore some of these wilder shores of medicine which at present tend to attract a motley collection of cognoscente, many of whom share only a keen eye for the bubble reputation of the mass media. It is not to these over-populated and over-televised littorals that I am referring, however, when I go along with Sir Geoffrey Vickers's opinion that psychiatrists are now entitled to look beyond the layman's madness to identify the larger part of mental disorder. In so doing I adopt a more sober stand, based squarely on the notion of psychiatry as a branch of medicine and with full awareness of the misleading discussions centred on the so-called 'medical model'—most of which would have been more accurately characterized as a 'medical muddle'. The orbit of the term 'psychological medicine', which is rarely employed outside Britain, should not, in my view, restrict the boundaries of psychiatry so much as enlarge those of medicine, and perhaps re-distribute some of its territory. In the process, the province and role of the psychiatrist must also inevitably change since, as Sir Aubrey Lewis has pointed out, 'The nature of psychiatry . . . could be expressed with some confidence when it was almost entirely concerned with those forms of insanity and defect to be met with in the special institutions variously known then as madhouses, asylums, or retreats. The neuroses were the province of the general physician or the neurologist; psychological anomalies in children were the paediatrician's concern. As specialization has increased, and the confidence of the psychiatrist (as well as other people's confidence in him) has grown, the field of action has become larger, the experience much wider, the responsibilities more heavy' (3). And, I would add, the need to define the tasks more urgent.

What then should be done? Rather than engage in further speculation about theoretical issues, it would seem more helpful to proceed by asking a triad of simple-sounding questions: (a) If the layman's madness is now to be regarded as a small part of mental disorder, with what other types of mental illness are we now being confronted? (b) How much illness is subsumed by these categories? (c) Where and how are the patients suffering from such disorders to be identified?

None of these questions can be approached without some agreement on definitions, for we cannot exclude 'madness' without facing the essential ambiguity of a term which to many, like Saint-Simon, is "nothing by extreme ardour . . . indispensable for accomplishing great things" and to others serves as a pretext for the contemporary verbal games of Dr Szasz and M. Foucault. It is, in fact, rather difficult to find 'madness' in a modern, specialized dictionary, but in one the word is defined simply as 'a non-technical synonym of insanity'. For heuristic purposes, then, the layman's madness would seem to be broadly synonymous with the psychiatrist's 'psychosis' and this, in the words of the World Health Organization's *Glossary of Mental Disorders* 'includes those conditions in which impairment of mental functions has developed to a degree that interferes grossly with insight, ability to meet some of the ordinary demands of life, or adequate contact with reality' (4). As the Glossary goes on to concede, psychosis is not 'an exact or well-defined term'. Nonetheless, it serves to cover the various organic and functional disorders (categories 290-9 in ICD 8) making up the first of the three large groups of conditions in Section V of the International Classification of Diseases which traditionally incorporates all forms of mental illness.

The psychoses can therefore be excluded from further consideration, and since with only minor modifications the same definition can be extended to cover many of the forms of mental retardation, the second of the two major groups in Section V falls outside our purview. We are left with the third group, comprising a large, heterogenous collection of categories under the heading of 'Neuroses, personality disorders, and other non-psychotic mental disorders'. Its ten sub-categories group themselves naturally into four, namely (*a*) the so-called 'minor' mental disorders, i.e. 'neuroses', 'personality disorders', 'behaviour disorders of childhood', 'sexual deviation'; (*b*) drug-associated disorders, i.e. 'alcoholism' and 'drug dependence'; (*c*) mental illness associated with somatic disease, i.e. 'physical disorders of presumably psychogenic origin' and 'mental disorders not specified as psychotic associated with physical conditions', and (*d*) 'other' conditions, including a rag-bag of 'transient situational disturbances' and 'special symptoms not elsewhere classified'. As we shall see, this list is still far from complete, but it helps to provide a partial answer to the first of our three questions.

The other two questions—How much? and Where?—call for empirical studies of a type which have been well-established in Great Britain since World War II. As early as 1943, a memorandum issued by the Royal Statistical Society indicated the way of things to come. 'Stastistics', it said, 'are no longer a by-product of administration or a useful index of the results of a course of action. The statistician is now not concerned mainly with post-mortems but with preventing post-mortems . . . the Government's demand for comprehensive statistical information during wartime will continue into the post-war period of reconstruction and beyond. It seems to us an inevitable social development that the State will intervene on an increasing scale in the life of the community in future years and, therefore, that an increasing amount of statistical information will have to be collected for Ministerial guidance'. During the war there were, in fact, a number of official enquiries directed at the extent of mental illness in industry and the services, and the post-war period has witnessed a growing role for the social statistician and his survey techniques in all spheres of corporate life, including physical and mental health. The lack of appeal made by morbidity statistics has been attributed by one eminent statistician to the fact that they do not bleed, but he might with equal justice have incriminated their unfortunate tendency to appear in the form of tabulated gravestones without so much as an epitaph to indicate their relevance to the living concerns of individual workers. Nonetheless, a large skeleton of information has been assembled on which it is not possible to add a little flesh to animate the issues under consideration.

There are, as we shall see, still some large gaps which point to the inadequacies and needs of psychiatry as a discipline but much information about the quantitative aspects of mental illness in this country is contained in the published national statistics. It is natural, therefore, to turn first to the data collected for the Mental Health Enquiry of the Department of Health and Social Security which utilizes the ICD for the purposes of classification (5). Figure 1 summarizes some of the data furnished by the report for 1971, excluding institutions for the mentally handicapped.

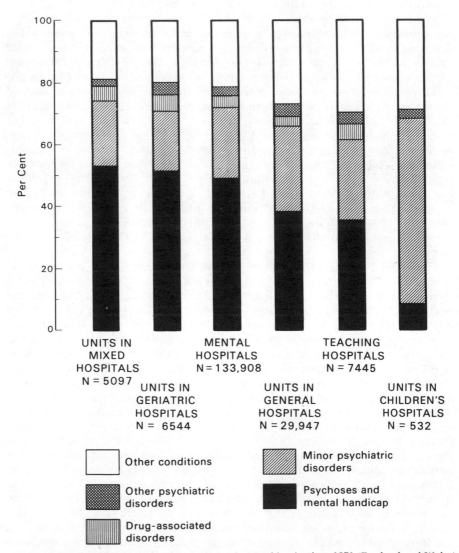

Figure 1   Admissions by diagnostic group and type of institution, 1971 (England and Wales).

A number of points stand out from this Figure. It is apparent, first, that the proportion of patients suffering from psychotic illnesses varies with the type of institution and that psychotic illness is most frequently encountered in the longer-stay mental hospitals. Even there the number of cases is not insubstantial, a finding which reflects a pronounced change in the distribution of patient-care; in my own detailed study of mental hospital statistics (which was carried out before such extensive national data were available and was focussed on one administrative area), for example, the non-psychotic population accounted for no more than about 1% of admissions and could only be categorized as 'unclassified' or 'miscellaneous' (6). Secondly, the so-called 'minor' mental disorders assume increasing numerical significance as we look to the general and teaching hospital as a source of information. Thirdly, the drug-associated disorders appear as numerically less prominent than the neuroses. Fourthly, mental disorder associated with somatic disease does not figure independently at all, the reason being that it comes under other psychiatric conditions. Finally, among 'all other conditions' which make up more than one-fifth of the total, it should be mentioned that about 90% are estimated to be suffering from 'depression not specified as neurotic or psychotic, epilepsy, undiagnosed cases and admissions for other than psychiatric disorders'.

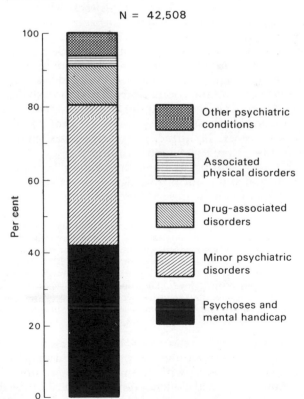

Figure 2 Estimated total discharges from all hospitals in England and Wales, 1971.

Clearly, however, such figures cannot be taken at their face value without regard to the possibility that cases are being admitted to other types of institution. Data from the Hospital In-patient Enquiry, which is conducted under the aegis of the Department of Health and Social Security and the Office of Population Censuses and Surveys, provide us with relevant figures, based on in-patient records from National Health Service Hospitals in England and Wales excluding hospitals confined to the treatment of psychiatric diseases and the psychiatric departments of general hospitals (7). The Enquiry, constructed on a one-in-ten sample 'of in-patients records, furnishes information relating to discharges and deaths which were estimated in 1971 as numbering 42,508 for all forms of mental disorder covered by Section V of the ICD. The breakdown into the simplified groups already presented in Figure 1 is again employed in Figure 2.

Here the marked shift towards a preponderance of 'minor' mental disorders is evident, though the number of psychiatric illnesses associated with somatic disease is still surprisingly small. In large measure, however, this finding turns out to reflect the unsatisfactory nature of the two relevant categories in the ICD. One of these, 'physical disorders of presumably psychogenic origin', accounted for only 1351 cases, of which the largest single sub-group is made up by young women with anorexia nervosa. As the wording implies, however, this category reflects a view of 'psychosomatic' illness which has become out-dated since the enunciation of Flanders Dunbar's 'two laws of emotional thermodynamics' in the mid 1940's (8). The first of these 'laws' was that psychic energy, when not expressed through higher levels, obtained its outlet through physical symptoms; the second stated that if such symptoms were the result of permanent structural damage, energy would be correspondingly dissipated and made unavailable. Somatic dysfunction was thus equated with 'a waste or dissipation of energy due to the faulty design of the personality', which led in turn to the quest for 'psychological profiles characteristic of specific disease syndromes'. So attractive an hypothesis led to the view that many somatic diseases were psychogenic in origin.

Since then the undermining of these high hopes by a large volume of intensive experimental and clinical investigations has been summed up by a well-qualified and sympathetic observer in the following terms:

'Psychosomatic medicine as an organized field of scientific enquiry', says Roy Grinker, 'began with an attempt to identify those psychological variables which promote the development of bodily disease. The early investigators focussed their studies on a group of conditions of unknown aetiology which they designated "psychosomatic disorders". That initial phase in the development of our discipline is over. It was productive of a body of aetiological hypotheses whose validation has largely bogged down. The concept of a psychosomatic disorder is fast becoming obsolete . . . psychosomatic medicine has become the study of the relationships among psychological and biological phenomena in humans, as they occur in and are influenced by the social and physical environment, both in health and disease' (9).

In this perspective it may reasonably be questioned whether clinical epidemiology and psychophysiology between them do not cover the field adequately enough to dispense with the need for so commodious a term, especially since much historical evidence now supports the view that the most appropriate fate for the naive concept of psychogenesis is a 'decent burial' (10).

In these circumstances the relatively small number of physical illnesses deemed to be 'of presumably psychogenic origin' is more readily understandable. The category 'mental disorders not specified as psychotic associated with physical conditions' apparently claims no cases at all, but the explanation turns out to reside in the fact that, in accord with a long-standing rule, the cases are classified primarily by the physical condition leading to admission. This process, however, must result in an underestimate of the psychiatric correlates of physical illness, and in particular depressive reactions whose detection calls for a clinical awareness not always present among general physicians. Some years ago I had occasion to discuss this question with a group of trainee internists at one of the major American medical centres where it was customary for would-be physicians to take a three months' psychiatric residency as part of their training. All of these men were hard-headed, physically-oriented doctors with no intention of taking up psychiatry as their chosen speciality and no fondness for 'psychosomatic' theorizing. Nonetheless, they were unanimous in their view of the value of the experience, partly as an educational opportunity, but principally because of its practical implications for their own work, specifically in the recognition and management of depression in relation to mental disorder. Empirical studies have provided support for this viewpoint. Thus in 1960 we took a close look at the psychiatric disorders calling for consultation in the wards of a general hospital, to find that about two-thirds of the cases, most of them suffering from clear-cut medical illnesses, were associated with a significant form of non-psychotic illness, some half of these being clinically depressed (11). Subsequent, more intensive studies have examined more representative samples of the in-patient population. Recently, for example, it has been estimated by direct examination that one quarter of medical in-patients are morbidly depressed during their stay in hospital (12) and another group of workers have shown that almost one quarter (23%) of 170 medical in-patients suffering from a variety of physical illnesses were suffering from coincident psychiatric disability, the large majority of them being depressed (13).

While the collections of such large-scale figures are clearly useful in themselves for administrative purposes, their value is much enhanced if a more detailed examination can be made of diagnostic sub-groups over time, though the marked change in the pattern of psychiatric care over the past twenty years makes it difficult to collate data from so many different sources. For such purposes, the more precise and reliable the clinical diagnosis the better and, consequently, it is most instructive to assess the relevant information concerning psychiatric morbidity associated with an unequivocally causal factor. One obvious example is alcohol. In 1949, when the figures were first published, fewer than five hundred alcoholic patients were admitted to National Health Service Hospitals and units; of these, about one half were said to be suffering from an 'alcoholic psychosis' and one half from 'alcoholism'. Nearly a generation later, in 1973, the number of admissions had risen more than twenty times to over twelve thousand. This sharp increase in numbers does not, of course, necessarily reflect incidence-rates accurately; we know, for example, that these rates exhibit regional variation which is positively correlated with the existence of special units for alcohol dependence and that only about 30% of cases admitted in 1970-72 were first admissions. More directly relevant to our present theme is the fact that over the years the ratio of alcoholism to alcoholic psychosis has risen to almost 6:1. Moreover, since a diagnosis of 'alcoholism' is, in the opinion of most authorities, incomplete it is significant that since 1964 'alcoholism' has been sub-classified as a primary and secondary diagnosis, the latter accounting for about a quarter of all cases and including a substantial number of patients diagnosed significantly as 'depressive not otherwise stated'.

The Hospital In-patient Enquiry supplements these data by revealing a comparable state of affairs in non-psychiatric beds, the numbers having risen at about the same rate to nearly 5000 in 1972. Of this population only three hundred were classified as alcoholic psychosis; there is a substantially higher proportion of women and a disturbingly large number of admissions under the age of fifteen. And, further, though three-quarters of these cases were treated in departments of general medicine, the figures do not include the various physical conditions related to excessive drinking such as malnutrition, polyneuritis myocarditis, gastro-intestinal disorders, accidents and, most overtly, hepatic cirrhosis, of which more than 5000 cases were treated in 1972, about one quarter being recorded as due to alcohol. At present such cases will be classified outside Section V of ICD 8. Cirrhosis of the liver, for example, will appear in Section IX under Category 571. In practice, therefore, it becomes necessary to adopt a system of double coding if one is to identify the psychiatric component of physical disorder. This principle, it may be noted, has been underlined in ICD 9, in which combination categories are to be eliminated so that only the psychiatric syndrome is to appear in Section V, while the associated physical conditions will appear elsewhere.

We must also go outside Section V if we are to record the importance of suicide in the general hospital. This issue has received much public attention and its outlines, at least in part, can be readily traced from the published statistics. In England and Wales the morbidity rate per 100,000 persons for suicide and self-inflicted injury was 8.1 in 1971, with self-poisoning the most frequently employed method. This figure is, of course, greatly exceeded by unsuccessful acts of attempted self-destruction, again comprising self-poisoning in the majority of cases, and the Hospital In-patient Enquiry suggest a disturbing rise: in 1970, 7% of all discharges (79,000) persons in all were so recorded, a figure which was under 20,000 twenty years ago. In view of the well-established association of attempted suicide with so-called neurotic depression and situational crises, the volume of psychiatric morbidity must be significant. However, although the act of suicide is associated with mental disorder in a high proportion of cases, the information published by the Registrar General falls outside Section V of the ICD and appears under the 'E' code, recorded as the external cause of death, and the 'N' code, recorded as the nature of the injury. The 'N' coding shows that four-fifths of the drugs employed are analgesics, psychotropic substances or hypnotics, all of them drugs often used for self-poisoning.

So much for in-patient statistics which, with all their limitations, take us some way towards an awareness of the extent of non-psychiatric illness leading to institutional care. The time has long since passed, however, when bed-occupancy could be regarded as an index of psychiatric morbidity, and the expanded forms of ambulant care for the mentally ill provided by the

Health Service might be expected to furnish a rich source of data, particularly from the out-patient departments wherever patients are seen. Unfortunately, large-scale statistics on this population are still lacking despite the huge volume of attendances, numbering almost two million in 1972. There is an evident need for a more detailed analysis of these figures which, in the case of childrens' disorders, account for the vast majority of cases. The few studies of individual centres or areas which have been undertaken by individual workers all show the numerical weight of the case-load carried by the mental health services at this level tilted sharply towards neurotic illness and personality disorder. It may also be added that the figures from psychiatric registers confirm that the great majority of non-psychotic patients are treated on an out-patient basis. The prevalence of alcoholic-dependence among psychiatric out-patients has still to be determined accurately, though in one study it was estimated to be as high as 6.8/1000 for men, and 1.52/1000 for women (14).

But if, in addition, the psychiatric aspects of illness referred to non-psychiatric out-patient departments are to be given due recognition, more elaborate enquiries will clearly be required. That the information will not be derived from a bare account of out-patient attendances was shown some years ago when we were able to assess psychiatric morbidity in a sample of two hundred consecutive out-patients in a general hospital, one hundred of them referred to medical and one hundred to surgical clinics (11). It had been recorded over a twelve-month period that the out-patient physicians, surgeons, and gynaecologists of the hospital had requested psychiatric opinions on 3.4% of all new patients in their clinics. On this basis one patient in thirty would be recognized as suffering from a psychiatric disability; this estimate, however, rises ten-fold when the figures from the out-patient survey are examined.

A closer examination of these findings proved to be revealing, for about 40% of the hundred patients attending the medical clinic and 5% of those referred to the surgeons exhibited no evidence of any form of physical disease, although somatic complaints were prominent. The majority of psychiatric illnesses among these patients were depressive and neurotic reactions and personality disorders: no more than one in three of the psychiatric patients suffered from a co-existent physical disorder, and when this was present the symptoms were those of exaggerations of or morbid reactions to organic disease. In essence, these patients were suffering from the same types of disorders as those referred for psychiatric opinion, differing principally in the severity of their symptoms. What stood out with equal force, however, was the significance of domestic and social problems in the matrix of their complaints and we were compelled to acknowledge that 'patients attending the medical and surgical clinics of a general hospital can present a relatively large number of minor psychosocial problems, the majority being found among the medical cases. Their management need not be elaborate; the great majority of these patients did not require more expert attention than could be expected reasonably from the combined resources of a general physician and a social worker.'

This conclusion bears directly on the mounting body of information indicating that hospital statistics, however complete they may become, cannot do justice to the dimensions of the problem of mental disorders in the community at large. Within the structure of the National Health Service the most compelling evidence has undoubtedly come from studies directed at the level of primary care. An overall view of the situation is provided by the two National Morbidity Surveys conducted by the Royal College of General Practitioners in 1955 and 1970-71, the first of these in collaboration with the Registrar General, the second with the Office of Population Censuses and Surveys and the Department of Health and Social Security (15, 16). A comparison of the results of these surveys reveals an apparently striking increase in the amount of mental disease presenting to the general practitioner the rate having more than doubled from the fifty patients per thousand population consulting at least once annually to 109.0, a figure which puts it in the forefront of disorders with which the practitioner has to deal. It cannot be maintained, however, that this statistic represents a true rise in the incidence of psychiatric morbidity, for a closer analysis of the figures shows the greater part of the increase to have been attributable to the much greater frequency with which the diagnosis of depressive illness has been made. The Director of the Research of the Royal College of General Practitioners has commented aptly:

'this increase in the rate for neurotic depression probably reflects an increased diagnostic awareness and reporting of depression by the patients. If the latter was the explanation, the increase should have been evident in all psycho-neurotic categories. This is probably also the explanation for the apparent increase for psychotic conditions for the bulk of this increase can be attributed to "affective" psychoses, usually depression. Also, we shall find that there has been a proportionate increase in the rates for "menopausal" symptoms, suggesting that the diagnosis of depression may have been used as an alternative diagnosis in the second survey' (17).

Independent confirmation of these findings have been furnished by our own more intensive studies of psychiatric illness in general practice, carried out over a one-year period on a sample of patients attending more than fifty practitioners (18). These estimates correspond very closely to the findings obtained elsewhere, when surveys have been carried out in comparable fashion in places as far apart as Australia (19), the USA (20), Austria (21) and Iran (22). Among what we called the 'formal' disorders (derived as simplified, collapsed categories from Section V of the ICD) the neurotic and personality disorders loom largest, but it was again the affective illnesses, with depression and anxiety or admixtures thereof, which assumed the greatest prominence. However, it became clear that such formal labels were inadequate to cover all the psychiatric conditions. The reason goes back to the nature of the primary doctor-patient contact since, as Kerr White has pointed out:

'Patients do not complain of diseases when they initially seek medical care. Terms such as arterio-sclerotic heart disease, multiple myeloma, duodenitis, and fractured femur are rarely used by patients, and only occasionally by first-contact physicians. Terms such as ache, pain, hurt, itch, rash, swelling, cough, blood, nervous, worried, tired, weak, "blue" and frightened are used. . . A diagnosis is merely an intermediate step in the process of resolving the patients' complaint and is of little interest and of no intrinsic utility to the patient' (23).

To incorporate these symptomatic complaints and problems in the total picture of morbidity, it is necessary to invoke Section XVI of the ICD where, under 'Symptoms and ill-defined conditions', we find such items as 'nervousness', 'debility', 'headache', and the ubiquitous 'depression', to which a formal diagnostic label cannot be applied with sufficient accuracy to justify inclusion in Section V. In our own study such complaints were labelled 'psychiatric associated' conditions, a group which increased the reported one-year consultation rate by almost 50%.

Even these figures do not, of course, do justice to the whole range of extra-mural psychiatric illness which comes to medical care. Alcoholism, for

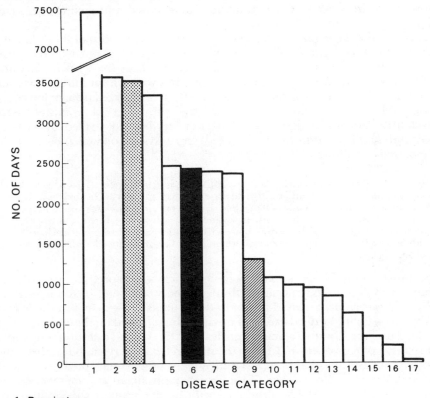

1. Respiratory
2. Circulatory
3. Symptoms, senility and ill-defined
4. Bones and organs of movement
5. Digestive
6. Non-psychotic mental
7. Nervous system and sense organs
8. Accidents, poisonings and violence
9. Psychoses
10. Genito-urinary
11. Infective and parasitic
12. Deliveries, complications of pregnancy, childbirth and puerperium
13. Allergic, endocrine, metabolic and nutritional
14. Skin and cellular tissue
15. Blood and blood-forming organs
16. Neoplasms
17. Congenital malformations, and certain diseases of early infancy

Figure 3   Total days of certified incapacity in 1967-68 (England and Wales).

example, is recognized much less often than it occurs, though it has recently been suggested that it might be screened effectively by the general practitioner (24). Further, though the interest in what was called 'industrial neurosis' forty years ago appears to have waned, there seems no reason to believe that it has decreased substantially, judging from the evidence available from the official claims for sickness and injury benefits under the National Insurance Acts, or those made in order to have contributions excused and credited (25) (see Figure 3).

It is, I think, legitimate to refer briefly to the implications of these data for that much-abused cliche, 'community mental health', about which a great deal has been written in recent years. In as much as the term retains any rational meaning, it appears to relate to patients with whom contact has been made at an institutional level but who have been discharged from or are being supported in the community. Thus the provision of comprehensive psychiatric care for a defined population has been described by Hill as 'hospital-based but community-oriented' (26), a system on which Bennett has elaborated as follows:

'there will be three psychiatrists . . . for the population of 60,000 persons. That is the basic unit in our planning. This population will yield about 500 patients who are in our care at any one time while approximately another 500 people . . . will come into care each year. They will be supported by hospital and public health nurses and by social workers. There will also be about 24 family doctors in the area. These doctors, however, cannot give psychiatrists much help for in our Health Service family doctors are already seeing the bulk of the patients with socioeconomic problems' (27).

It must surely be questioned whether such a perspective can only be obtained by looking at the scene through the wrong end of the telescope. When the instrument is used properly the conclusions reached in the WHO report on primary medical care and mental illness, based on the experience of twelve European countries, stand out clearly: 'The crucial question is not how the general practitioner can fit into the mental health services but rather how the psychiatrist can collaborate most effectively with primary medical services and reinforce the effectiveness of the primary physician as a member of the mental health team. . . The primary medical care team is the keystone of community psychiatry' (28).

There is, it should be emphasized, little new in this conclusion. It was anticipated by C.P. Blacker when he published his remarkably prescient study of the principles of mental health planning in the National Health Service thirty years ago (29). And it was nearly a hundred years ago that Andrew Wynter advanced the argument in favour of bringing psychiatry into the general practice of medicine:

'We believe ourselves', he said, "that the separation of one organ, and that the highest, the brain, from general medical study, is the most fruitful cause of incipient insanity being suffered to degenerate into confirmed lunacy. The sentinel who is at every man's door, be he rich or poor— the general practitioner—is the one who should be able to foresee the approach of an attack. But he has never studied, or has the slightest possible knowledge of, psychological medicine; the danger goes on from day to day, the chance of averting the evil is lost, and when the patient has become an outrageous lunatic, he is taken to a "mad doctor"—that is, if he has the means to pay his fees, if not he is allowed to linger on making his home miserable and sinking every day into deeper disease, when he is taken to the asylum.'

'The loss to the community by reason of this defect in the knowledge of the general practitioner is not the only evil of this separation of psychological medicine from general medicine. The error which underlies all special study and experience, even if it makes the vision keener in a limited area, is far more serious where mental afflictions are concerned than in other diseases. A surgeon may with advantage devote himself to particular manipulative arts. A man who is drawing teeth all day makes a far better dentist than a general practitioner. The operation of lithotomy requires special skill, which practice alone can secure. But to treat mental illness properly, not only the condition of the brain but of the whole body must be taken into account, as in all cases madness arises from morbid bodily conditions, some of which the specialist overlooks, or rather he is so engaged in looking for one thing, that he overlooks another which may be of equal or greater importance. Of course, there will always be physicians eminent in mental disease, leading men whose genius in their own departments over-rides all other short-comings, but these will necessarily be few. Otherwise we are convinced that; for the good of general medicine, this particular study, dealing as it does with so many complex problems, should be merged in the general routine of medical practice' (30).

It would seem that these sentiments are at last finding favour with general practitioners in Britain, and even with some psychiatrists. The first goal for the future primary care physicians as formulated in the forward-looking document brought out under the aegis of the Royal College of General Practitioners five years ago is: 'To make diagnoses about his patient which are expressed simultaeously in physical, psychological and social terms' (31). And, the report goes on: 'he will need to know, therefore, psychological and social norms as well as physical ones, and to consider these three dimensions when defining the causes, effects and management of an illness. . . This wider approach does not imply that the diagnoses of physical diseases is of reduced importance.'

But the document proceeds still further in extending the boundaries of mental disorder by making a somewhat idiosyncratic distinction between 'disease' and 'illness'. By 'disease' it includes any of the ICD categories, including the symptoms and ill-defined conditions in Section XVI. 'Illness', by contrast, covers the patient's total experience of being unwell and includes not only disease but a 'wide variety of maladaptive responses to the patient's total environment'. The report then furnishes two examples of such 'maladaptive responses':

1. 'symptoms of anxiety in an immature unmarried mother who is having difficulty in coping with an over-active sleepless child'.
2. 'a childless widow's loneliness, expressed in frequent visits to the doctor about a variety of minor physical complaints'.

The significance of this approach for my theme emerges from the conclusion that: 'A more common strategy for dealing with "illness" that lies outside the concept of "disease" is to translate these manifestations into some sort of psychiatric language, in other words to identify them with a "disease" label. Words like "functional overlay", "inadequate personality" or even "hysteria" or "neurotic" mask the fact that the doctor really has no useful way of describing the manifestations of what he sees.' Here the logic of the argument is difficult to follow, for in practice the mental status of the patient must always be considered if a full assessment is to be made. Even if this should be deemed normal, the ICD can still cover the situation adequately through its 'Y' code of supplementary classifications, in particular category

Y.11.0, 'Social maladjustment without manifest psychiatric disorder'. The distinction can, of course, be a delicate matter in practice, and, as we shall see, becomes a central issue when we turn to the complex question of defining and detecting mental disorder in the community at large.

In going beyond the layman's madness so far we have remained close to the identification of mental disorder at different levels of medical care. This task is much facilitated in Britain by the knowledge that more than 97% of the population is registered with a general practitioner, and there is some evidence indicating that sooner or later most sick people make contact with representatives of the primary medical care system (32). In theory, of course, the physician who lives and works in a community small enough to bring him into contact with the entire population is well-placed to pronounce on this question, and occasionally such individuals take advantage of their special position to furnish useful information. Inevitably, perhaps, the areas covered tend to be geographically isolated, often in islands or remote regions. In the United Kingdom, for example, Primrose described some years ago a twelve-month period prevalence study in a small Scottish community of some 1700 persons to whom he provided the medical and many of the social services (33). His figures, as he pointed out, were surprisingly high, the rates for 'neurosis' being 91/1,000, the next largest category being chronic alcoholism at 10/1000. Psychosis, by contrast, was a negligible category. But Primrose emphasizes that these rates must be assessed against the background of his patients' living conditions. Though his own description of these conditions would be unlikely to satisfy a sociological purist, it provides a pithy summary of the situation as 'a moderately prosperous and stable population of Calvinistic traditions, with tendencies to shotgun weddings and excessive consumption of alcohol, in transition from harder times to the sophistication of modern gadgetry'.

Such accounts are, unfortunately, all too rare and in assessing psychiatric morbidity which fails to come to the attention of or is not recognized by the medical services, some form of population enquiry is usually required, since the chain which leads from awareness of symptoms to recognition of illness can be a long one, the links comprising in an awareness of distress of discomfort, the identification of this state as morbid, the belief in the need and value to seek medical treatment, the overcoming of possible obstacles to such a step, e.g. fear, expense, inconvenience; further account must be taken of private and public attitudes towards health and the health professions. In the sphere of public health and clinical epidemiology the spur to such investigations is customarily designated 'screening'. As this currently fashionable term has now come to be extended to embrace mental as well as physical disorders, it is necessary to specify as clearly as possible what is in question. Thus, according to Wilson and Jungner (34), the introduction of a 'screening' programme *in sensu strictu* should meet ten criteria:

1. It should be an important public health problem;
2. There should be an acceptable form of treatment for recognized conditions;
3. The natural history of the conditions should be understood;
4. There should be a recognizable latent or early symptomatic phase during which

5. A suitable test should be available and acceptable;
6. Any facilities required for diagnosis and treatment of untreated cases should be available;
7. Early treatment should favourably influence outcome;
8. Agreement should be reached on whom to treat;
9. The cost of screening should not be excessive; and
10. The case-finding should be a continuing process.

Only the first of these categories—the size of the public health problem—can justifiably be applied to most forms of mental disorder. However, as several authors have pointed out, many so-called screening programmes would be better described as morbidity surveys (35) and, all too often, the strategy of screening becomes identified with the concepts and techniques of case-identification which, in the field of mental disorder, presents particular difficulties. While these are not in some respects different from those which confront the investigator of, say, diabetes or hypertension, the lack of relatively objective criteria has proved a major stumbling block to a number of strenuous but largely misdirected ventures. As Taylor and Chave have commented, 'the "over-enthusiastic diagnostician" can find evidence of psychiatric ill-health in most human beings; such findings perhaps tell us more about the observer than about those observed' (36). It would, perhaps, be more accurate to direct the charge at the instruments employed by the observers, for the definition and detection of the psychiatric case has turned, in large measure, on questions of the techniques employed, which in medical hands consist principally in psychiatric interviews, psychological tests and scales, and assessments of symptoms, illness and disability.

Yet whatever method be chosen, an obvious practical difficutly resides in the need to interview large numbers of people in a standardized manner. To overcome this hurdle there is much to recommend a two-stage approach, using a relatively simple questionnaire to identify vulnerable individuals who can then be interviewed as a whole group or in samples. This is the procedure which we have followed in our own studies (37, 38) and a number of investigations have been carried out along these lines. The results show an uncomfortably large proportion to demonstrate abnormal responses, most of them characterized by dysthymic mood-state, comprising such features as depression, anxiety, preoccupation with health, irritability and insomnia. The designation of these phenomena has raised, and continues to raise, problems of classification, for to include them with the neurotic depressive disorders of Section V of the ICD can serve to extend an outworn concept to breaking-point. They are more adequately covered by the description of depression in Section XVI as a 'decrease of functional activity, not psychosis or psychoneurosis'. The same conclusion has found some theoretical support from Foulds' analysis of the classification of psychiatric disorder in hierarchical terms (39). According to this schema, 'dysthymia' takes its place as a category of reaction below neurotic depression, and the existence of a large pool of individuals with dysthymic states in the general population is of potential clinical significance since there is some evidence to suggest that it contains many of those vulnerable individuals who are prone to develop more overt signs of frank mental disorder (40).

It is, however, possible to approach case-finding in another way, as Blum explicitly pointed out some years ago: '. . . in practice', he said, 'the psychiatric evaluation remains the primary means for making judgments for the purposes of case identification. It will probably continue as the ultimate criterion either until a more reliable, demonstrably valid and practical alternative is developed, or until confidence wanes in the value of medically oriented investigations into those kinds of human behaviour which, when labelled as psychiatric disorder, are not considered to fall within the medical domain' (41).

Since those words were written there has been, not so much a waning of medically-oriented studies as the emergence of alternative frameworks inspired by the social sciences related to medicine. A charter for this approach was provided in 1960 by the proposal of a WHO Committee that '. . . a "case" be defined as a manifest disturbance of mental functioning specific enough in clinical character to be consistently recognizable as conforming to a clearly defined standard pattern *and* severe enough to cause loss of working or social capacity, or both, to a degree which can be specified in terms of absence from work or the taking of legal or other social action' (42). This statement appears to imply that a social dimension must be deemed indispensable to the definition of mental disease; and by so doing it acts an an open-sesame for the many social investigators who have tended to incorporate ill-health into their framework of enquiry.

That much mental disorder is closely associated with social dysfunction has, of course, been recognized for some time and is underlined by the substantial numbers of mentally ill people under the care of the local authority services. Both medical and non-medical investigators may be concerned with the study of aggregates and groups, and major advances have undoubtedly been made by social statisticians in outlining the principles of sampling for population surveys so that the techniques and methods of much social science enquiry overlap closely with those of psychiatric epidemiology. But this community of interests has too often concealed a fundamental difference in objectives which bears directly on the issue of case-definition. Essentially the psychiatrist, working in the extended medical tradition, continues to take the individual as the ultimate unit of his concern. For the social scientist, however, this is not the case. When Karl Marx developed his concept of *Homo economicus* he commented that 'Society does not consist of individuals, but represents the sum of those relationships and affinities which these individuals have with one another.' More than a century later so influential a contemporary figure as Professor Ralf Dahrendorf makes exactly the same point: 'Man basically figures in sociological analysis only to the extent that he complies with all the expectations associated with his social positions. This abstraction, the scientific unit of sociology, may be called *Homo sociologicus*' (43).

If, then, *Homo sociologicus* is the direct descendant of Marx's *Homo economicus* he is genealogically unrelated to *Homo sapiens*. Unfortunately, this distinction is not always apparent in the work of many medical sociologists and perhaps especially from those with an interest in mental disorder. Brown has recently put the case in these terms: 'Sociology has been concerned not only with the workings of social systems as a whole, but also on the impact they have on the individual caught up in them; and in the long run one does not seem to me to make sense with the other. I therefore begin by asking, how successful have we been in relating "personal troubles" to wider social systems?' (44). This type of conceptual diplopia comes to assume some significance when we come to look at case-identification in the perspective of social investigation. The current vogue for constructing all-purpose social concepts which embrace psychological states exemplifies the process well. Thus the suspect metaphor of the 'sick society' creeps back, in the modern guise of 'social malaise' as presented by Flynn, who includes 'adults mentally ill' along with disinfested dwellings, Electricity Board entry warrants, numbers of debtors and of deloused children as 'malaise indicators' in his statistical paella (45). Even more striking is the rash of social indicators which have been devised to measure that most elusive of concepts, the 'quality of life'. While the notion of indicators was originally introduced to cover such relatively objective phenomena as economic attributes, its extension to include so-called 'subjective' indicators has opened the way for the incorporation of such notions as satisfaction, well-being, happiness, alienation and annoyance, all of which are widely employed in social investigations and impinge on mental health, especially through the altered mood-state which is commonly reported by those investigators who have bothered to look for it (46).

It is against this background that we must evaluate the large-scale surveys which have been conducted to furnish facts about mental ill-health. The most ambitious inqury in this country has been the British Survey of Sickness which ran from 1943 to 1952 (47). It was initiated because of the interest developed in minor ailments and general ill-health as an index of national well-being in the Second World War. The information was derived extensively from questionnaires administered to a sample of 2500 people who were asked about illnesses during the preceding trimester. The essentially subjective nature of this judgment, however, is contained in the expressed view that 'a person is ill if he feels ill'. Accordingly, the amount of formal mental disorders recorded is much less prominent than the rubric of 'nervousness and debility' and 'headache' which were consistently exceeded in frequency only by 'muscular and unspecified rheumatism' and the 'common cold'.

Much of the methodological experience acquired during the period of the Survey of Sickness has been incorporated more recently into the health section of the multi-purpose General Household Survey conducted by the Office of Population Censuses and Surveys (48). Here the questionnaire has been expanded to cover the limitations of activity caused by illness, the use of health and personal social services, consultations with doctors and visits to hospitals. As the authors of the report take pains to emphasize, 'morbidity information obtained from sample surveys is not equivalent to clinical diagnosis', and they are correspondingly cautious in presenting diagnostic data. Nonetheless, their tabulation of the rate per 1000 persons reporting conditions leading to consultation with a National Health Service general practitioner in a two-week period shows mental disorders, at 10.5/100, to rank third, following behind only diseases of the upper respiratory tract and 'symptoms and ill-defined diseases'. The proportion of mental disorders is in fact rather smaller than that recorded in the National Morbidity Survey. The reason, say the authors, is that they are 'typically disorders which the doctor may ascribe to a category without telling the patient, or which, in the case of the informant who has been told, she may not confide to the interviewer'.

A major survey focused on the mental health of the general population has still to be mounted in Britain, but in the United States the Health Examination Survey of the National Health Survey has yielded some information, derived from a probability sample of 7710 persons aged 18 to 79 years (49). It emerged that almost 5% of the adult population reported what they called 'nervous breakdowns', a term ascertained as covering an extreme emotional reaction to various factors, most prominently an illness of the respondent or a close friend or relative, an enforced separation, occupational or financial difficulties and inter-personal problems. It was further established that almost three times as many more adults complained of feelings of an impending nervous breakdown defined in this way.

The argument emerging from this attempt to tackle my three questions rests, therefore, essentially on four principal points. First, it is apparent that in going beyond 'madness' or 'psychosis' it becomes necessary to go beyond Section V of the International Classification of Diseases to incorporate categories from the Section on 'symptoms and ill-defined disorders', from the Sections on 'accidents, poisonings, and violence', and from the supplementary classifications. Second, in so doing we encounter involvement with both physical illness and social dysfunction. Third, in numerical terms dysthymic mood-states represent the largest clinical category. And, finally, as a major public health problem much, if not most, mental disorder is to be detected extramurally and so escapes the attention of the specialized mental health facilities.

Which brings me full circle to the second of Sir Geoffrey Vickers' papers to which I can appropriately refer by way of conclusion. This is his address, delivered nearly twenty years ago and entitled 'What sets the goals of public health?' (50). As he pointed out, the question is more complex than it might appear since it calls for not only a clear outline of the dimensions and nature of disease and ill-health, but also for an examination of the influence of such factors as needs, techniques and ideologies. And, in addition, public health itself can make distinct contributions to the setting of its own goals. In Sir Geoffrey's own words: 'It can evaluate health by the criteria which we currently use. It can criticize these criteria and thus help to deepen and refine them. And it can explore those processes of decision by which public-health policy is defined and implemented.' In this paper I have developed the first two of these themes from the standpoint of mental health and, in so doing, I have tried to prepare the ground for a rational approach to the third. To do justice to this, however, would call for an extended consideration of who should intervene, how intervention should be carried out and in what ways it should be evaluated.

References

(1)   Vickers, G. (1962) Mental disorder in British culture. In *Aspects of Psychiatric Research*, Eds. D. Richter, J.M. Tanner, Lord Taylor and O.L. Zangwill, p. 1. London, Oxford University Press.

(2)   Pines, M. (1974) Psychotherapy outside the National Health Service. In *Psychotherapy Today*, Ed. V. Varma, p. 274. London, Constable.
(3)   Lewis, A. (1963) Medicine and the affections of the mind. *Br. med. J.*, *2*, 1549-57.
(4)   World Health Organization (1974) *Glossary of Mental Disorders and Guide to their Classification*. Geneva, WHO.
(5)   Department of Health and Social Security (1973) Psychiatric units in England and Wales. In-patient statistics from the Mental Health Enquiry for the year 1971. *Statistical and Research Report Series No. 6*. London, HMSO.
(6)   Shepherd, M. (1957) *A Study of the Major Psychoses in an English County*. Maudsley Monograph No. 3. London, Oxford University Press.
(7)   Office of Population Censuses and Surveys (1974) *Hospital In-patient Enquiry, 1972*. London, HMSO.
(8)   Dunbar, H.F. (1943) *Psychosomatic Diagnosis*. New York, Hoeber.
(9)   Grinker, R.R. (1973) *Psychosomatic Concepts*. New York, Aronson.
(10) Lewis, A. (1972) 'Psychogenic': a word and its mutations. *Psychol. Med.*, *2*, 209-15.
(11) Shepherd, M., Davies, B. and Culpan, R.H. (1960) Psychiatric Illness in the general hospital. *Acta Psychiatrica et Neurologica Scandinavica*, *35*, 518-25.
(12) Maguire, G.P., Julier, D.L., Hawton, K.E. and Bancroft, J.H.J. (1974) Psychiatric morbidity and referral on two general medical wards. *Br. med. J.*, *1*, 268-70.
(13) Moffice, H.S. and Paykel, E.S. (1975) Depression in medical in-patients. *Br. J. Psychiat.*, *126*, 346-53.
(14) Hughes, J.N.P. (1966) Alcoholism in Cardiff. *Medical Officer*, *115*, 161-3.
(15) Logan, W.P.D. and Cushion, A.A. (1958) *Morbidity Statistics from general Practice Vol. 1. Studies on Medical and Population Subjects No. 14*, London, HMSO.
(16) Collaborative Study RCGP, OPCS, DHSS (1974) *Morbidity Statistics from General Practice—Second National Study 1970-71. Studies on Medical and Population Subjects No. 26*, London, HMSO.
(17) Crombie, D.L. (1974) Changes in patterns of recorded morbidity. In *Benefits and Risks in Medical Care*, Ed. D. Taylor, p. 17. London, Office of Health Economics.
(18) Shepherd, M., Cooper, B., Brown, A.C. and Kalton G.W. (1966) *Psychiatric Illness in General Practice*. London, Oxford University Press.
(19) Stoller, A. and Krupinski, J. (1966) Psychiatric disturbances. In *Report on a National Morbidity Survey*, Ch. 6, p. 48. Canberra, NHMRC.
(20) Locke, B.Z., Finucane, D.L. and Hassler, F. (1967) Emotionally disturbed patients under care of private non-psychiatric physicians. In *Psychiatric Epidemiology and Mental Health Planning. Psychiatric Research Report 22*. Washington, American Psychiatric Association.
(21) Strotzka, H. (1969) *Kleinburg*. Vienna, Österreichischer Bundesverlag für Unterricht, Wissenschaft und Kunst.
(22) Bash, K.W. and Bash-Liechti, J. (1974) Studies on the epidemiology of neuropsychiatric disorders among the population of the city of Shiraz, Iran. *Soc. Psychiat.*, *9*, 163-71.
(23) White, K.L. (1970) Classification of patient symptoms, complaints and problems. Paper to *Expert Committee on Health Statistics (Statistical Indicators for the Planning & Evaluation of Public Health Programmes)*. Geneva, WHO.
(24) Wilkins, R.H. (1974) *The Hidden Alcoholic in General Practice*. London, Elek Science.
(25) Department of Health and Social Security (1974) *Digest of Statistics Analysing Certificates of Incapacity, June 1969-May 1970*. London, HMSO.
(26) Hill, D. (1968) Introduction. In *The Treatment of Mental Disorders in the Community*, Eds. G.R. Daniel and H.L. Freeman, p. 1. London, Bailliere Tindall and Cassell.
(27) Bennett, D. (1973) Community mental health services in Britain. *Am. J. Psychiat.*, *130*, 10, 1065-70.
(28) Report of Working Group (1973) *Psychiatry and Primary Medical Care*. Copenhagen, WHO.
(29) Blacker, C.P. (1946) *Neurosis and the Mental Health Services*. London, Oxford University Press.
(30) Wynter, A. (1875) The role of the general practitioner. In *The Borderlands of Insanity*, p. 156. London, Robert Hardwicke.
(31) Report of Working Party of the Royal College of General Practitioners (1972) *The Future General Practitioner*. London, British Medical Association.

(32) Kalton, G.W. (1968) The contribution of research in general practice to the study of morbidity. *J. R. Coll. Gen. Pract., 15*, 81-95.
(33) Primrose, E.J.R. (1962) *Psychological Illness.* London, Tavistock.
(34) Wilson, J.M.G. and Jungner, G. (1968) Principles and Practice of Screening for Disease. *WHO Public Health Papers, No. 34*, Geneva, WHO.
(35) Sackett, D.L. and Holland, W.W. (1975) Controversy in the detection of disease. *Lancet, 2*, 357-9.
(36) Taylor S. and Chave, S. (1964) *Mental Health and Environment.* London, Harrap.
(37) Goldberg, D.P. (1972) *The Detection of Psychiatric Illness by Questionnaire.* Maudsley Monograph No. 21. London, Oxford University Press.
(38) Goldberg, D.P., Cooper, B., Eastwood, M.R., Kedward, H.B. and Shepherd, M. (1970) A standardised psychiatric interview suitable for use in community surveys. *Br. J. prev. soc. Med., 24*, 18-23.
(39) Foulds, G.A. and Bedford, A. (1975) Hierarchy of classes of personal illness. *Psychol. Med., 5*, 181-92.
(40) Price, J. (1969) Personality differences within families: comparison of adult brothers and sisters. *J. biosoc. Sci., 1*, 177-205.
(41) Blum, R.H. (1962) Case-identification in psychiatric epidemiology: methods and problems. *Milbank Memorial Fund Quarterly, XL*, 253-88.
(42) Expert Committee on Mental Health (1960) Epidemiology of mental disorders. *WHO Technical Report Series No. 185.* Geneva, WHO.
(43) Dahrendorf, R. (1973) *Homo Sociologicus.* London, Routledge and Kegan Paul.
(44) Brown, G.W. (1974) Sociological research—how seriously do we take it? Unpublished manuscript.
(45) Flynn, M., Flynn, P. and Mellor, N. (1972) Social malaise research: a study in Liverpool. *Social Trends, 3*, 42-52.
(46) Abrams, M. (1973) Subjective social indicators. *Social Trends, 4*, 35-50.
(47) Logan, W.P.D. and Brooke, E.M. (1957) The survey of sickness. 1943-1952. *General Register Office Studies on Medical and Population Subjects. No. 12.* London, HMSO.
(48) Office of Population Censuses and Surveys (1973) *The General Household Survey.* London, HMSO.
(49) Vital and Health Statistics. Data from the National Health Survey (1970) *Selected Symptoms of Psychological Distress.* National Center for Health Statistics, Series II, No. 37. Rockville, US Department of Health, Education and Welfare.
(50) Vickers, G. (1958) What sets the goals of public health? *The Lancet, 1*, 599-604.

11. Biological differences and social justice

Eliot Slater

This subject takes us into three sensitive areas: differences in intelligence between individuals, differences between Negroes and Whites, and differences between men and women.* These differences may lead to discrimination, and discrimination to injustice. But if we wish to avoid injustice, we need to look at its causes; it does not help to maintain that a biological difference does not exist, or that it is merely a social artefact. I believe we can find a way to social justice, when all the uncomfortable facts have been allowed. In the very contentious terrain we shall be entering we shall need a guiding principle. This has been given us by Bertrand Russell (1): 'Ethical considerations can only legitimately appear when the truth has been ascertained: they can and should appear as determining our feelings towards the truth, and our manner of ordering our lives in view of the truth, but not as themselves dictating what the truth is to be.'

Biological differences between individuals and between groups are a constant source of distress, and we tend to handle them symptomatically. We try, in fact, to relieve our own feelings, and do not consider whether that is the best way to deal with the problems. We have, for instance, been so impressed by the sufferings of the young, deprived of adult status for so many years of waiting, that by a stroke of the lawgiver's pen we have transformed infants of eighteen, nineteen and twenty years into full citizens. There are massive statistics to show the perils of early marriages, and the high risk they face of years of unhappiness for whole families before final shipwreck. Nevertheless, because the young complained, we thought fit to cut short the golden period of their childhood, and to push them three years earlier into the rough seas of responsibility. Perhaps it is partly because they are made responsible so prematurely, and take their responsibility so deadly seriously, that our young people see the society that did this to them as fundamentally unjust.

Where there is a difference, between individuals or between groups, one side will probably be at an advantage. Then we are likely to see amicable relationships between the two sides poisoned by envy. In his great work on envy, Helmut Schoeck (2) has pointed out the motive force of this rather ugly emotion in bringing about social change. On the side of the envier there is a

---

*These are not all of the same kind. Differences in intelligence (or, better, in IQ) between individuals are differences between points on a single unimodal curve; differences between Negroes and Whites involve differences between means, and taking both together, the distribution is bimodal; with men and women we have to bear a qualitative difference in mind.

The Sir Geoffrey Vickers Lecture of 21 February 1973, an abridged version of which was published in *New Statesman*, 6 April 1973.

vindictive, inwardly tormenting displeasure, combining feelings of aggression and impotence; the advantages of the other cause him anguish; he would rather destroy those advantages than obtain them for himself. The envied, aware of the feelings he is arousing, feels guilt; he wishes only to be invisible; he feels the existence of an injustice, and may even begin to punish himself. Envy provides the dynamic for every social revolution. It is one of the necessary foundations for the development of law and order, for combining individuals into groups for political action, and for building a social organization. It opposes, with its egalitarian drive, the pressures caused by individuals constantly striving to advance themselves and improve their personal lot.

Schoeck is surely right in thinking that what constitutes an injustice is the emotions aroused by an inequality, not the inequality itself. There has to be polarization, resentment on one side provoking guilt on the other, or vice versa. No polarization, no injustice. By and large, old people accept as inevitable the disabilities that creep up on them in an increasing load from year to year. After all, there is going to be a way out. For the physically and mentally handicapped there is no escape. Nor is it possible to give them any adequate reparation, even if it is measured in tens of thousands of pounds. Our guilt provokes their resentment. And here, as elsewhere, our guilt leads us into actions directed more towards soothing our own distress than towards tackling the problem in a rational way. If seriously damaged babies did not survive birth their families would be more helped than by any measures of social support.

Differences in IQ

Mental handicaps do not have to be pathological to cause distressing social inequalities: normal people show a very wide range. When measured by psychometric tests, we speak of an intelligence quotient, or IQ, with a population mean of 100 and a standard deviation of 15. Both genetical and environmental factors enter into the causes of this great span of variation, going all the way from below 55 up to, say, 200. In a given population at a stated time it is possible to estimate the fraction of the total variance which can be attributed to hereditary factors on the one hand and to environmental ones on the other. For instance, for the British population of school children about ten years ago, it was estimated that about 75% of the total variance in IQ was due to heredity, and 20% to the environment, with 5% for error. Since then times have changed. The gene pool has been greatly enriched by immigration from the Commonwealth, and with the provisions of the welfare state some of the environmental inequalities have been evened out. One would expect that new estimates today might rate the importance of heredity even higher than ten years ago. If we ever achieve a completely egalitarian society, those IQ differences will still be there, but will be 100% hereditary. The social reformer will have worked himself out of a job, but will the social injustice be cured?

The simplified picture I have given would probably be found acceptable (within its modest limits) by most psychologists, but not by all. Some of them, deeply committed to the welfare of the underprivileged, go to opposite extremes. One of the most distinguished, Professor Liam Hudson, believes in the prepotence of social and psychological factors over genetic ones and flatly denies Russell's principle (3). Facts can be full of subjectivities, he thinks, and what matters is knowing the extent of one's own commitment. He denies that 'any one child's ability to benefit from teaching has a fixed limit'. 'Logically', he says, 'we can set limits to children's capacity to learn only if every permutation of their environment, every method of nurturing them, has been exhausted.' This is nailing the flag to the mast, declaring that there will be no surrender, however the facts or the arguments may go. He is saying that, given the right education, any and every child has the potentialities of developing the command of language of Shakespeare, the mathematical powers of Newton, and the artistic genius of Turner. And he declares that no evidence will convince him to the contrary, or should convince us, since of the nature of things we shall never be able to exhaust all the permutations of the environment and every possible method of nurturing and teaching. If one allows ethical considerations to control one's view of the truth, one arrives at absurdities; and those who believe absurdities will commit atrocities. The view that there are no inborn weaknesses also implies that there are no inborn strengths. The danger hidden in Hudson's views is that children, with all their infinite diversity of strengths and weaknesses and aptitudes and tastes and enthusiams will be subjected to a uniform processing.

We must not lose sight of the fact that, barring those who have a monozygotic twin, each one of us is genetically unique. So unique, in fact, that there will never be a repeat until the end of time.* Each of us is, then, unique in our genetical predisposition to our particular combination of strengths and weaknesses, intellectual, characterological, temperamental. This is one of those brute facts which cannot be surmounted by tendentious argument. It is one that should be built into the foundation of any just society. A society of individuals should be designed for individuals.

Some sociologists go further even than Professor Hudson. They deny the validity of the concept of intelligence. They deny the relevance of genetical variation in individual potentialities for intelligent behaviour. And they present the academic and occupational significance of test results, as exhibited in the IQ, as something like a self-fulfilling prophecy. Some maintain that psychometric tests are all socially, and indeed politically, loaded, and are the instruments of ethnocentric, elitist and inhumane policies. By passing the test, one child is given advantages from which, on the same test, another child is excluded. Here, they say, is injustice.

Now there is much to be said in criticism of the extremely inflated value

---

*Neel and Schull (4) give as a minimum estimate 100,000 loci encoding for protein structure. At many of these loci there will be an alternative gene available, allowing a genetic polymorphism. If we take as a genetic polymorphism one in which 2% or more of the population belong to the rarer genotype(s), then mankind's polymorphisms extend to about 30% of the available loci, and the average single individual is heterozygous at about 16% of his loci. Using Neel and Schull's figures, what is the most standardized product we can obtain? Let us suppose that all those polymorphisms are dichotomizing at the extreme 98:2 relative frequencies; then the most frequent possible combination, an individual belonging to the 98% class at each and all of his 30,000 loci, has a probability of 10^{-270}. Any other genotype would be still rarer. If this least improbable of individuals were once thrown up, the chance of getting a repeat out of a billion (10^9) births a year for a billion years would be the hardly less astronomically infinitesimal probability of 10^{-252}.

which has been given to the IQ, a point to which I come in a moment. But one should remember that when IQ tests were introduced in the 11+ examination, it was with the purpose of aiding justice. Grammar school type education was available for only a minority of children, and it was necessary to select children who would be best able to take advantage of it. Tests of educational attainment favoured children from middle-class homes. The introduction of the IQ at last gave a chance to the bright child of low achievement coming from the underprivileged home. And it at once showed up the fact that the majority of high IQ children came from working-class homes. In fact, the IQ test helped to even out higher-level schooling across the social classes. Its success was enough to cause it to fail. The drive behind the move for comprehensive education, and away from grammar schools and streaming and differential education, has come from prosperous, literate middle-class parents. They reacted in this way when they found their children scoring too low on IQ tests to gain entry to the privileged schooling whicy they felt was their due. Envy of the working-class families and others whose children did gain such entry led to the demand that schooling must be the same for all.

Now one must not fall down and worship IQ, as some have done. As Ruth Hubbard has said, IQ tests ignore much that is artistic, contemplative and non-verbal. They were constructed to predict success in the kind of schools that have prevailed in Europe and the United States. Many of us have been losing faith in what these schools have done to us, and are currently doing to our children (5). High IQ for a man is rather like high horse-power for an engine. While it provides the capacity for doing a lot of work, it does not mean that the work done is socially valuable; it can just as well be exploitative, or even directly antisocial. Moreover, the high-powered engine is suitable for some purposes, but for others a lower-powered engine may be more economical and more efficient. Societies do not run themselves harmoniously merely by trying to solve problems by the application of IQ; kindness, consideration for others and unselfishness are a great deal more important, in directing where the intelligence should be applied and which are the solutions to be chosen.

However, IQ does not take one all the way, even in terms of worldly success. One of the surprises that emerged from Terman's studies of 'genius' was the mediocrity of the careers achieved by high IQ people. Terman followed up approximately 1000 American children with IQs averaging 151 both for boys and for girls. For the most part these children came from a superior family background, with parents better educated than the average. Their performances at school were good, but were not matched by their grade placements. The educational system tended to hold them back rather than fully to develop them. At the follow-up, conducted in middle-life (6) they had become, in order of choice: lawyers, executives in business and industry, college and university faculty members, engineers, executives in banking, finance and insurance. Only a sprinkling had become journalists or authors, or were in the arts. The extreme poverty of truly creative workers was noteworthy. The best achievements were in science, and 70 of the 577 males secured listing in *American Men of Science*. When the group were asked what they thought of themselves, only 4% could say that they had fully lived up to their abilities.

Very significant is the fact that the IQ ratings of those who were not successful were just as high as those of the successful.

One might say that the value of the high IQ man depends on the values of the society in which he lives. In our western societies, with their degraded view of the purpose of human existence, the high IQ man is a lowly order of creature. He has become the servant of the technological machine.

What do we want from our really gifted people? Surely it is more than mere worldly success, more than the kind of service that just keeps the world's machinery moving, especially when that movement is in its present self-destructive direction. What we want from them is an entry on the credit side of the ledger, something that two generations later will be recognizable as a benefaction to mankind. When we look at what humanity in the past has done for humanity now, we see that what really endures are the achievements of the human spirit. Viewing the human procession from this vantage point, we see the uncountable millions disappearing traceless into the shadows. The captains and the kings depart. What has been given us by the artists and writers remains for ever.

What can be said about this immensely esteemed high IQ? What is its contribution to the spiritual capital of mankind? We note:

1. The highest achievement is possible with a very average IQ; but a high IQ is an aid to certain kinds of high achievement.

2. The range of abilities in the general population, very insufficiently measured by the IQ, is such as to provide a very much larger number of potential high achievers than ever achieve.

3. Potential high achievers run into every kind of environmental frustration, both at home and at school.* These frustrations would be less important in a setting in which every child was encouraged in the pursuit of all manner of excellencies, and given the opportunities to discover the field in which he might excel.

4. As things are, the fate of the high IQ individual is to get directed up one of the standard ladders; to be pushed into a competitive race for advancement, that is, a race in which the other abilities which rounded out his IQ are likely to wither. He can expect to work too hard in too narrow a field, and to sacrifice his leisure and domesticities for material rewards and spiritual starvation. Competitive striving encourages the will to power, and builds up a ruthless aggressive life-style. As the American aphorism has it, *nice guys finish last.* Everyone, even the man himself, hates the guy who finishes first; in fact, we can very well do without him. What we want and need are the nice guys. There are never enough of them.

Race

In Britain, there is no evidence known to me that Negroes are any less

*Kellmer Pringle (7) studied a group of 103 able misfits, children with IQs between 120 and 200. She concluded that the school fails to provide a second chance to highly gifted children whose ability has been undernourished at home. The able child 'whose potential has remained largely dormant may get by, performing at an average or possibly below average level for his age. Or he becomes so bored by methods and curricula geared to the average that his interest and curiosity are never aroused; consequently he opts out altogether, becoming not only a misfit but a failure.'

intelligent than the rest of us. Circumstances are different in the United States. The relation there between race and IQ is ground that has been fought over for a considerable time. At last some agreement is emerging about the facts, though not about their interpretation. The observation that the IQ mean for Negroes is about one standard deviation, or 15 points, lower than for Whites seems to have been established. The difference could be caused by genetical factors, or environmental ones, or by an additive combination of both, or by their interaction. Genetical differences do cause IQ differences, and Negroes and Whites do differ genetically. But if one were to conclude that the genetical differences accounted for the difference between mean IQs, the argument would be fatally flawed by the logical solecism of the undistributed middle term. In fact, Arthur Jensen, who has come under such virulent attack for his views, has disclaimed (8) the idea that within-group heritability can prove between-group heritability. What he did say in his much celebrated article in the *Harvard Educational Review* in 1969, was that the evidence available made it 'a not unreasonable hypothesis that genetic factors are strongly implicated' in the Negro-White average intelligence difference. This is, surely, not unreasonable; and, as a working hypothesis, it has been the starting point of some very interesting research.

American Negroes suffer under economic disadvanages. As IQ is correlated with socio-economic class, it has not unreasonably been suggested that their IQ deficit might be attributable to this cause. However, this can only be a part of the answer since, when Negro and White children are balanced against one another in social class, the Negro children still average a lower IQ. The difference now is not 15 but about 11 points. The genetical hypothesis is, then, to some extent sustained. But this fact can be stood on its head and looked at another way. As Biederman has pointed out (9), it also means that IQ for IQ the Negro does better socio-economically than the White.

According to Jensen, this is confirmed by clinical impressions. He contrasts the low IQ children coming from middle-class homes with low IQ children from disadvantaged homes. The disadvantaged children, he says, seem much brighter than their IQs, and brighter than the middle-class children of the same IQ, though not better in scholastic performance. Their brightness shows in their quickness in orienting to the school environment, in learning the names of their playmates and in learning their games.

Jensen's researches led him to identify two ways of learning. They might be called associative and cognitive respectively; but he prefers the non-committal names of Level I and Level II learning processes. Level I learning is the first to develop, and we do not know fully how far it could take us. Jensen is convinced that all the basic scholastic skills can be learned by children with Level I learning ability, provided the instructional systems are suitably chosen. Unfortunately, they are not. Instead, demands are made on g, the IQ general factor, that is on Level II learning abilities. This can be disastrous for the Negro child. He is called on to learn by methods that do not suit him; and if he does learn in his own way, the teacher makes it plain that getting the right answer the wrong way is not acceptable. The teacher rewards effort rather than success, and tells him to try harder. The behaviours that promote learning are not reinforced, so that they are actively extinguished. The teacher, the books, paper, pencils, all become conditioned inhibitors.

Incomprehensible training leads to catastrophic reactions, anger, rebellion, school phobia, truanting.

Jensen thinks it possible that there are different polygenic systems for Level I and Level II learning, and that the Negro is better endowed with the former. Patterns of ability are different for Chinese, Jewish, Negro and Puerto Rican children. The difficulties that face the Negro child could then be, in large part, ones forced on him by the educationist.

Jensen is a sharp critic of the IQ mystique. He does not accept a unidimensional concept of intelligence. Learning is based on sub-abilities, and the pattern of sub-abilities varies from child to child. It is the pressure for uniformity instead of diversity in teaching aims and methods that does the damage; and it is the disadvantaged child who is the worst sufferer. Once the slow learner has been left behind, he may remain stranded for good. Many skills have to be learned in a one-to-one tutorial situation. This is provided by the parents in a middle-class home, but may be nearly lacking at a lower socio-economic level. If this were recognized, an alternative might be provided, e.g. by automated teaching, or perhaps by one-to-one tutoring between older and younger pupils.

Jensen is contemptuous of our present methods, and describes them as 'a largely antiquated elitist-oriented educational system, which originally evolved to serve only a relatively small segment of society... It seems incredible that a system can still survive which virtually guarantees frustration and failure for a large proportion of the children it should intend to serve.' One does not help the disadvantaged child by trying to turn him into a typical middle-class child. It is unfair to teach children cognitively who can best learn associatively. One would do better to teach specific skills directly rather than to try to boost overall cognitive development. Schools must find ways of using the strengths of children whose main strength is not cognitive. In a few words, Jensen's recommended reforms would involve: (*a*) full allowance for individual variation in learning strengths and weaknesses; (*b*) task analysis of what is taught; (*c*) diversification of educational methods, programmes, goals and occupational opportunities to a range as wide as the range of human abilities.

It will be seen that Jensen's genetic hypothesis, informed by his liberal, humane and compassionate disposition, has led him to valuable research results, and to lines of attack on the educational difficulties of the Negro which look promising. This cannot be said of the environmental hypotheses, which postulate various types of psychological or sociological vicious circle from which there is no way out.* There does not seem to be any objective

---

*For example: Negroes carry, publicly displayed, their identification as members of a lower social class. The Negro child has absorbed the idea of his inferiority by the time he is old enough to be tested; he is taught from birth that he has no chance, no opportunity. The Negro thinks badly of himself; even Black children think better of Whites. As the Negress is more acceptable to Whites than the Negro, she quickly learns to regard the male as her inferior. Even Negro schoolteachers may be hostile to lower-class Negro children. The Negro has been overwhelmed by the destructive forces of the White supremacist society. The era of slavery has left the Negro dependent and unable to mature. The Negro is culturally deprived, with inadequate language development, and starts school with a handicap that is never overcome. Most of these are cited by Proshansky and Newton (10).

evidence in favour of them, and most of them are so vague that it is difficult to see how relevant evidence could be gained. Others again, e.g. that it is all due to the past era of slavery, are of their nature untestable.

The only idea that has come up from the environmental psycho-sociological angle has been that movement, inspired by the generosity of the American temperament, known as 'Affirmative Action'. This is racism in reverse. The movement calls for disrimination by race and sex in the hiring of employees, but in the opposite direction to the prevailing trend, e.g. an increased representation in university staff of racial minority groups and of women until they reach specified fractions of the total faculty. This might, indeed, provide a breakthrough against prejudices which show signs of only very slow erosion. The principle is not unknown in other fields. In Britain, large employing agencies are under an obligation to empliy registered disabled persons up to a quota of their employees, a measure which infringes several of the egalitarian principles on which our society runs itself: those of equal opportunity, advancement by merit, and let the best man win. More widely applied, such infringements might make winning rather less important than it is. It would be another step away from the free towards the planned society, but perhaps none the worse for that.

Genetical theories suppose the Negro is different; psychosocial theories suppose he is damaged. If one consults the Negro, one finds the psychosocial theories are no less objectionable to Negroes, and no less wounding to their self-respect. In fact there is no current attitude on the part of Whites that is not objectionable. To regard the Negro as an individual damaged from whatever cause is in itself insulting. To pretend to what has been called 'colour blindness' is perhaps the most insulting attitude of all, since this is a denial of Negro ethnic loyalty and personal identity. If they examined it carefully, Negroes might find Jensen's genetic hypothesis a more satisfactory way of seeing themselves. If they see themselves as differing from Whites not only in colour and in all the other anthropometric particulars in which they do differ, but also in the genetic basis of cerebral organization, and so in temperamental and cognitive style, the way is thrown open to that pride in their own nature which is what they need.

If my neighbour invariably beats me in a game of chess, I do not think myself an inferior human being to him. If American Negroes are surpassed by American Whites in IQ tests, let them regard it as the bagatelle it is. And if the Negro is at a disadvantage in the acquisitive competitive societies of the west which the White man has built for himself, then let him see that as a good reason for him to reject those ways of life, and to demand a better ordering of the societies in which he lives. Pluralistic societies can and do get on perfectly well, as has been demonstrated in the Caribbean. Trinidad, with a population of East Indians, Negroes, Portuguese, Chinese, Whites, Amerindians and others, has managed itself very peaceably under Negro domination (11).

The Black Moslems have found a recipe for Negro self-respect, when living as an underprivileged minority in an adverse White society, that of separatism, For those Negroes who do not feel rejected by the white man, and who wish to integrate, the path to integration is by genetic mixture, by intermarriage. The Negro who does reject the white man's rejection should reject also White customs and religions, prestige symbols and White styles in hair and dress. Let him foster his own music, dance, drama and art, for which his genetic constitution provides the talent, as for no white man. Let him build up his own communities, his own way of life, his own nexus of family relationships, his own racial independence. These are all things which he will have to do for himself; and in doing them, even against White resistance, he would set himself beyond the reach of derogatory classifications.

Sex

The last of my three themes is the nature of the biological differences between men and women, and the social injustice to which women have been and still are subjected. If the facts were not so familiar as to be taken for granted, we would be staggered by the irrationality and unfairness with which we subject women to legal incapacities, procedural handicaps, occupational bars and financial degradation. It is painful for a biologist to have to admit that this oppression has actually been supported, though never justified, by arguments based on the biological differences between men and women, their different roles and different needs.

These specious and misleading arguments have had a most unfortunate effect. Women liberationists, instead of showing that the premises do not justify the conclusions, have tried to undermine the premises. They have pointed out the common humanity of men and women, and have minimized psychological differences. They caught at the idea, promoted by some psychologists on the basis of work done by Money and the Hampsons, that gender role is not inborn but is learned by the infant and young child from the way he or she is brought up, once the original distinction has been made from the appearance of the external genitals. It was found that intersexual individuals successfully adjusted to the sex role to which they were allocated, although it might be contrary, say, to their chromosomal sex. A deeper understanding of the embryonic processes leads to a quite opposite conclusion.

Fertilized egg-cells are either male or female according to their chromosomal constitution. Developing embryos take a common line of development up to the appearance of a primitive gonad. At about the seventh week in the male embryo, the Y chromosome steps in for the first and only time in the life of the individual and starts the gonad developing into a testis. If nothing happens, then a little later the gonad of its own accord develops into an ovary. All the male reproductive system is developed from the Wolffian system under the control of the testis, and further development of the Mullerian system is inhibited. If there is no control by the testis, then the Mullerian system develops into the female reproductive organs. Between the 60th and the 120th day the testis hormone starts influencing the organization of the hypothalamus in the brain. If there is no testis hormone, then the hypothalamus is programmed along female lines. So by the time it is born the infant is already equipped with a male brain or a female brain. The big difference is that the female hypothalamus works cyclically, the male hypothalamus acyclically. Both hormonal balances and their phasing differ in the two sexes (12, 13, 14).

Male sex hormones also have an anabolic effect, so that the male grows bigger and stronger than the female, in skeleton and musculature. Not only does the male carry a lot more muscle than the female, but in his case the muscle fibres are intrinsically more efficient, especially under stressed or hypoxic conditions (15). The fact that men are physically so much stronger than women has been a prime factor in the oppression of women, because it has made that oppression, not justifiable, or reasonable, or even adaptive, but simply, possible.

Intellectual differences between the sexes are very interesting, though they do not appear to affect dominance. Men are more variable than women, with a shift towards male preponderance in the sex ratio, both among mental defectives and at a highest intellectual peak. There is no difference between means, so that for society's normal purposes neither sex should be at an advantage. There is also a difference in cognitive style. Women do better than men in tests of verbal intelligence, men better than women in spatio-temporal tests. On that basis one might expect men to provide more than their share of engineers, and less than their share of politicians. If things don't work out that way, maybe it is because we are not selecting our politicians on their merits.

None of what we know about male-female differences in any way justifies or excuses the oppression to which women have been subjected. We have, then, to look not for rational reasons but for irrational motives. Looked at in this way, we see how deep in the unconscious these motives take their root. We are struck at once by the ferocity with which the oppression has been conducted. Perhaps we have now reached a kinder age, but in past eras, at least in Christendom, women have been loaded with every sort of disparagement, denigration, vilification. This is in spite of the fact that, although of course asperities do arise at times, in the main women provide for men a warm loving supportive environment. They are the source of tenderness and care which he cannot expect from other men. Why then have the prophets and saints, theologians and philosophers heaped on womankind every imaginable insult? Typical of the male hatred and fear of an earlier Christian anti-feminism is the sulphurous pit opened up by Shakespeare in *King Lear*.* What unleashes this fury is woman in her sexual aspect, a subject on which women themselves do not open up very much, an aspect which has remained for the male perpetually beyond his empathy, or his comprehension, or his conquest.

Here there is an asymmetry, even though male and female sexuality are matched against one another. The female is liable to find male sexuality, when it is not wanted, a nuisance or even a danger, but not a pretext for despising the whole male sex. The male, on the other hand, is very

---

* Behold yond simp'ring dame
  Whose face between her forks presages snow,
  That minces virtue and does shake the head
  To hear of pleasure's name,
  The fitchew nor the soiled horse goes to't
  With a more riotous appetite.
  Down from the waist they are centaurs,
  Though women all above.
  But to the girdle do the gods inherit,
  Beneath is all the fiend's.
  There's hell, there's darkness, there is the sulphurous pit,
  Burning, scalding, stench, consumption. (Cambridge edition, 4.6.118-29).

uncomfortable with his own lust, tends to be rather ashamed of his libidinal satisfactions, and to find those of the female inexcusable. There must be a reason.

According to an ancient myth,* the blind prophet Tiresias in his youth changed his sex by a miracle, and lived for seven years as a girl, during which time he married. Later on he was asked by the gods to settle a dispute, which of the two sexes received greater pleasure in copulation. When he replied that the pleasure received by the female was ten times greater than that of the male, the goddesss struck him blind.

The truth that lies in this old story has been fully confirmed by recent scientific investigation. The researches of Masters and Johnston have shown that the orgasm capacity of the female is a whole degree of magnitude greater than that of the male: whereas he can manage one, two or three orgasms, she is good for ten, twenty or thirty. Such a difference must be based on differences at the organic level, and this is what we find. The clitoris in the female is a very richly innervated sense organ. The male has nothing to compare with it. Indeed, the penis has a poor nerve supply, and is nearly anaesthetic. One never finds a well-innervated peripheral sensory apparatus without corresponding central representation. The female must have a mass of circuitry in the subcortical centres in an activated state, which in the male has been shut off by the testis hormone and has remained latent. This organization in the female will also have its chemical support system. We may suppose that the neuro-transmitting substances, which are so rapidly exhausted in the male, are in much larger supply in the female and allow her the higher level of performance of which she is capable.

One might ask, what selective advantage could it have for the female to be so much better endowed than the male? Surely, it is because the tasks nature demands of her are so much heavier. Since any coitus is capable of causing her a nine-months' pregnancy followed by a perilous confinement, sexual activity might have become extinguished unless its immediate rewards had been very great. Even now maternal mortality stands at 14 per 100,000 still- and live-births, and in past ages must have been a hundredfold greater. Paternal mortality, on the other hand, is and must always have been zero; and it was not necessary for nature to provide the male with anything much more than an irritable persistent itch to make sure the job was done. The female, indeed, has been further rewarded by blooming health during pregnancy, and, after the difficult confinement, compensations in suckling, caring for, responding to and playing with the infant. All this has been a closed book to the male.

*Tiresias, a celebrated prophet of Thebes, lived to a great age... It is said that in his youth he found two serpents in the act of copulation on mount Cyllene, and that when he struck them with a stick to separate them, he found himself suddenly changed into a girl. Seven years after he found again some serpents together in the same manner, and he recovered his original sex by striking them a second time with his wand. When he was a woman, Tiresias had married, and it was from those reasons, according to some of the ancients, that Jupiter and Juno referred to his decision a dispute in which the deities wished to know which of the sexes received greater pleasure from the connubial state. Tiresias, who could speak from actual experience, decided in favour of Jupiter, and declared that the pleasure which the female received was ten times greater than that of the male. Juno, who supported a different opinion, and gave the superiority to the male sex, punished Tiresias by depriving him of his eyesight.' (Lemprière's Classical Dictionary, 1949).

Down the ages, then, the stronger, more muscular, more aggressive male has had to try to compensate himself for these biological deficiencies. The female might be frigid, though all that meant was that she had not been adequately aroused. But the male, deprived of a specific sense organ, was sexually blind, and not only blind but, all too often, paralytic. It is the male sex that is the impotent sex. In the flower of his youth, it is just where he is tempted to pride himself, in his virility, that the male finds himself weakest, matched with a partner with ten times his powers. No wonder he sometimes turns to homosexuality.

With the male at such disadvantage, if he did not dominate the female by muscular strength and aggressive drive, he might easily become enslaved. Above all, for his pride and security against invidious comparisons, her faithfulness had to be maintained. This was most easily done by the institution of monogamous marriage. This is a male supremacist arrangement about which women have not been consulted. In matriarchal societies it is not thought necessary. Monogamy serves the invaluable social purpose of providing a female for every male, even the most inadequate. Its evolutionary effects for the male sex have not been entirely satisfactory. There has been no counterselection against relative impotence, when all but the absolutely impotent have been able to propagate their kind.

Male supremacist attitudes, then, can be plausibly accounted for by the human urge to envy those better endowed than ourselves, and if possible to take their advantage from them. Freud went astray with his concept of penis envy; Adler's ideas on organ inferiority and masculine protest are more to the point. We can see sex-envy in the male as a powerful motive force in determining male domination over women, the social contract of marriage, and the organization of societies. When power is wielded by the envious, who still cannot right their wrongs, it can lead to savage and appalling aberrations. Perhaps the most typically symptomatic is seen in the clitoridectomy practised by some primitive peoples.

Suffering under such an incurable disadvantage, how can the male be purged of his envy? Surely, only by recognizing it for what it is and learning to accept it. Men do accept with a good grace many other disadvanages—their lessened life expectation, their greater morbidity and mortality at all ages, their complete expendability as biological units in warfare and hazardous enterprises. If the male could learn to think of himself as the less gifted partner in love-making, and could take his mate for his mistress and his teacher, the psychosexual relations of men and women would be put on a sounder basis. He would have his superiorities and she would have hers. Then perhaps he could start to allow her an equal place in the world. The coming decrease in the proportion of their lifespan spent in reproduction will release women for more mentally active lives. Their contribution is very urgently needed.

There are many obstacles in the way, not least in women's own attitudes, their educational deprivation and their commercial exploitation. We can be sure that Women Liberationists will not get far without male help. They must accept the help of men, and try to persuade them how necessary the liberation of women is for the welfare of men themselves, and for us all. The world in which we live has grown distorted by the institutionalization of male drives. Aggressive striving, ruthless competition between institutions and individuals, the mindless urge for material wealth, for prestige, and above all for power, these things are masculinity run mad. We are looking at our problems with one eye only, and miss all the perspective. We have the equipment for binocular vision, for a female as well as a male view-point; and we should ensure that the information reaches the decision centres. Women, they say, are more nurturative than men. Sharing the power, they would surely turn us into looking along gentler pathways. If the American Constitution had provided for a change of sex in each successive Presidency, we can be sure that such pathological phenomena as the Vietnam war would never have gone on.

The trouble about political power is that it goes to those who seek it, and so gets into the wrong hands. Those who wish for power are, above all others, those whose intentions are most to be feared. It is only the rare woman who seeks for political power; and yet the future health of our world demands that political power should be shared equally between the sexes. If this can be achieved, we shall have found a way to divert power from the power-hungry into more responsible and altruistic hands.

Conclusion

To summarize, human diversity provides not only an infinity of individual difference, but also group differences of great social importance. Where they exist, one group will be more powerful than the others, and will tend to oppress them. This is a precondition for social injustice. But the injustices are not to be remedied by denying the differences. Biological differences will always be with us. They are not to be ironed out, and it would be unwise to try. The genetical heterogeneity and biological diversity of a species are its capital and its insurance against environmental catastrophe. Differences of all kinds, genetical and cultural, are the source of our mental and spiritual wealth. If we could give up our puerile notions of superiority and inferiority, we might start to appreciate our differences for the colourful things they are. If we could put the facts first, and then see how the best use can be made of them ethically, we might start solving our problems instead of fudging them. Biological differences are basic; what we need to do is to adjust our world to make the utmost of them, and to enjoy them.

References

(1) Russell, B. (1954) *Mysticism and Logic*, pp. 13-14. Harmondsworth, Penguin.
(2) Schoeck, H. (1969) *Envy: A Theory of Social Behaviour*, trans. M. Glenny and Betty Ross. London, Secker and Warburg.
(3) Hudson, L. (1972) *The Cult of the Fact*. London, Cape.
(4) Neel, J.V., and Schull, W.J. (1968) On some trends in understanding the genetics of man. *Perspectives in Biology and Medicine*, 2, 562-602.
(5) Hubbard, Ruth (1972) Letter in *Science*, 178, 229-40.
(6) Terman, L.M. and Oden, Melitta, H. (1959) *The Gifted Group at Mid-Life*, vol. 5 of *Genetic Studies of Genius*, Ed. L.M. Terman. London, Oxford University Press.
(7) Pringle, M.L. Kellmer (1970) *Able Misfits*. London, Longman.
(8) Jensen, A.R. (1972) *Genetics and Education*. London, Methuen.
(9) Biederman, I. (1970) Testing Negro intelligence: comments on Eysenck. *The Humanist*, Jan-Feb, 34-7.
(10) Proshansky, H. and Newton, Peggy (1968) The nature and meaning of Negro self-identity.

In *Social Class, Race, and Psychological Development,* Eds. M. Deutsch, I. Katz and A.R. Jensen, pp. 178-318. New York, Holt, Rinehart and Winston.

(11)   Oxaal, I. (1969) Race, pluralism and nationalism in the British Caribbean, *J. biosoc. Sci.,* Suppl. 1, *Biosocial Aspects of Race,* Eds. G.A. Harrison and J. Peel, pp. 53-62.

(12)   Harris, G.W. (1971) Coordination of the reproductive processes. *J. biosoc. Sci.,* Suppl. 3, *Biosocial Aspects of Human Fertility,* Eds. A.A. Parkes, J. Peel and Barbara Thompson, pp. 5-12.

(13)   Hutt, Corinne (1972) *Males and Females.* Harmondsworth, Penguin.

(14)   Taylor, D.C. (1973) The influence of sexual differentiation on growth, development and disease. In *Scientific Foundations of Paediatrics,* Eds. J. Davis and J. Dobbing. London, Heinemann Medical.

(15)   Marshall, W.A. (1970) Sex differences at puberty. *J. biosoc. Sci.,* Suppl. 2, *Biosocial Aspects of Sex,* Eds. G.A. Harrison and J. Peel, pp. 31-41.

12 Inequality and the Health Service

Peter Townsend

Many histories of the evolution of health services are based on the naive assumption of continuous progress. Sometimes progress is assumed to be steady and sometimes, after a dramatic discovery in medical science, the introduction of a new method of treating disease or the introduction of legislative and administrative reform, is assumed to be rapid. The establishment of the National Health Service in England and Wales, and of the parallel services in Scotland and Northern Ireland, tends to be regarded as a glorious achievement which will endure forever. But the truth is more complex, the achievement less certain, and the future less optimistic. If achievement means just the pieces of paper which are approved by Parliament it must logically be final. If it means a living reality serving certain principles of care and distribution of resources better and better as the years pass on, it is more contentious.

Social institutions of health

Health services are social institutions, and as such they can change relatively to their own past, to other institutions, and, most important of all, to the health needs of the community. This must include the possibility of retrogression as well as progression. Sociology is only beginning to trace the implications for medicine, nursing, and public policy of a thorough social analysis of the provision of health services in these three distinct senses. That is partly because sociologists are only slowly becoming aware of the close relationship that exists between the form of the health services, definitions of the need for such services or even definitions of health, and social structure and values. That same awareness has also been slow to take root in medicine. Despite the distinguished history of epidemiology (1) the proportion of resources devoted to research and teaching in that subject remains miserably small. To take one small example, there were the whole-time equivalent of only seven specialists in social medicine among 8500 consultants attached to hospitals in England in 1972 (2).

Until very recently sociological work, notably in the United States, has taken the restricted forms of study of professional and patients' roles; of particular conceptions of illness, such as mental illness; and of particular organizations such as general hospitals for the acutely ill and mentally ill. Now the need to study the entire system of health care and its internal

A revised form of the Sir Geoffrey Vickers Lecture of 6 February 1974, the original version of which was published in the *Lancet*, 1974, *1*, 1179-90.

structure as well as its external relationship to other systems, like the economy and the polity, and particularly its relationship to national and international systems of social stratification is better recognized as providing the right framework for specialist study. This means, first, study of the structure of public and private health services through the various tiers of central Government, regional and area health authorities and local government, and hospitals, health centres, and general practice; industrial, voluntary and private agencies and services; the structure and distribution of professions, their training, and recruitment; the social and other characteristics of the different occupational groups concerned with the health of the individual and of local communities; the allocation and control of resources; and the experiences, attitudes and conditions of patients. But, second, this 'internal' system cannot be separated from its national, cultural, economic, and social setting. How far are health-care values and practices shaped by the general structure of inequality in society? Or, to put this type of question the other way round, how far has the development of the medical and other professions within the structure of health services positively contributed to the conceptions of status and rewards generally held in society? Does the system of health services help to shape the structure and values of society in general, or is the direction of influence the other way? Can one, indeed, be disentangled from the other? Can equality in medicine, like equality before the Law, be practised on a kind of island remote from the cruel inequalities of the rest of social life?

The development of health services takes place not only, of course, within a national but also, third, in a world setting. Through social means knowledge about scientific discoveries, methods of curing, preventing and controlling illness, and new types of health services is diffused. But we tend to dwell on the promotional and apparently constructive features of international relations between health systems instead of their exploitative and destructive features. Some uncomfortable facts about inequalities between nations are, it is true, revealed. Thus the statistical yearbooks of the United Nations and the World Health Organization have called our attention to the fact that while there are between 120 and 200 doctors per 100,000 population in Britain, the United States and much of Europe, there are only thirty-two in Taiwan, twenty-two in India, nineteen in Pakistan, four in Indonesia and Tanzania, two in Malawi and Nepal and one in Ethiopia (3). Too often such information is presented without any attempt to explain that some of the privileges of the rich countries are gained at the expense of the poor countries. A large proportion of Britain's hospital medical staff has been drawn from the Commonwealth. In the twelve months ending October, 1969, 164 of 169 new general practitioners moving into underdoctored areas came from overseas (4). Foreign doctors account for 20% of the annual addition to the American profession, and it has been calculated that the United States gains more in dollar value of medical aid from the rest of the world than it provides in aid to foreign countries, publicly, and privately (5). The third world is also disadvantaged in some respects by attempts to introduce inappropriate Western concepts of medicine and treatment and by the profit-seeking operation of the drug companies. The international profit-and-loss account in relations between health service systems requires searching scrutiny, not just because systems in the third world remain deprived but because inequalities in care in Western systems may be reinforced and because Western conceptions of health care may be culturally insular if not smug. There may be instructive lessons to be drawn from health services in developing countries.

This analytic framework, although very sketchily drawn, has implications for any evaluation of change. I have spoken of conceptions of illness or health, the structure of the health care system, and the pattern of health needs in society. Any one, or all, of these three may change significantly over time. If our definition of what constitutes illness and states of health is greatly extended and complicated, our expectations of the health services and the standards by which we judge them change correspondingly. By this test the health services may fall further short of expectations. Even if our definition remains roughly constant we may find that the reduction in the prevalence of some diseases has to be weighed against the growth in prevalence of others. The reasons for disappointing as well as encouraging trends have to be sought in the structure and operation as much of the health care system as in society generally. I am alluding not simply to changes, for example, in the number, distribution, and quality of health personnel, compared with the past, but also their responsiveness to present patterns of need.

The development of health services, therefore, has to be measured in relation to changing conceptions of illness or health and to patterns of need. Conceptions are constantly being amended or revised. There are substantial cultural differences between developing and market or planned societies, and also among the latter. Revisions are made not just in response to the recognition and communication of social discovery and innovation, or to professional judgments of objective needs and of the status of different diseases and treatments, but also in response to the pressure of vested interests, and the level and type of public anxiety and demand. Pain, discomfort, debility and different forms of incapacity may come to play, in relation to prospective sudden death or physiological malfunctioning, a more prominent part in social and medical conceptions. Types of human behaviour may be shifted into the territory labelled 'illness' and controversies about the demarcation of the boundaries may be settled. The boundary is continually being redrawn and disputed. This could be illustrated from the history of so-called 'fringe' medicine, the history of the treatment of madness, and the diverse history in different countries of the treatment of severe mental handicap. Fundamentally, all societies distinguish between those abnormal, conditions and actions requiring sympathetic indulgence and expert aid, and those conditions and actions regarded as deviant and requiring reprobation and correction. Inevitably medicine is drawn into the argument by virtue of its responsibility for definitions of illness or disability. In this debate, we may observe, medicine is by no means necessarily on the side of the humanitarian or radical values. While some types of criminals have been reclassified as sick and have as a consequence received rehabilitative rather than custodial or punitive forms of treatment, some types of healthy people, who happen to have been critical of Government or an embarrassment to the community, have been classified as sick and removed from view.

Just as the scope of the conception may change, elements within it may be accorded different weight or priority. Views are reached about the seriousness of certain states of health. The construction and priorities of the health services follow suit. The relative scale and importance of different services tend to get distorted whether, for example, as a result of willingness on the part of consultants and general practitioners to accede to requests for certain forms of treatment and surgery (cosmetic surgery is a case in point) or as a result of the disproportionate esteem in which certain types of specialist roles are held within the medical profession (as in the unequal value accorded to acute as compared with chronic sickness, physical as compared with mental illness or handicap, surgery as compared with preventive health). Health personnel, patients, and organizations come to be divided up more for purposes of status differentiation than mere convenience or efficiency. Once institutionalized, an unbalanced structure affects the behaviour of participants. It affects priorities, for example, by influencing the number and urgency of referrals and distorts professional as well as public judgments of medical need, and hence what is believed in society to be the nature of illness itself. In short, conceptions of illness or disability and therefore also of severity of condition are shaped socially. They are institutionalized in medical practice and the organization, subdivisions, and administration of services.

That is why, under the aegis of the medical and social sciences, there has to be an unremitting search for independent, detached, or objective standards of measurement or evaluation. As I have suggested, this can be done to a large extent by systematic application of the comparative method; conceptions of health standards of care and investment of resources can be compared cross-culturally, resources and quality of service can be compared regionally and locally, between short-stay and long-stay patients, between services in institutions and those in the community, between rich and poor, people of different age, the employed and the non-employed, and people with different types of disease or disability. Like the scientist's use of the randomized control trial (6), this approach represents one of the social scientist's methods of attempting to escape subjectivity and convention and so to comprehend the subtle operations of prejudice and privilege in our midst.

The National Health Service (NHS)

Some of these ideas can be applied to the NHS. Its creation has deeper roots than is often supposed (7). The vast majority of hospital patients, for example, were treated free long before 1948. Paying patients had never accounted for more than a small fraction, perhaps 5%, of all hospital patients (7). As elsewhere in Europe there was a long history of the sponsorship and control by consumers of prepayment methods of meeting medical costs. In 1804, long before the British Medical Association (BMA) was founded, there were about a million members of friendly societies in Britain and, in 1900, seven million (8). Between 1918 and 1939, beginning with the Dawson Report in 1920, a succession of studies and reports recommending a comprehensive health service were issued by a wide range of different organizations, including the BMA. The Emergency Medical Service and the extension of national health insurance in the 1939-45 war preceded the declaration of principle in the Beveridge Report and the Coalition Government's white papers. A

Conservative Government would have been obliged in 1945 to sustain the momentum. But despite this propitious history and a national consensus about the desirability of a service, political courage and staying power were still required to resolve the contest between different interest groups and create a more or less unified structure. Weaker or less astute men than Aneurin Bevan would have settled for a lot less than he did. Like other overseas historians, Almont Lindsay concluded that 'the Health Service cannot very well be excluded from any list of notable achievements of the 20th Century' (9). In his biography of Aneurin Bevan, Michael Foot pointed out that in July 1960 even the *British Medical Journal* paid tribute to the 'imagination and flexibility' of 'the most brilliant Minister of Health this country has ever had' (10). Foot quoted Lord Hill to suggest that certain major features of the final plans for the service—the fusion of voluntary and local authority hospitals into one nationally coordinated hospital scheme, and the abolition of the ownership of medical practices—owed much to Bevan (11).

Even now the immediate social effects are difficult to disentangle. In 1938, 20% of general practitioners in their forties earned under £700 per annum and the average GP only £938. The Spens Committee recommended a 13% increase in the average, before adding any increase for inflation between 1938 and 1948 (12). There are, therefore, strong grounds for arguing that the profession as a whole, and poorer doctors especially, gained in income as a result of the introduction of the Service. Again, middle-class families could be said to have been freed for the first time from the crippling financial prospects of paying for care during a serious disabling illness. But working-class women and children also gained in the sense that they had not previously been covered by health insurance for GP consultations and prescriptions, though many obtained free or subsidized care through the voluntary hospitals. Certainly the Government's *Surveys of Sickness* showed an increase in the use of GP services by lower-income groups between 1945 and 1952 (13). The question 'Who gained?' is still worth debating, in order to break down the myths and stereotypes which too easily circulate and to lay the basis for searching analysis of who gains today.

Suppose, then, we try to pursue the question of the achievements or effects of the introduction of the NHS. After an initial period of panic about high and growing costs the Government and the profession were educated, especially by the Guillebaud Report and the measured evidence assembled by Abel-Smith and Titmuss, into more positive support of its operation and needs. The pronouncements of the two major medical journals afford significant illustration. From the start *The Lancet* was a powerful advocate. Ten years after the Act was passed the journal announced (14): 'For our part we think the National Health Service one of the biggest improvements in the life of this country since the war. . . It has done much to better the conditions of medical care, especially in hospital, and it has been an immense comfort to the public.' But, 'Any jubilation must be at best provisional.' Morale was 'not high'; the status of the doctor was 'depreciating'; administration had to be made 'more appropriate to its purpose, and more efficient'.

Not surprisingly, in view of its unremitting campaign against the introduction of the Service, the *British Medical Journal* was more critical (15): 'The end of the first decade of a social revolution finds the profession in no mood for jubilation ... whatever benefits it has received the public is beginning uneasily to wonder whether the price has not been too high in this free-for-all scramble for medical attention. . . A plebiscite today (among the profession) would undoubtedly show a majority to be highly critical of the Service in favour of reform.' The prophets of gloom and disaster were already qualifying their criticism heavily. Note the implicit acknowledgment of a 'social revolution', 'benefits' to the public, and 'reform' rather than dismantlement. The *BMJ* went on: 'most people would agree ... that from the point of view of the public the Health Service has been a success. Many barriers that existed before have been removed, especially for those of moderate means. There has been a more even distribution of consultants throughout the country and a general increase of hosptial facilities. But many of the benefits laid at the door of the NHS more properly could be credited to the advances of modern medicine' (15).

Twenty years later *The Lancet* acknowledged the continuing criticisms of administrative structure and inadequate resources, but concentrated on the issues of economizing on resources by building upon collaborative experiments between different arms of the Service, group practices and health centres, the need to bridge the widening division between consultant and family doctor, and much better communication between doctor and patient. It maintained the view that 'the first principle and chief strength of the NHS was that good medical care is a right and not a privilege and, in application, is a powerful safeguard of standards of efficiency and courtesy' (16).

These views call our attention to the diverse nature of evaluation and the problem of monitoring changing expectations, performance, and need.

Measures of health

Estimates of the effect or value of the Health Service depend of course on the kind as well as availability of information used to measure such effect or value. There are measures of health, as such, which depend on conceptions of health, and there are measures of utilization and provision of services, each of which is needed to assist explanations of trends in health, and of social differences in mortality and morbidity.

Measures of the health of populations can take many different forms. Among the most familiar are mortality rates, prevalence or incidence morbidity rates, sickness-absence rates, and restricted-activity rates. Each is limited as an indicator of health and involves problems of measurement. If we were to concentrate too much attention on mortality we should imply that health services can adopt the goals of death in life or medicated survival, and if on medically identifiable morbidity that some conditions of listlessness, depression, sleeplessness, and anxiety can be discounted or at least be treated relatively lightly. It was to bring wider conceptions of states of health into the picture that the World Health Organization adopted the sweeping goal of positive physical, mental and social wellbeing rather than the absence of disease. This posed problems not only of measurement in research and the collection of statistical data but of the practical use of such measures in preventive and curative health policies. Attempts are indeed being made to construct more sophisticated health indicators. Thus, one 'state of health' indicator combines the two dimensions of pain and restricted activity (17). The problem here is that the pursuit of novel methods can lead to an arrogant disregard of the valuable lessons that can be drawn by continuing to apply the simpler methods used in pioneering studies, like Titmuss's *Poverty and Population.*

Let me give a few examples. By the test of trends in mortality rates, critical questions have to be posed about the performance of Britain's health services. The test can be made in different ways. First, reduction in mortality rates has been slower in Britain than in some other advanced industrial societies. A Scottish study pointed out that despite a continuing reduction of infant mortality over the past twenty years England and Wales slipped from fifth to eighth place, and Scotland from eighth to twelfth in the ranking of the countries (18). Table 1 gives illustrations of the differential rates of improvement, including remarkable improvements in the Netherlands, Belgium, France, and especially, Japan.

TABLE 1   Infant mortality: rate per 1000 live births

Country	1950	1960	1970	1971
Netherlands	25.2	17-9	12.7	11.1
USA	29.2	26.0	19.8	19.2
United Kingdom	31.4	22.5	18.4	17.9
Canada	41.3	27.3	18.8	17.6
France	52.0	27.4	15.1	14.4
Belgium	53.4	31.2	20.5	19.8
USSR	—	35.0	24.4	22.6
Germany (Fed. Rep.)	55.5	33.8	23.6	23.2
Japan	60.1	30.7	13.1	12.4
Italy	63.8	43.9	29.2	28.3

Source: UN Statistical Yearbook 1972.

The same trends can be followed, though less reliably, at later ages. Even a cursory scrutiny of the United Nations *Statistical Yearbook* shows, for example for men, that while the expectation of life at birth has lengthened in England and Wales by 2% or 3% in twenty years, it has lengthened more dramatically in other industrial nations, some of which have now surpassed, and others almost attained, our figure.

The explanation of the figures can be pursued by examining inequalities between the sexes, age groups, classes, areas, types of disease, and disability. Over a period of twenty years the ratio of female to male expectation of life in England and Wales has increased at all ages. While female expectation of life has lengthened at all ages male expectation has increased to only a modest extent among those in their twenties and thirties, has barely increased among men aged forty-five, and has decreased marginally among older men (Table 2).

The trends are different for people of different class, and, in terms of probing constructively the operation of the Health Service, are perhaps the

TABLE 2   Expectation of life (years), England and Wales

Age	Males		Females	
	1948-50	1968-70	1948-50	1968-70
0	66.3	68.6	71.0	74.9
5	64.2	65.3	68.4	71.3
25	45.3	46.0	49.4	51.7
45	27.0	27.1	30.9	32.6
55	18.8	18.7	22.4	23.8
65	12.2	11.9	14.6	15.8

Source: DHSS (41), Table 1.6.

most important of all to examine. Between 1949-53 and 1959-63 inequality between social classes in mortality experience appears, from data published by the Registrar General, to have widened. Indeed, 'the social class gradient increases with successive censuses so that in 1959-63 the Standardized Mortality Ratio for social class I is only about half that of social class V' (19). The trouble is that the figures do not represent the real trends very accurately, because of changes introduced in 1960 in the classification of occupations, possible changes in the number and extent of discrepancies between the recording of occupations on death certificates and on census schedules, and the fact that occupations in the Census of 1961 were based on a 10% sample.

Statisticians and social scientists have therefore been slow to utilize the data, dismayed perhaps by the Registrar General's statement that 'It is impossible to disentangle real differential changes in mortality in this context from apparent differences due to changes in classification' (19). But the Registrar General must bear responsibility for failing to disentangle these elements, for example by working out the SMRs for each class in 1959-63 according to the 1950 Census of Occupations and not only for social class V, which he did as a kind of partial addendum. Specialist analysis and anxiety, and public comment, have been inhibited.

Yet the data are of immense significance. Further examination suggests that even if its exact extent remains debatable the trend of growing inequality is securely established. For example, the Registrar General points out that among the closed professions the data are 'substantially free from the effect of classification changes, and errors due to mis-statement of occupation or change of occupation must be few', and between 1951 and 1961 the mortality rates for middle-aged lawyers, teachers, and clergymen fell more sharply than those for all men. So 'not all the improvements in social classes I and II is due to differences in classification'. Moreover, he finds that 'the most disturbing feature of the present results when compared with earlier analyses is the apparent deterioration in social class V. . . . whilst the mortality of all men fell at all ages except 70-74, that for social class V men . . . rose at all ages except 25-34. *Even when the rates are adjusted to the 1950 classification,* it is clear that class V men fared much worse than average' (my emphasis) (19). An adjusted figure for class V as a whole is not given, but the adjusted figures for particular age groups (Table D6) suggest that if the old classificaton had been used the figure of 143 in Table 3 for social class V would still be around 128, representing a clear deterioration between 1949-53 and 1959-63.

TABLE 3   Standardized mortality ratios by social class

Social class	Men (15-64)			Married women (15-64)	Single women (15-64)
	1930-32	1949-53	1959-63	1959-63	1959-63
I. Professional	90	86	76	77	83
II. Managerial	94	92	81	83	88
III. Skilled manual and non-manual	97	101	100	102	90
IV. Partly skilled	102	104	103	105	108
V. Unskilled	111	118	143	141	121

(1) Information about occupations in the 1961 Census with which information from death
  certificates for 1959-63 was compared, was based on a 10% sample.
(2) Occupations in 1961 were reclassified on a new basis with the result that approximately 24%
  would have been allocated to a different class if the 1950 basis of classification had been used.
  However, the vast majority of these (92%) were reclassified to the next ascending or descending
  class in rank order.
(3) The SMRs for 1949-53 in column 2 have been adjusted by the Registrar General from the
  figures first published to correct certain errors.

Source: Registrar General's Decennial Supplement (19), Tables D4 and 4.

For ten separate causes, mortality rates for all age groups of class V
improved less or deteriorated more than the equivalent rates for all men. In
1959-63 more class V men died at every age than in 1949-53 from cancer of the
lung, vascular lesions of the central nervous system, arteriosclerotic and
degenerative heart disease, motor vehicle accidents, and other accidents. Some
diseases, like lung cancer, and duodenal ulcer, which showed no trend with
social class, or, like coronary disease, an inverse trend forty years ago, are now
producing much higher mortality in social classes IV and V than I and II (20).
In his latest report the Registrar General found that for 49 out of 85 separate
causes of death applying to men, and for 54 out of 87 applying to women,
standardized mortality ratios for social classes IV and V were higher than for I
and II (Table E1). For only four causes of death in each instance was the class
gradient reversed. It would seem from this evidence that undue attention has
been given in recent years to the so-called diseases of affluence.

Inequality between the classes in mortality experience is roughly the same
among married women, but rather less pronounced among single women,
than among men (see Table 3). The disadvantages of membership of class V
for women as well as men are striking. Inequalities tend to be most
pronounced not among the oldest age groups but among men between 25 and
44, among married women between 15 and 44 and among single women
between 15 and 34 (Table 4).

These data need to be related to changes in types and conditions of work,
income, nutritional status, environmental conditions, and styles of living.
There remain, for example, big differences in death rates by area, with the
urban industrial areas of the North and of Wales on the one hand, and the
county towns, seaside resorts, and metropolitan suburbs of the South and
South-East on the other, continuing to represent the inequality of national

TABLE 4 Comparative incidence of social class mortalities in different age groups for men, married women, and single women (1959-63)

	Social class	15-19	20-24	25-34	35-44	45-54	55-64	65-74
Men	I	72	59	73	69	76	78	86
	II	106	85	72	73	77	84	94
	III	97	90	89	97	100	102	116
	IV	118	100	107	104	104	101	105
	V	142	149	181	181	158	134	123
Married	I	(38)	(79)	83	75	78	76	74
women	II	(41)	64	76	79	82	85	93
	III	97	97	99	102	102	102	111
	IV	(88)	92	103	106	104	106	107
	V	(159)	159	163	153	144	136	128
Single	I	97	79	(67)	82	86	83	103
women	II	103	70	56	65	82	99	144
	III	78	72	74	73	86	104	144
	IV	95	98	93	97	104	116	166
	V	197	213	145	132	105	119	130

Source: Registrar General's Decennial Supplement (19), Tables 3 and 4.

industrial and social structure. Thus in 1959-63 the death rate of infants under one year was between 30 and 33 per 1000 live births in Bootle, Merthyr Tydfil, Preston, and Oldham and only 17 or 18 in Oxford, Ipswich, Exeter, Hampstead, and Croydon. For the same years the death rate of men aged 45-64 was between 18 and 20 per 1000 of that age in Salford, Manchester, Bootle, Burnley, Dewsbury, and Merthyr Tydfil and only 11 or 12 in Ipswich, Oxford, Great Yarmouth, and Southend.

Taking all adults of both sexes between the ages of 15 and 64 the disadvantages during the five years 1959-63 can be summarized. If the mortality experience of social class I had applied to social class V, only just over half of them would have died; 40,000 lives would have been spared.

This disturbing trend has to be judged in the context of a wide variety of other data. Although maternal mortality among married women has continued to fall, the differences between the social classes have widened (19). Trends in infant mortality are harder to establish. As Morris and others have shown, the differential between the classes narrowed between 1930 and 1950 but this was during a period when the differential was greater than it was in the case of adult mortality (20). By 1959-63 the differential seems to have come to correspond more closely with that for adults (see Table 5), but separate data for each social class and for different occupations for the three Census periods have not been published (21). This is a serious gap in medical and social knowledge, as Hart has eloquently argued (22).

In the early 1960s the Department of Health became concerned about the slow decrease in the death-rate for infants at ages between one month and one year and undertook a study in three areas to try to identify avoidable factors contributing to deaths. Two paediatric assessors estimated that there were

TABLE 5 Comparative incidence of infant mortality by social class

Social class	Ratios of actual to expected deaths of infants		
	1930-32	1949-53	1959-63
I	53	63	} 73
II	73	73	
III	94	97	98
IV	108	114	} 119
V	125	138	

Source: Estimates derived by Hart (22) from Spicer and Lipworth (21).

avoidable factors in 28% of cases, in about a third of which social factors, another third parental factors and a quarter of which general practitioner or hospital factors were believed to be responsible. The GP factors included diagnostic delay or failure, slowness in reference to hospital, failure to realise severity of the situation, and delay in visiting. The hospital service factors involved diagnostic failures or delay, hospital acquired infection, and faulty management (23). This was a pilot inquiry and it is likely that more rigorous research on a comparative basis would come better to grips with all the factors involved and demonstrate inadequacies not only of income, environment, and education, but of health services too.

A good start has been made in parallel work in hospitals. A number of research studies have demonstrated sharp differences among hospitals in the outcome of treatment for specific conditions, some types of hospital, for example, having much higher rates of case fatality (24). This type of work begins to call attention to inequalities in the distribution of resources, and quality of care, in the hospital service.

To what extent are the patterns produced by analyses of mortality a misleading representation of patterns of illness? One source of information is sickness absence rates. While pointing out the unusual degree of care that has to be exercized in interpreting sickness absence statistics, some studies show, for example, high correlations between mortality and inception rates of sickness, and between mortality and days of sickness (25). Various reservations have to be made about particular types of diseases and causes of mortality. Thus, diseases of the respiratory system 'cause a considerably larger proportion of sickness than of mortality, but the average length of such spells of sickness is comparatively short. On the other hand, arteriosclerotic and degenerative heart disease cause over a quarter of male deaths in the age range 15-64, but only a very small part of the total sickness is recorded against them, but where such sickness does occur, it is of long duration' (25) But in compiling mortality and sickness absence ratios both for specific occupations and for social classes, such factors tend to balance out, and there are high correlations between the two, especially between mortality and days of sickness. Table 6 compares mortality with sickness absence ratios by social class. The sickness absence ratios were derived from claims for sickness benefit in Britain for the period June 5, 1961, to June 2, 1962, as analysed in a Government report (26). Spells of notified sickness lasting less than four days

TABLE 6 Comparative ratios for mortality (1959-63) and sickness absence (1961-62) for males by social class

Social class	All males 15-64	Employed males 15-64 sickness	
		Comparative inception figure	Comparative duration figure
I and II	80	64	50
III	100	100	93
IV	103	109	117
V	143	124	154

Source: Daw (25).

were excluded, since very few such spells are reported. Some long-term sickness was excluded because those who had been ill for a long time were less likely to be on an employer's payroll.

A second measure of morbidity has been developed recently. For 1972 the General Household Survey found that in England and Wales nearly three times as many unskilled as professional men and more than three times as many females suffered, by their own account, from 'limiting long-standing illness, disability or infirmity' (27) (Table 7). For 1971, according to the same source, nearly 2½ times as many unskilled as professional men reported absence from work due to illness or injury during a two-week period and they lost an average of 4½ times as many days from work in the year (28). Like mortality ratios, both sickness absence ratios and measures of 'limiting long-standing illness' demonstrate the disadvantage of the partly skilled and unskilled occupational classes.

Another, indirect, measure of state of health is of physique. Careful measures of differences in height and weight in a population can be valuable

TABLE 7 Morbidity: limiting long-standing illness, 1972 rates expressed as a percentage of those for all socio-economic groups

Socio-economic groups	Males				Females			
	All ages	15-44	45-64	65+	All ages	15-44	45-64	65+
Professional	64	89	63	—	55	71	65	—
Employers and managerial	79	94	62	84	69	94	60	75
Intermediate and junior non-manual	89	91	98	82	81	75	88	90
Skilled manual	95	96	101	101	96	122	102	100
Partly skilled	126	109	129	115	137	112	134	111
Unskilled	164	177	160	124	166	137	132	113
All	100	100	100	100	100	100	100	100

Source: Social Trends, 1973, no. 4, Table 69.

indicators of trends in health. In the mid-1960s data from the National Child Development Study for seven-year-olds showed that there had been 'little if any change in Social Class differences' since 1953. The actual figures derived from the two studies show a slight widening of the gap—though this could be attributable to sampling and slight differences in method. An average difference in height of 3.3 cm between children from social class I or II and those from social class V was found, compared with 2.8 cm between 'upper middle class' and 'lower working class' children in 1953 (29, 30).

Inequalities in the development of services

I am painfully aware that these measures of health are incomplete and that a more comprehensive picture might be built up patiently from the rich literature which we possess, even if, in the end, the aim to develop in precise terms a balanced index of the health needs of the population remained unfulfilled. But the measurement of inequalities in need by class or by income is, I believe, central to that task and to the evaluation of the Health Service.

The role of the Health Service is by no means the only or even the crucial factor in determining social differences in mortality or morbidity. Explanations for inequalities in health have complex aetiologies. The quality and distribution of different health services could improve relative to other social institutions as well as the past and yet, because of a relative growth in other forms of inequality of incomes or wealth, work conditions and physical arduousness, home, family and social conditions and life styles, the effects of such improvement on trends in mortality, morbidity, and states of health could be cancelled out. But trends in the organization and utilization of the health services must themselves be summarized and understood.

We must proceed from the general to the particular. Britain devotes a

TABLE 8   Total expenditures for health services as a percentage of GNP and average percentage rate of increase, seven countries 1961-69

Country	Early 1960s		1969	Average annual rate of increase in real terms (%)†
	Year	% of GNP	% of GNP	
Canada	1961	6.0	7.3	7.7
United States	1961-62	5.8	6.8	9.0
Sweden	1962	5.4	6.7	8.7
Netherlands	1963	4.8	5.9	8.7
Germany				
(Fed. Rep.)	1961	4.5*	5.7	4.7
France	1963	4.4	5.7	6.5
United Kingdom	1961-62	4.2	4.8	5.1

* Estimate made by the US Social Security Administration.
† Health expenditures adjusted by the US Social Security Administration according to average consumer price index and wage index changes.

Source: Simanis (34) and Abel-Smith (32).

smaller proportion of its total resources to the health services than several other advanced industrial societies, and this proportion is growing less swiftly (Table 8). Earlier studies for WHO (31, 32), and by the Canadian Royal Commission on Health Services (33) had shown that Britain's percentage of gross national product devoted to health had remained fairly static in the first years after the establishment of the National Health Service in 1948, while that of other countries had been growing. The latest comparative study shows that although Britain's figure grew in the 1960s, it grew relatively slowly: 'Three countries, France, Canada, and Sweden, have the most rapid adjusted rate of growth in health expenditures, ranging from 8.7 to 9.0 per cent. In contrast, Germany and the United Kingdom show the slowest growth rate, 4.7 and 5.1 per cent, respectively' (34). The rate of growth was approximately the same under the Labour Administration of 1964-70 as under the Conservative Administration of 1959-63, and was distinctly smaller than the rate for other social services (e.g. education) (35, 36). According to the latest public expenditure programme for the years up to 1977-78, this pattern is unlikely to change—indeed, proposed expenditure on health for the next five years has been cut back from what was envisaged in the previous white paper (37).

Although Britain spends relatively less than, say, the United States, this is partly because its health services are less expensive, and partly because its rates of admission to hospital and rates of surgery are lower (38). There is evidence too that, from a smaller cost base, services are in some respects more equally distributed. Thus, utilization of medical services by different status groups, by the acute and chronic sick or mentally ill and handicapped, and by adults below and above pensionable age, is more unequal in the United States than in Britain (39, 40). On the other hand, services in some Eruopean countries, such as Czechoslovakia and Sweden, are less unequally distributed in some respects than in Britain, for example, between the acute sick and the chronic sick, mentally ill or handicapped in hospital (31, 32).

The hospitals have more than maintained their share (more than half) of total expenditure on health services. Against a slightly lower total number of in-patient beds (though with much higher admission and discharge rates) has to be set a doubling of both hospital medical and nursing staff between 1949 and 1971. But the number of general medical practitioners has not changed substantially. In 1959 there were 38% more general practitioners than hospital medical staff in England and Wales; in 1971 there were 8% less. This suggests the power or predominance of the hospital in the British system, the increasing location of clinical expertise outside local communities, and the evolution of a better developed status hierarchy in medical practice, consultants obtaining enhanced power.

In total the number of physicians in the UK has been growing less swiftly than in countries such as Sweden, France, Belgium and the United States, and it has substantially fewer doctors per 100,000 population than a wide range of countries (Table 9). We can note in passing that there are countries like the Netherlands and Japan which have achieved striking reductions in the infant mortality rates in recent years without major addition to their medical manpower. Britain's heavy dependence on medical personnel from overseas makes comparison on the other hand with other countries, especially the third world, all the more poignant. In 1971, 33.5% had been born in overseas

TABLE 9   Numbers of physicians per 100,000 population in selected countries 1960-1970

Country	Year	Number	Year	Number
Czechoslovakia	1962	185	1969	200
Austria	1962	182	1970	185
Hungary	1961	164	1969	192
Italy	1961	164	1970	181
Germany (Fed. Rep.)	1962	149	1969	168
Belgium	1962	139	1968	155
United States	1962	132	1969	149
Denmark	1960	123	1969	145
Spain	1962	122	1969	132
Netherlands	1961	112	1970	120
Japan	1962	111	1969	111
England and Wales	1960	104	1969	117
Sweden	1961	100	1969	130

Source: UN Statistical Yearbooks, 1964 and 1971.

countries other than Ireland; however, the figure is only 13% for consultants, compared with 55% for registrars and 61% for senior house-officers. Between 1969 and 1971, 35% of the net addition of 2038 to the total medical personnel of England and Wales had been born overseas, including 76% of the 500 medical practitioners (41). The net addition in these two years of 714 from overseas represents more than the entire medical manpower of Guinea and Congo, nearly the same as that of Kenya or the Sudan, and more than double that of Ethiopia.

Is medical manpower better distributed as a consequence of the operation of the Health Service? Let me quote one authority, Sir George Godber, in his valedictory report in 1973 as Chief Medical Officer, *On the State of the Public Health* (42):

'Although Britain's relatively low health expenditure may be partly due to more economical delivery of our centrally financed services . . . it is still true that there is great unevenness in the distribution of the funds we have in proportion to population in Great Britain and within England. Some areas started with greater resources of people and of things and a higher level of finance than others. The South-East of England has substantial advantages over the North-East or the Midlands and Scotland has substantial advantages over England and Wales as a whole in manpower and money. At the end of 25 years these differences, particularly in the distribution of medical manpower, still exist.'

The sociologist might only comment that discussion of inequalities between regions and areas is too often sealed off from discussion of the underlying inequalities of class, income, and housing and living conditions created in our market economy and that these underlying inequalities are even more important to attend to if the claim that the NHS 'has preserved more successfully than most of the other systems both freedom of access to medical and allied care at times of need and the availability of a personal medical attendant' is to be justified (42). Neither social class nor income level features as a variable in analysis or even as a term so far as I can discern anywhere in the 182 pages of the Chief Medical Officer's report *On the State of the Public*

Health for 1972, or for that matter in the reports of the previous three years, and there is no discussion of the decennial supplements and other reports on the relationship between mortality and class.

In some respects long-term improvements in the distribution of medical manpower cannot be demonstrated. Since 1948, areas with too few GPs have been designated and mild inducements introduced for doctors to practise there. Up to 1958 the proportion of doctors working in areas with high average lists of patients fell, then fluctuated, and in the mid- and late 1960s increased rapidly. A recent careful study concluded: 'The National Health Service has not brought about any dramatic shift in the location of GPs. . . The broad patterns of staffing needs have not changed dramatically over the last twenty to thirty years. Areas which are currently facing the most serious shortages seem to have a fairly long history of manpower difficulties, whilst those which are today relatively well supplied with family doctors have generally had no difficulty in past years in attracting and keeping an adequate number of practitioners. . . . Certain areas of the country are medically deprived in the sense that the existing services are unable to cope with the demands placed upon them, while others have a relative abundance of medical resources in relation to their needs' (43). In planning health services, deprived areas have to be identified more precisely, though in relation to the more fundamental problem of deprived strata.

According to some specialists evidence about consultation rates by social class broadly suggests an equitable distribution of services (44, 45). However, the evidence is limited either because in scope it does not allow precise analysis by individual class, age group, and type of area, (46), or because sufficient account cannot be taken of the place, type, length and content of consultation (47). Data about large lists in industrial areas (43) and the tendency of middle-class patients to be on small lists or the lists of practitioners with further qualifications and easy access to diagnostic and special therapeutic facilities (40) do in themselves suggest unequal outcomes. For social classes IV and V the latest evidence suggests relatively low utilization under the age of five, relatively high utilization in late middle

TABLE 10 Consultation rates per person per year, for males only, 1971 expressed as a percentage of those per person for all socioeconomic groups

Socio-economic group	Age					
	All	0-4	5-14	15-44	45-64	65+
Professional, employers and managers	100	113	105	100	91	100
Intermediate and junior non-manual	97	111	95	100	88	96
Skilled manual	103	107	95	104	100	107
Partly skilled and un-skilled manual	109	65	105	117	132	96
All	100	100	100	100	100	100

Source: General Household Survey (28).

age, and just under average utilization over the age of 65 (Table 10).

But most important of all is the fact that utilization is not standardized by need. For all age groups utilization of medical services by class does not correspond with measures of need, at least as expressed by those of mortality, sickness absence and limiting long-standing illness (as in Tables 3-7).

In pursuing measures of utilization by social class or income level, two distinctions are necessary. If the number of consultations in a year are aggregated for each of two categories which are to be compared, differences between the proportions in each category not consulting at all and those consulting frequently because of some long-standing disability may be obscured. Consultations for acute episodes and among the chronic sick need to be distinguished. Again, some effort has to be made to standardize for type of consultation. Some consultations may be more for 'social control' or administrative purposes than to meet a specific health need, for example, medical certification for bad housing or sickness insurance.

I am arguing that measures of utilization have to be related to measures of need. This principle has been applied imaginatively in Britain by some writers lately (49, 50) but no opportunity seems to have been taken to apply it as systematically as in some other societies. For example, a Finnish study published in 1968 showed that the average number of consultations per 100 days with a physician was higher in the lowest than in the highest income group, but when consultations were standardized in respect of days of sickness, the trend was reversed. Moreover, the advantage of the relatively rich was shown for both the acute and chronic sick: 'The lower the income, the higher the morbidity and the lower the utilization of medical services in relation to morbidity.' Incidentally, and this has important implications for the development in Britain of group practice, health centres, and district general hospitals of substantial size, the use of a physician's services was found to decrease with increasing distance to physician for all groups (51).

In building up a picture of utilization of different health services it must not be supposed, because some services are heavily utilized by the poorer working classes, that this is necessarily contributory evidence of equitable provision of health services as a whole. Like other major institutional systems of society the health system is organized in a hierarchy of value and status. No one today would argue that the heavy utilization of secondary modern schools by the working classes constitutes evidence of equality of education provision. Despite the scarcity of data the point can be made for health institutions. In a national study of the elderly in institutions in the mid-1960s I found that more of those from non-manual than unskilled or partly skilled manual backgrounds were in geriatric hospitals than in psychiatric hospitals, even when some attempt was made to standardize among patients by degree of incapacity, confusion, and lucidity, and were also in the better endowed hospitals within these sectors—defined by furnishings and shared spaces as well as staffing ratios. The same applied to the populations of private, voluntary, and newly built local-authority residential homes, when compared with the populations of older local-authority homes (52-4). At least to some extent, clinical and administrative decisions seem to be influenced both by the status of institutions and the social class of patients. More, too, of the poorer working classes may stay longer in certain health and residential institutions

TABLE 11 Weekly cost per patient of different types of hospital as % of cost per patient in acute non-teaching hospitals (England and Wales)

Type of hospital	1955- 56*	1958- 59*	1966- 67	1970- 71	1971- 72†
Teaching hospitals (London)	153	145	143	150	147
Teaching hospitals (outside)	121	120	127	136	130
Maternity	109	103	104	101	102
Mainly acute	92	86	88	88	89
Chronic sick	45	43	42	41	40
Mental illness	30	29	31	33	33
Mental handicap	28	27	27	29	31

* Based on limited coverage of hospitals.
† England only.

Source: DHSS (41), Table 2.9. Cost per inpatient week of acute non-teaching hospitals was £17.75 in 1955-56, £23.85 in 1958-59, £43.13 in 1966-67, £65.03 in 1970-71 and (for England only) £76.65 in 1971-72.

for social reasons, either because there is no easy alternative mode of life for them in the community (they cannot find homes, have no capital and little income) or because the institutions in which they live develop a functional need for their labour, their lack of demand upon a hard-pressed medical and nursing staff or their value for teaching.

That there is a hierarchy of status and quality of care can be illustrated from the hospital costings returns and new statistical studies of the distribution of services published by the DHSS. First, the structure of expenditure and staffing in different types of hospital is hard to defend. Table 11 shows that cost per patient in long-stay, chronic, mental illness and mental handicap hospitals ranges from only under a third to about two-fifths of that in acute hospitals. This is attributable not just to greater need for, and provision of, medical and nursing staff in the latter, as Table 12 demonstrates. Even the costs of domestic services, catering, laundry, and general cleaning, for example, in the low-status hospitals are substantially below half the comparable costs in the acute hospitals. The differences are not easy to explain simply as reflections of differences of staffing, space, and the presence of equipment. And the pattern is even more astonishing when costs and staffing ratios for individual low-status hospitals are examined. The average number of medical staff in mental illness hospitals in 1971 was 1.8 per 100 patients, but among hospitals with 200 beds or more it varied from 0.75 to 8.7. The average number of nurses was 36.3, but varied from 22.5 to 70.6. In mental handicap hospitals the range per 100 patients was between 0.05 and 2.55 for medical staff and between 15.4 and 59.2 for nursing staff. It seems unlikely that different composition of patient populations can explain such pronounced inequalities (55). Comprehensive official statistics can be used in this way to confirm the more elaborate findings of independent research surveys (56, 57).

Second, the structure of inequality has not changed much over the years.

TABLE 12 Cost per inpatient-week of different services in different types of hospital as a percentage of the cost of non-teaching hospitals, England, 1971-72

Type of service	Acute hospitals (over 100 beds)		Maternity	Long-stay	Chronic	Mental illness	Mental handicap
	Amount (£)	%					
Medical	4.48	100	65	27	13	26	13
Nursing	20.81	100	152	66	66	45	40
Domestic	3.76	100	143	58	60	27	27
Catering	7.39	100	100	55	48	45	43
Laundry	1.45	100	163	63	62	38	46
Power, light and heat	2.43	100	115	65	57	50	42
Building and engineering maintenance	3.11	100	92	60	50	60	54
General cleaning	0.74	100	182	68	55	35	32
Total net costs	78.58	100	100	44	39	32	30

Source: DHSS and Welsh Office, National Health Service, Hospital Costing Returns, year ended March 31, 1972, HM Stationery Office.

Especially depressing is the failure to raise expenditure per patient in long-stay and mental illness hospitals and to raise it more than marginally in mental handicap hospitals, relative to that in hospitals for the acute sick, despite a succession of investigations of bad conditions in the late 1960s and early 1970s in different long-stay hospitals (58-63), widespread publicity and concern, and the introduction of new Government policies aimed at promoting rapid improvement. Examination of the whole episode—of the failure of the health system to respond to the new policies, or perhaps of the policies themselves to effect change—would be more likely than examination of any other sequence of events in recent years to yield insights into the general deficiencies of Health Service planning.

The problems of professionalism, managerial control, and privileged access to knowledge

I have pursued the twin themes of inequality in health conditions or needs and of provision of services. The evidence invites searching reappraisal of the whole development of our health system. There are problems of identifying performance, understanding the interconnections within the health system of different branches of service and defining its boundaries, and explaining why policies designed to lead to more equitable distribution of services have been frustrated. A deeper analysis of the persistence and even the widening of inequality may be required.

Of course, however widely the health system is conceived and drawn, its potentiality is restricted. The system is not the only determinant of mortality or morbidity. States of health depend on peace or war, nutrition, living standards, education, and the working environment. One illustration might be given. Whereas staffing ratios for health visitors, consultant obstetricians, paediatricians, and general practitioners are all slightly higher in Scotland than in England and Wales, the infant mortality rate in Scotland remains relatively high. Scotland has a legacy of poor housing, especially in the major cities, and a Scottish Health Service study found, for example, that the infant mortality rate was directly proportional to the degree of overcrowding (64).

The interdependence of services within the system also deserves to be better understood. Measures of adequacy and efficiency must be developed not just for particular services, because that implies they are isolated from one another, and isolated in their effects. They must be designed to represent that interdependence. General practice complements and is interconnected with hospital and specialist medicine on the one hand and with the public health and welfare or personal social services on the other. The relative scale, balance, and working functions of each part of the system have to be identified for local communities as well as for the nation as a whole.

This functional interdependence has been recognized in the plans for the reorganization in 1974 of the NHS. The trouble is that reorganization takes a hierarchical form, stressing the virtues of managerial control or efficiency, the superior status and power of the upper reaches of the medical profession, and the exclusivity of knowledge. I believe it conflicts not only with democratic conceptions of health services, but with comprehensive conceptions of health needs, equitable and inexpensive deployment of resources and the long-term advance in standards of health education. What is wanted is not a long and remote chain of command but access to, and involvement in, strong community health, welfare and housing services. The problem is far from being just that of establishing the consumer's right to comment on the operation of the structure. It is whether a hierarchical managerial model derived from industry is likely, in the end, to promote or retard 'freedom of access to medical and allied care at times of need' for all members of the population. Although the structure is complex and embodies attempts, through multi-disciplinary district management and health care planning teams, to delegate certain powers to the different health care professions working locally, its hierarchical form remains marked. Alternative models have received scant attention (65, 67), but the criticisms now being expressed about recent reorganization, (68, 69) from the adoption of the Salmon Committee's recommendations on nursing in 1966 (70) to the culminating Act of 1973, are likely to bring them to the forefront, or encourage others to be devised.

One might argue that the Labour Government's second green paper on reorganization did not go far enough in devolving power and strengthening the community services (71). But its proposed regional health councils were intended to wield control only over the blood transfusion service and the organization of postgraduate education and research, and only a third of the members of the strong area health authorities were to be appointed by the Secretary of State. On the grounds of managerial efficiency the Conservative Government introduced a multi-tier organization almost totally controlled from above. The 14 regional health authorities in England have powers to plan the regions and allocate resources to and supervise area health authorities. They are responsible to the DHSS. All the members are appointed by the Secretary of State, and few of those who have been appointed are manual workers or consumers. Nearly a third are businessmen—bankers, company directors, business executives, property developers, and brokers. The next largest section comprise doctors, and the next, solicitors and accountants (72). Below the 14 RHAs are 90 area health authorities, each of them having 15 members. The chairman is appointed by the Secretary of State, and, except for four members who represent local authorities, the remaining members are appointed by the RHAs. Below this management structure community health councils have been formed. These councils have minimal rights and no executive powers. Each council will consist of between eighteen and thirty members, of whom about half will be appointed by the local authorities and about a third will represent voluntary organizations—the remaining members being selected by the RHAs who finance the councils. Although the councils were made more democratic during the passage of the 1973 Act they are still incapable of acting effectively as 'public watchdogs'. Critics of the structure have fastened on the failure to provide for informed public criticism of the needs of the health services (73).

It is in such a managerial system that the consultants can exert greatest influence—on the DHSS through professional pressure-groups and all kinds of central departmental committees and working-parties, and on the RHAs, where all the vital planning decisions about the hospital service are taken. Moreover, the change from regional *hospital* boards to regional *health* authorities indicates the increased scope of their influence over planning decisions which also affect the general practitioner and other community health services.

The accommodation of the health and other social service professions to the structure and operating assumptions of corporate management, whether of industry or State, represents the largest single threat to free access to health care and the aim of a healthy society. In the history of all the professions there has been the problem of reconciling the acquisition or practice of 'skills presupposing willingness to enter into social relations on a basis apparently incompatible with noble rank' with the ascription or temptation to secure high status as a guarantee of autonomy (74). On the one hand there is the obligation to stress altruistic values, to serve the community, consider the individual without regard to his social background or status, be available at all reasonable times, and put the needs of clients, patients, or consumers before self-interests. Professional codes of conduct have been developed with the intention of prescribing duties to the public and guaranteeing quality of service. Qualifications, training schools, and conditions of entry to the profession have been introduced with the intention of ensuring conformity and high standards of practice. Humanistic and individualistic creeds have been established as a protective social force independent of the exercise of political power and impersonal bureaucracy. On the other hand there have been simultaneous tendencies to monopolize technical know-how, establish dogmas of omniscience, omnipotence or infallibility, protect members against outside criticisms, use power to secure excessively privileged conditions of remuneration and work, and resist change.

The development and significance of this contest have to be reviewed in different contexts. On the debit side might be listed the recent history of the medical profession's insistence, above all else, on high remuneration and privileged terms of service, including the expensive charade of merit awards (75, 76); the failure to institute effective complaints procedures (77-80); the failure to broaden medical education and to admit greater numbers of women and manual workers' children to medical training (81); the failure to introduce greater control over, and supervision of, the pharmaceutical industry, as exemplified in the Sainsbury Report (82); and the failure to understand the implications of trends in patterns of disease and mortality for the wider control of industry (in the case of the tobacco and vehicle industries), the value of health education and the importance of the social aspects of disease to the practice of medicine.

On the credit side might be listed the belated creation of a large number of health centres, the growth of group practice with ancillary workers and diagnostic facilities, the signs of a critical spirit among new entrants to the medical profession (83), the increase, though slow, in numbers of district nurses and home helps; the reduction in number of mental hospital patients and the beginning of alternative services, such as sheltered housing and workshops and day centres, for the mentally ill, mentally handicapped, elderly, and disabled in the community. Although these trends are overshadowed by the reinforcement of consultant power and status in the hospitals, and in themselves are not above criticism, they provide the potentiality for the organization of the health services of the future.

The right of the sick to free access to health care, irrespective of class or income, remains to be firmly established. The treatment in particular of many of the aged, chronic sick and disabled, mentally ill and mentally handicapped, remains scandalously poor and can in the long run be dramatically improved only by a redefinition of health and health needs, and by a reconstruction of professional values and organization, the education and involvement of the patient, and the establishment of social equality.

Acknowledgements

I am grateful for help and comments by Professor Brian Abel-Smith, Dr A.M. Adelstein, John Bond, Harvey Goldstein, Dr Julian Tudor Hart, Elizabeth Monck, Professor J.N. Morris, Joy Skegg, Adrian Sinfield, Professor Margaret Stacey, and Professor J.M. Tanner.

References

(1) Morris, J.N. (1964) *Uses of Epidemiology*. London, E. & S. Livingstone.
(2) Department of Health and Social Security (1973) *Health and Personal Social Services Statistics for England 1973*, p. 39. London, HMSO.
(3) *United Nations Statistical Yearbook, 1971*.
(4) Department of Health and Social Security (1970) *Annual Report for 1969*. London, HMSO.
(5) Titmuss, R.M. (1969) *Commitment to Welfare*, p. 126. London, Allen and Unwin.
(6) Cochrane, A.L. (1972) *Effectiveness and Efficiency*, chs 4 and 6. London, Nuffield Provincial Hospitals Trust.
(7) Abel-Smith, B. (1972) *The Hospitals 1800-1948*. London, Heinemann.
      Hart, J.T. (1972) *International Journal of the Health Services*, 2, 349.
(8) Abel-Smith, B. (1964) *Bulletin of the New York Academy of Medicine*, 40, 545.
(9) Lindsey, A. (1962) *Socialised Medicine in England and Wales; the National Health Service, 1948-61*. Chapel Hill, North Carolina, University of North Carolina Press.
(10) Foot, M. (1973) *Aneurin Bevan 1945-60*, p. 216. London, Davis-Poynter.
(11) Hill, C. (1964) *Both Sides of the Hill*, p. 99. London, Heinemann.
(12) Forsyth, G. (1966) *Doctors and State Medicine; a Study of the National Health Service*, pp. 26 and 34. London, Pitman Medical.
(13) Logan, W.P.C. and Brook, E.M. (1957) *Survey of Sickness 1943-52*. London, HMSO.
(14) The Partnership (editorial), *Lancet*, 1958, 2, 27.
(15) Ten years (editorial), *Br. med. J.*, 1958, 2, 33-4.
(16) Twenty years hard (editorial), *Lancet*, 1968, 1, 1411-12.
(17) Culyer, A.J., Lavers, R.J. and Williams, A. (1972) In *Social Indicators and Social Policy*, Eds. A. Shonfield and S. Shaw. London, Heinemann.
(18) Joint Working Party on the Integration of Medical Work (1973) *Towards an Integrated Child Health Service*, p. 8. Edinburgh, Scottish Home and Health Department.
(19) Registrar General's Decennial Supplement, England and Wales (1961) *Occupational Mortality Tables*. London, HMSO.
(20) Morris, J.N. (1959) Health and social class, *Lancet*, 1, 303.
(21) Spicer, C.C. and Lipworth, L. (1966) *Regional and Social Factors in Infant Mortality*, G.R.O. Studies on Medical Population Subjects, no. 19. London, HMSO.
(22) Hart, J.T. (1972) Data on occupational mortality 1959-1963, *Lancet*, 1, 192.
(23) *Public Health and Medical Subjects* (1970) no. 125, pp. 10-23.
(24) Ashley, J.S.A., Howlett, A. and Morris, J.N. (1971) Case fatality of hyperplasia of the prostate in two teaching and three regional board hospitals, *Lancet*, 2, 1308.
(25) Daw, R.H. (1971) *Journal of the Institute of Actuaries*, 97, 17.
(26) Ministry of Pensions and National Insurance (1965) *Report on an Enquiry into the Incidence of Incapacity for Work; part 11, incidence of incapacity for work in different areas and occupations*. London, HMSO.
(27) *Social Trends 1973* (1974) No. 4, table 69. London, Central Statistical Office.
(28) Office of Population Censuses and Surveys, Social Survey Division (1973) *The General Household Survey*, p. 304. London, HMSO.

(29) Goldstein, H. (1971) Factors influencing the height of seven-year-old children—results from the National Child Development Study, *Hum. Biol., 43*, 92.

(30) Douglas, J.W.B. and Simpson, H. (1964) Height in relation to puberty, family size and social class, *Milbank Memorial Foundation Quarterly, 42*, 20.

(31) Abel-Smith, B. (1963) *Paying for Health Services; a Study of the Costs and Sources of Finance in Six Countries.* Geneva, WHO.

(32) Abel-Smith, B. (1967) *An International Study of Health Expenditure.* Geneva, WHO.

(33) Report of the Royal Commission on Health Services (1964) Vol. 1, pp. 482-93. Ottawa, Queens Printer.

(34) Simanis, J.G. (1973) *Social Security Bulletin, 36,* March, p. 41.

(35) Townsend, P. (1971) *The Times.* London, 11 March.

(36) Townsend, P. (1975) *Sociology and Social Policy.* London, Allen Lane.

(37) *Public Expenditure to 1977-78* (1973) Cmnd. 5519, pp. 6, 96-7. London, HMSO.

(38) Mechanic, D. (1971) The English National Health Service: some comparisons with the United States, *Journal of Health and Social Behaviour, 12,* 18.

(39) Mechanic, D. (1968) *Medical Sociology; a Selective View,* pp. 266-70. Illinois, The Free Press.

(40) Townsend, P. (1968) Medical Services. In *Old People in Three Industrial Societies,* E. Shanas, P. Townsend, D. Wedderburn, H. Friis, P. Milhoj and J. Stehouwer, p. 97. London, Routledge and Kegan Paul.

(41) Department of Health and Social Security (1973) *Health and Personal Social Services Statistics for England* (with summary tables for Great Britain), table 3.9. London, HMSO.

(42) On the State of the Public Health (1973) Annual report of the Chief Medical Officer of the Department of Health and Social Security for the year 1972, p. 2. London, HMSO.

(43) Butler, J.R., Bevan, J.M. and Taylor, R.C. (1973) *Family Doctors and Public Policy,* pp. 41-42, 153. London, Routledge and Kegan Paul.

(44) Rein, M. (1969) Social class and the Health Service, *New Society, 14,* 373, 807-10 (20 Nov.).

(45) Rein, M. (1969) *Journal of the American Hospitals Association, 43,* no. 13.

(46) Cartwright, A. (1967) *Patients and their Doctors: a Study of General Practice,* p. 34. London, Routledge and Kegan Paul.

(47) Logan, W.P.D. and Cushion, A.A. (1958) *Morbidity Statistics from General Practice, No. 2, G.R.O. Studies on Medical Population Subjects,* no. 14. London, HMSO.

(48) Cartwright, A. (1964) *Human Relations and Hospital Care,* p. 191. London, Routledge and Kegan Paul.

(49) Morris, J.N. (1970) In *The NHS: Three Views,* Fabian Research Series, no. 287. London, Fabian Society.

(50) Morris, J.N. (1973) Four cheers for prevention, *Proc. R. Soc. Med., 66,* 225.

(51) Purola, T., Kalimo, E., Sievers, K. and Nyman, K. (1968) *The Utilisation of the Medical Services and its Relationship ⋅ ⋅ Morbidity, Health Resources and Social Factors,* p. 144. Helsinki, Research Institute for Social Security.

(52) Townsend, P. (1973) In *Needs of the Elderly for Health and Welfare Services,* Eds. R.W. Canvin and N.G. Pearson. University of Exeter.

(53) Townsend, P. (1962) *The Last Refuge,* p. 580. London, Routledge and Kegan Paul.

(54) Carstairs, V. and Morrison, M. (1972) *Scottish Health Service Studies,* no. 19, p. 40.

(55) Department of Health and Social Security and Welsh Office (1973) *The Facilities and Services of Psychiatric Hospitals in England and Wales 1971,* tables 3, 18, 27. London, HMSO.

(56) Morris, P. (1969) *Put Away.* London, Routledge and Kegan Paul.

(57) Wing, J.K. and Brown, G.W. (1970) *Institutionalism and Schizophrenia.* London, Cambridge University Press.

(58) *Findings and Recommendations Following Enquiries into Allegations Concerning the Care of Elderly Patients in Certain Hospitals* (1968) Cmnd. 3687. London, HMSO.

(59) *Report of the Committee of Inquiry into Allegations of Ill-Treatment of Patients and Other Irregularities at the Ely Hospital,* Cardiff (1969) Cmnd. 3957. London, HMSO.

(60) *Report of the Farleigh Hospital Committee of Inquiry* (1971) Cmnd. 4557. London, HMSO.

(61) *Report of the Committee of Inquiry into Whittingham Hospital* (1972) Cmnd. 4861. London, HMSO.

(62) *Report of the Professional Investigation into Medical and Nursing Practices on Certain Wards at Napsbury Hospital, near St. Albans* (1973) London, HMSO.

(63) Annual reports of the National Health Service Hospital Advisory Service for 1969-72 (1971-73) London, HMSO.

(64) Richards, I.D.G. (1971) *Infant Mortality in Scotland.* Scottish Health Service Studies, no. 16.

(65) Strauss, A. *et al.* (1963) In *The Hospital in Modern Society,* Ed. E. Friedson. New York.

(66) Strauss, A. *et al.* (1964) *Psychiatric Ideologies and Institutions.* New York.

(67) Hunter, T.D. (1971) *Hospital,* April.

(68) Draper, P. and Smart, T. (1972) *The Future of our Health Care.* Department of Community Medicine, Guy's Hospital Medical School, London.

(69) Draper, P. (1973) *Community Medicine,* 23 Feb.

(70) Ministry of Health and Scottish Home and Health Department (1966) *Report of the Committee on Senior Nursing Staff Structure.* London, HMSO.

(71) Department of Health and Social Security (1970) *The Future Structure of the National Health Service.* London, HMSO.

(72) Hart, J.T. (1973) Industry and the Health Service, *Lancet, 2,* 611.

(73) Abel-Smith, B. (1971) The politics of health, *New Society, 18,* 461, 192 (29 July).

(74) Aubert, V. (1962) *Transactions of the 5th World Congress of Sociology,* vol. III, p. 244.

(75) Townsend, P. (1970) Revolution in community care, *Lancet, 1269,* 513.

(76) *Twelfth Report of the Review Body on Doctors' and Dentists' Remuneration* (1970) Cmnd. 4352. London, HMSO.

(77) *Report of the Committee on Hospital Complaints Procedures* (1973) London, HMSO. See *Lancet* (1974) *1,* 52.

(78) Rose, H. (1972) General practice complaints, *New Law Journal,* August 24 and 31.

(79) Klein, R. (1973) *Complaints Against Doctors.* London, Charles Knight.

(80) Stacey, M. (1973) *Consumer Complaints Procedures in the British National Health Service.* Society for the Study of Social Problems (unpublished).

(81) *Report of the Royal Commission on Medical Education (1965-68)* (1968) Cmnd. 3569. London, HMSO.

(82) *Report of the Committee of Enquiry into the Relationship of the Pharmaceutical Industry with the National Health Service.* (1967) Cmnd. 3410. London, HMSO.

(83) Robson, J., Iliffe, S. and Le Fanu, J. (1972) *Lancet, 2,* 648.

13. The promotion of psychiatric research

Sir Geoffrey Vickers

I

Research workers are commonly regarded as geese who occasionally lay golden eggs. The three main ways of encouraging them to do so reflect different views of the extent to which this odd process can be either stimulated or directed.

One way is to cosset any goose which actually has laid a golden egg, in the hope that it will lay some more. A second way is to specify the golden eggs required and offer rewards for them, hoping thus to move still unidentified geese to egg-laying. The third way is to go on increasing the goose farm, in the hope that some statistical law will ensure that the number of golden eggs laid rises roughly in proportion to the number of birds capable of laying eggs at all.

Each of these methods has much to be said for it and much to be said against it. Personally, I favour them all and believe them to be complementary; for the first and second, useful in themselves, make little sense apart from the third, and indeed are themselves part of the total design of the goose farm.

The first, or personal, approach has been highly developed by the Medical Research Council (MRC). The second I will call the institutional approach, because it usually involves setting up an institute devoted to producing the particular golden eggs required. The specification may be general or specific. The most specific example in the medical field is probably the Institute of Cancer Research. This was born of a widespread popular wish to promote research in the cure of cancer. Though it is now an Institute of the Postgraduate Medical Federation of the University of London and receives a substantial grant from the Medical Research Council (£435,000 in 1967), its main support still comes from the public. Psychiatry has nothing so specific as that; but it too has an Institute, which is part of the same Postgraduate Medical Federation.

I shall have more to say later about the Institute of Psychiatry and about the MRC; and, more generally, about the merits and limitations of the personal and the institutional approaches. I want first to talk about what I have called the design of the farm. For I believe that the way to promote research in general, and psychiatric research in particular, is to explore very carefully the system which throws up both questions to be answered and men and resources to answer them; and then to shape this system so as to keep it lively and self-exciting and to direct it to whatever extent may be found to be both possible

---

A lecture given at the Annual General Meeting of the Mental Health Research and Trust Fund on 7 November 1967, with a Supplementary Comment written in 1974. The original lecture was published in the *British Journal of Psychiatry*, 1968, *114*, 925-34.

and desirable. The giving of personal support and the creation of new institutes and institutions are among the various ways of intervening in the system, so as to improve its input or its output or both.

Psychiatric research is, of course, far wider than research by psychiatrists. More, perhaps, than any other branch of medical research, the questions which it tries to answer lead through all the basic sciences on the one hand and all the psychosocial sciences on the other. Yet the psychiatrist is central to the picture because these questions are *his* questions, and his patients' also. What is the matter with this man? How did it happen? How can it be cured or prevented? These are the classical, clinical questions which a doctor asks himself when confronted with a patient. If he does not ask them, no one else will. The answers may involve neurophysiologists and biochemists, psychologists and sociologists, epidemiologists and computer theorists; but none of these is likely to try to answer such questions unless the questions are being constantly asked by doctors who need the answers to abate human disorder and distress.

So we need first to consider the system by which research psychiatrists are evoked and evolved.

Every October, a stream of young men and women flows into the medical schools of this country—in 1966 about 2500. Within a decade or so, this stream will divide itself between the main branches of medicine, the hospital service, general practice, public health and so on; and one of these streams will further divide itself between more than a dozen clinical specialities, including psychiatry. At the same time, another differentiation will be taking place, between the activities of therapy, teaching and research, representing as they do, the three main responsibilities of medicine or any other profession—to practise its skills, to increase them, and to pass them on. The present state of psychiatric research reflects the forces, which over recent decades have guided the present occupants into the posts in which psychiatric research can be practised. Its state over coming decades will reflect these forces as they are today and tomorrow—for most of these influences operate with a substantial time lag. To promote psychiatric research means influencing, in one way or another, the individual choices which lead an adequate proportion (in number and quality) of these newcomers to choose research, rather than other activities, and psychiatry rather than specialities.

This is to operate in one of the most obscure fields of human behaviour; but one aspect of it is reasonably clear. The paths which open before the feet of these newcomers are paved with posts, with pay and prospects. These posts limit the intake; for no one can operate without a post. They also attract or repel intake, by what they offer in opportunity, pay, prospects and prestige, when compared with other paths which are open at the same time.

Thus the architecture of the career structure is of cardinal importance; for it both limits and attracts the incoming stream to each career. It needs to be sensitive both to professional and public needs and to the interests and aspirations of incoming individuals. Let me draw a summary picture of this architecture as it exists today, first in medical and then in psychiatric research.

II

There are about 65,000 doctors active in the United Kingdom (1). Of these about 26,000 are in the hospital service and about the same number in general practice. Of the remainder, the number engaged in teaching, research and postgraduate study is something over 5000, perhaps substantially more. These figures, especially the last, are rough, but they serve to indicate the relative orders of magnitude of these various streams today.

The three main employers of doctors are the National Health Service (NHS), the universities through their medical schools, and the MRC. The three functions of therapy, teaching and research are not tidily distributed between these three employers, because the three functions are not mutually exclusive or even wholly separable. A clinical teacher teaches largely by demonstrating his therapeutic skills and supervising the exercise of these skills by others; so therapy is a necessary incident of teaching, just as teaching is of therapy, whenever juniors work under a consultant's responsibility. Similarly, much clinical research is done in the course of therapy, and some of it can be done by a doctor carrying a normal therapeutic load, especially if he is provided with appropriate help. (After all, every diagnosis and treatment involves formulating and verifying an hypothesis and this is also the essence of research.) So research and teaching are not always incompatible with a post of which the official duties are wholly therapeutic.

On the other hand, much clinical research needs more time than therapy in itself allows, and some research needs to be done by medical researchers who are relieved of clinical responsibility. So the career structure of research needs posts which provide time and facilities for these and are correspondingly protected from the claims of therapy. These relatively 'sheltered' posts are the focus of my inquiry. They are to be found in non-teaching hospitals; in undergraduate medical schools and their associated teaching hospitals; in postgraduate teaching institutions; and in research organizations more or less independnent of the university system. They vary both in the degree of permanence they provide and in the degree of shelter they afford.

Some of these posts are 'established'; when they fall vacant, no new authority is required to fill them. Some are filled by permanent but personal contracts, and are reconsidered when the holder leaves. Some are temporary. Most of the established posts are provided by universities. Most of the personal posts are provided by the MRC. The temporary posts are provided by a great variety of sources, including the MRC, the NHS, the endowment funds of hospitals, foundations here and abroad, and fund-raising bodies like the Mental Health Research and Trust Fund. The relations between all these are so important that I will examine them a little more fully.

The NHS provides few, if any, *permanent* posts which impose any *obligation* for anything but therapy. It allows its employees to teach in medical schools and to do research consistent with their therapeutic duties; and it provides research funds through Regional Hospital Boards— commonly known as the decentralized research scheme—to finance research projects in its hospitals. Further, since its doctors can serve on part-time contracts, they can keep part of their time available for other purposes, including research, for which they may seek support from other sources; and this they often supplement by that elastic resource known as 'spare time'. So a substantial amount of research is, in fact, done by doctors on NHS contracts, in posts in which research is not an obligation.

University-supported posts in medical schools are supposed to be concerned with research no less than with teaching; but teaching, with its associated therapy take most of the time. The load is supposed to be adjusted (in quantity, and to some extent in character) so as to leave some time and opportunity for research. How much time and opportunity is in fact available for research varies widely. It depends partly on the weight of teaching and therapy in relation to the staff, partly on the composition of the staff, and partly, of course, on the energy and research interest of the professor. The staff, effectively, includes not only the holders of the established university posts (which are commonly full-time) but also, usually, part-time teachers drawn from the NHS doctors on the hospital staff, and attached research workers, medical and non-medical, usually with whole-time but temporary support from outside sources. Some of these may be working for postgraduate degrees. The NHS teachers sometimes contribute to research directly, more often indirectly, by easing the teaching load; but the research potential depends largely on the number of posts (if any) in which research can be primary responsibility.

Postgraduate schools and institutes are usually larger, and are able to devote rather more of their time to research, partly because research is more closely related to postgraduate education.

The MRC supplements these university establishments by forms of support which range from fully institutional to temporary personal. In the non-clinical field it maintains the largest medical research laboratories in the country; and it is in process of establishing a clinical research centre of its own, which will be in effect a hospital designed primarily for research and which is to contain a psychiatric component. In addition to these institutional activities, it maintains over eighty research units, which are usually at least as permanent as their directors, sometimes more so. Some of these are sited near non-teaching hospitals or other facilities which they need; and even when they are established within teaching departments, they are formally independent. The MRC also maintains groups of research workers as part of teaching departments, designed to be taken over by the university in due course. It maintains individuals on permanent contracts, whole or part time, as members of its external staff. And it is much the largest single source of temporary grants and fellowships.

This description reverses the order in which the MRC has conceived its function. Its approach has been personal, and it aims (at least in the clinical field) to become as little institutional as may be. It supports individuals first by temporary grants; it builds up its units round established workers and reconsiders their future whenever the director vacates office. Its aim is that universities should institutionalize the development of new disciplines and lines of inquiry, so soon as the need to teach them becomes substantial enough to warrant the founding or extension of university departments.

Time will, I think, continue to press the MRC to support an increasing number of established posts, both in universities and in its own institutions, and I hope that it will continue to respond to this demand. This, however, should not mask the extreme value of the MRC unit as a type of organization which can be quickly created, developed and if need be curtailed and even disbanded, and which is yet sufficiently substantial and enduring to pursue weighty objectives over extended spans of time.

This then is the broad pattern of posts within which incoming doctors who engage in research at all will choose or stumble on the patterns of their individual careers. It makes provision for careers, whole-time and part-time, whole-life and part-life, in which therapy, teaching and research may be pursued in various combinations. It provides opportunities both for specialization and for cooperation between departments and between disciplines. It also provides varying degrees of rigidity, from the established departments and instituions of universities of the MRC, through the personal security of the MRC's permanent contracts, to the constantly varying stream of temporary grants.

It thus provides what seem to me to be the main ingredients for the design of that combined activity of which research is one aspect and one outcome. Whether these elements are in fact combined in a successful design in any particular field is, of course, another matter. We should need to ask whether in that field there is an appropriate number and relation of institutional posts, personal posts and temporary posts; whether these are sufficiently attractive, relative to other alternatives, to secure the requisite intake of talent; and whether these posts are so grouped as to secure the optimum output for the resources expended.

To answer these questions in regard to psychiatry, let me briefly draw the corresponding picture of psychiatric posts. Most of the figures which follow have not been collected before, so far as I know. They are approximate, but I believe they give a substantially correct impression.

III

The NHS employs about 2600 psychiatrists of all grades in the United Kingdom (2). Of these something over 150 are engaged in research, mostly part-time, under its decentralized research scheme or otherwise. The psychiatric departments of undergraduate medical schools provide about eighty established psychiatric posts. The Institute of Psychiatry adds a further fifteen or so. There are thus rather less than 100 established academic posts in psychiatry in the United Kingdom. Very few of these are primarily for research. To be exact, one undergraduate medical school has six such posts and will soon have seven. The other sixteen departments, so far as I can discover, have only one among them all. I will explain this oddity later.

The MRC supports nine units directly concerned with psychiatry (3). These employ at present about thirty psychiatrists. It also supports as members of external staff another eight doctors who qualify as psychiatrists by the definition I am using. If we regard all these as 'permanent' posts (which they are not) and add them to the previous count, we find that there are about 135 more or less permanent posts in which research is expected of psychiatrists, and that research is the primary activity in about forty of them.

The departments, the Institute and the units contain also attached workers, supported by various sources. Of these, the medically qualified ('psychiatrists', by my liberal definition) number in all about fifty. Those attached to the departments number twenty-four, of whom five are supported by the

MRC, four by the Nuffield Foundation and 3½ by the Mental Health Research and Trust Fund.

I will describe the organization of these posts in greater detail later. Let us first consider the total figures.

Only about one-tenth of the doctors in the hospital service are psychiatrists; 8% in general psychiatry, 1% in child psychiatry, and a further 1% in mental subnormality. This seems a small proportion, when we remember that psychiatric beds still form about 47% of all hospital beds. I do not suggest that the number of psychiatrists should be proportionate to the number of beds, since more of these than in other categories of illness are still occupied by long-stay patients, for many of whom doctors can do relatively little. But a growing proportion of the mentally ill demand and repay the expenditure of *more* than average time; and as domiciliary care grows, the load on hosptial doctors as well as on GPs must grow. It would seem that the total number of psychiatrists is still substantially too low.

The proportion of psychiatrists primarily engaged in teaching would seem to be even lower. In medicine generally, professors and medical teachers number over 1500, of whom no less than 450 are professors (4). The corresponding numbers for psychiatry, so far as I can identify them, are eighty and twenty. The number of university teaching posts open to psychiatrists is only about 7½% of the total, probably less, while the proportion of professorial chairs is only 3½%. There are over six teaching posts for every one-hundred doctors in the hospital service, but under four for every one-hundred psychiatrists; more than two professors for every one-hundred doctors, less than one for every one-hundred psychiatrists.

Evidently, the teaching departments in psychiatry are still weak, even in relation to the present numbers in the speciality.

This is not surprising; for all these figures are one frame in a rapidly moving picture. In 1947 there were two professors of psychiatry in the United Kingdom. In 1955 there were five chairs, of which two were vacant. Today (1967) there are seventeen departmental chairs (5) and three in the Institute of Psychiatry. This is a most welcome and rapid expansion; but it leaves no doubt, I think, about the interpretation of the figures.

Until recently, psychiatry was a subject neglected as a field of practice, of study and of research. For this there are historical, as well as medical reasons; notably the fact that until recently the teaching hospitals did not admit psychiatric patients. The three aspects of this branch of medicine, therapy, teaching and research, were caught up in a mutually restricting system, from which they have only recently begun to emerge. In our university system, changes of emphasis come slowly, especially at times of financial restriction, when one discipline can only grow at the expense of another. Psychiatric departments have grown in stature and prestige in the last ten years as quickly as I would have expected. We need not be surprised, but we should not forget that they have not yet caught up.

None the less, the relative weakness of university departments of psychiatry and their overload with teaching and therapy remain, I believe, a serious defect in the design of that part of the goose farm which it is my task to examine. To appreciate its effect, we need to bear in mind the sequence in which the medical student and young doctor make contact with psychiatry and psychiatric research and the points in that sequence at which their choices must be exercized. For these also are important factors in deciding how apt the resulting pattern can be expected to be.

IV

The medical student in his pre-clinical days studies the basic sciences governing that 'order' which illness disturbs. This course is less relevant to mental than to physical disorder, for the good reason that our understanding of order and of the ordering process is much less in the mental than in the physical field. It is none the less evident that the pre-clinical years usually cover much too little basic science in the psychosocial field. It is a welcome, but a novel development in medical education to allot a substantial number of pre-clinical hours to these sciences. The number so allotted today in the medical schools of the United Kingdom varies from ninety hours to none (6).

In his clinical years, the medical student is briefly exposed to all medical specialities, including psychiatry. The time allotted to psychiatry and psychosomatic disorders ranges from three months full-time to thirty hours (7). In so far as he is given any training in general practice—another welcome development which is not yet universal—he has some introduction to the pervasive influence of mental illness and more generally of human psychological difference in experiencing and responding to sickness of all kinds. It remains true at present that, at the time when he qualifies, mental illness is generally little more for the medical student than the subject of one among many medical specialities, distinguished largely by the inadequacy of its base in pre-clinical science and the empirical nature of its treatments. The amount of time devoted to it could be increased, and I hope will be increased, but it has much leeway to catch up in most medical schools, as these figures show.

After graduation, the student will spend his pre-registration year in a general hospital. He will then be free, if he wishes, to seek an appointment in a mental hospital. Unless he serves as registrar and senior registrar in a mental hospital at this stage, he will have to do so later, should he decide subsequently to specialize in psychiatry; so his choice in favour of psychiatry will be more costly, if it is not made soon after registration.

All these factors at present combine to restrict the choice of psychiatry as a career.

Among those who choose psychiatry, the decision to embark on research is also restricted. The opportunities have increased, especially since the decentralization research scheme was introduced; but the decision to embark on even temporary research work is a serious choice, because though it favours a research or, slightly less, an academic career, it is likely to delay progress towards a clinical consultancy. How serious the delay depends primarily on the extent to which it diminishes the intensity and variety of the worker's clinical experience. But, by and large, years spent in research count for less, in qualifying for consultancy, than years spent in clinical work. This may not be true of consultancies in teaching hospitals; but in the more numerous non-teaching hospitals some consultancies stand vacant today for lack of suitable applicants.

Thus the worker who embarks on tempoary research takes a path which may quickly become canalized towards an academic or a permanent research career. Because the academic departments are still inadequately staffed, those who embark on temporary, whole-time research work have no sufficient assurance of reaching an established academic post.

They have even less assurance of reaching an established research post. This would matter less if the academic structure were adequate. It is greatly to be prized that MRC research units can grow, shrink or change direction more quickly than academic departments. It means, however, that permanent appointments with the MRC are obtained later in life than university appointments, and that these appointments, when they fall vacant, are not advertised or automatically refilled, as are established academic posts. An outstanding researcher is more likely to be provided with a new unit by the MRC than with a new chair by some university; but he is correspondingly less likely to inherit a directorship from someone else.

V

This survey of psychiatry and psychiatric research posts as they stand today leads me to this conclusion. The further promotion of psychiatric research calls for action in three main directions—to increase the established posts in the academic departments; to expose medical students and young doctors to a much greater amount of psychiatry and psychiatric research before they take their first registrarship; and to increase both within these departments and outside them (or beside them) the number of psychiatric posts in which research is the primary responsibility.

On the first and second of these I need add little. The paths by which university establishments are increased and their teaching syllabuses changed are steep and stony but well known. Both needs, I believe, are recognized. The second was underlined in the General Medical Council's recommendations on basic medical education in 1967. But I would like to express my views about the third of these needs—the ways in which specifically research posts can be increased.

By far the most powerful agency is the MRC. Its most direct influence on academic departments is by creating groups, maintained within a department at MRC's expense, until such time as the university can take them over. The singularly happy position of one among the seventeen undergraduate departments of psychiatry, as I described it earlier, is due to the fact that in mid-1967 it thus absorbed a group. You will appreciate that this radical change was imperceptible at the working level; the only change was that five people's salaries would in future swell a different column in the budget of the same Department of State. What matters is that, through the MRC's provisions, they had been at work for years before the academic bit of the budget would have provided for them.

The MRC can also support whole-time and part-time external staff, who can have honorary appointments or further part-time appointments with a department—or, for that matter, with the NHS. This is a most effective way of integrating a research psychiatrist into a medical school or hospital staff, while safeguarding the primacy of his research interest. One professor of psychiatry relies for his research potential almost entirely on a group of three external MRC staff based at a nearby hospital.

MRC units also have great flexibility. One way to associate them with a department is to place them under the honorary directorship of a Professor; or, more usually, to allow the director to accept a professorship while remaining as honorary director. Of the nine psychiatric units, two are directed by professors of psychiatry and two by professors of pharmacology. (Not all professors agree with this policy, which means that the unit's director is the only member of it who cannot give it his undivided attention. But it remains an often valuable possibility.)

Thus the MRC has great and flexible powers to reinforce the research resources of university departments; or, for that matter, of any hospital or place of work which it wants to fortify. Of its nine psychiatric units, two are situated at the Institute of Psychiatry, four in medical schools, one at the London School of Economics, one in a non-teaching mental hospital in Sussex and one in its own laboratories at Carshalton, close to the large concentration of mental hospitals in Surrey.

Some foundations are sufficiently large and permanent to play somewhat similar roles, establishing within a department a post or even a group of posts, to be taken over at some future date. The Nuffield Foundation has done so in psychiatry. The endowment funds of hospitals are sometimes used for the same end on a smaller scale. Grant-giving bodies are commonly reluctant to do this, unless they have a firmer assurance than they can usually get that the post so provided will be taken over by a fixed and reasonably early date. To do otherwise would risk tying up funds indefinitely for what is regarded as a university responsibility. The Mental Health Research and Trust Fund has had arduous experience in this field, but has one success to its credit. The funds available for short-term grant-giving are not so large that much of them can be risked in this way.

This raises what I believe to be a very important point concerning university responsibility for research.

It is generally agreed that research is still an essential, though not an exclusive, responsibility of universities, especially in association with post-graduate education (8). It is clear, none the less, that in clinical departments, teaching and therapy will exclude research unless *either* the staff is large enough for all three functions *or* some of them are partly sheltered from clinical and teaching demands. It is equally clear that when a speciality is undermanned and growing, as psychiatry is, the increasing demands of therapy and teaching are likely to offset increases in staff, perhaps for several years; and that at such a time it is especially difficult for universities to provide 'sheltered' posts, when the unsheltered posts are crying out for reinforcement.

In such a situation (and it is the situation in psychiatry today), if research is not to suffer unduly, outside agencies must do more than their normal share to provide the 'sheltered' posts. But this is checked by reluctance on both sides. Universities often hesitate to accept from outsiders posts which they may soon be pressed to take over; and outsiders hesitate to offer posts which will only relieve, rather than supplement, what they regard as the universities' proper responsibilities. I would plead that both these hesitancies be abated.

Departments of psychiatry, like other clinical departments, need *some* permanent posts in which research is the primary responsibility. These are needed at two levels—near the top, where the senior man can help to sustain the impetus of research, despite the overload and distraction of the professor; and near the bottom, where a relatively junior man can help his seniors, and especially the professor, to keep their research going. Posts at the higher level can best be supplied by the MRC, as they have been in the examples I have given; for the MRC is best placed both to negotiate with universities for their ultimate absorption and to carry them in the meantime. Some useful help might be expected from the foundations, and indeed, from the Mental Health Research and Trust Fund, when its revenues from the public get anywhere near the public support for cancer research—and why should they not? Posts at the lower level are less easily supplied by universities. Yet it is a common complaint of professors that they lack precisely this form of assistance—a man not tied to a project or a programme but available for general research purposes, preferably occupying a post which can be refilled when he goes on to other work. It may be that this need has at least as good a claim on the resources of grant-giving bodies as those for more specific projects.

This survey of psychiatric research as it is today raised the question whether the resources now available from all sources are appropriately divided between the various locations at which research should be going on, and between different types of research requiring different concentrations of resources and different expectations of continuance. So let me conclude by describing briefly the ways in which these resources are now disposed.

The amount of psychiatric research which is being done in non-teaching hospitals by psychiatrists on NHS contracts is clearly substantial. The information supplied to me by Regional Hospital Boards lists over 150 projects, involving about the same number of psychiatrists. This is certainly not all; for only about half the Boards have full information about the research going on in their hospitals apart from what they are themselves financing; and it is clear from these that more than half the current projects require no financial help or get what they require from other sources. Many schemes may be slight, but the resultant involvement of psychiatrists is none the less wide. It includes many consultants; for though consultants may not be supported full-time under the decentralized research scheme, they derive help from it both for part-time support and, more often, for assistance. The amount being done appears to vary widely between regions, the projects listed ranging from over thirty to none. One region devoted between 40 and 50% of its research budget to psychiatric projects.

In addition, the Ministry of Health controls a substantial fund for operational research, under which at least thirty-four psychiatric projects are under way; though some of them do not involve psychiatrists.

The amount of research in undergraduate teaching departments varies vastly. The largest department has ten established posts, all medical, and eighteen attached workers, of whom five are medical, a total of twenty-eight. Another has ten established posts, eight of them medical and eleven attached workers, five medical, a total of twenty-one; and also a MRC unit numbering thirteen, directed by the professor. At the other extreme are departments, sometimes newly established, which have scarcely any established posts except the professorship, and no attached research workers.

My impression is that departments vary greatly also in the extent of their collaboration with NHS consultants in their own teaching hospital and elsewhere in their region. This may well be a factor of importance on which comparisons would be illuminating.

Medical schools which have as yet no professorial department of psychiatry provide teaching by the part-time service of NHS psychiatrists. These sometimes manage to carry out some research, although these schools usually have no established university posts.

The Institute of Psychiatry has the largest concentration of resources. It has at present fifteen medical and thirty-three non-medical posts; and it has attached to it a further fourteen medical and fifty-one non-medical workers, a total of 113. The proportion of medical to non-medical posts is much lower there than in the undergraduate departments.

The nine MRC units vary, with from twenty-one to seven posts. The proportion of medical to non-medical workers in these is even lower than in the Institute.

Is this the pattern in which we should choose to dispose these resources, if *output* were our only concern? How, in any case, should we wish to vary this pattern as more resources become available? These questions are not wholly relevant; for, as I mentioned earlier, therapy, teaching and research are not wholly separable. What matters is that none of these variables should be allowed to distort more than is absolutely unavoidable the responses needed by the demands of the other two.

The therapeutic load, for example, is very uneven; and it will certainly grow. The teaching load is also uneven and will grow in response to different demands and limitations. Research activity is even more uneven and will be stimulated by at least three different needs. One is the need to maintain in every teaching centre enough research to stimulate teaching and make students aware of the attractions and difficulties of research—and equally, in every hospital, enough research to keep alive the spirit of inquiry. Another is the need to back men with ideas, wherever they emerge, and to bring them together with the resources which they require. A third is the need to provide some institutional centres in which research may develop a momentum of its own and a continuity not wholly dependent on an individual. These three research needs are not easy to combine with each other or, collectively, with the needs of teaching and therapy.

None the less, the machinery for relating teaching institutions with the general body of working psychiatrists on the one hand and with research resources on the other seems to me to be generally well suited to dealing with these three variables, without letting them interfere unduly with each other. But the machinery needs to be used wisely, firmly and continuously if so complex a system is to be well regulated. I hope this may be furthered, however slightly, by this general analysis of the state of the system and its inherent dynamics.

It raises many questions that I cannot answer and some that I have not even posed. I offer it with the humility proper to an outsider. This is not my goose farm. But the approach which I have illustrated is not confined to research or to psychiatry. In all fields of activity we do well, from time to time, to ask ourselves what we are trying to do and how we could most effectively go about it; and to compare it with what we are doing and with the results to which that familiar pattern is likely to lead. And such often disturbing questions are sometimes most easily framed and asked not by a busy participant but by a concerned and sympathetic spectator.

Supplementary comment written in 1974

In view of the years which have passed since the foregoing paper was published, it needs a supplementary note. Ideally this should give the latest available figures corresponding to each of the figures given in the paper, record other relevant information and draw such conclusions as may seem justified.

The first of these needs I can supply only to a limited extent. I have been unable to collect figures sufficiently complete to compare with all those earlier figures, which were aggregates of details collected by me. And some of the figures which I have drawn from collated statistics or which have been supplied to me by the kind help of those I have consulted are not precisely comparable with those quoted in my earlier paper. These uncertainties weaken some of the conclusions which I might otherwise have drawn, especially as regards research supported from university funds. I confine what follows to areas of relative assurance. In these, with two significant exceptions, the picture drawn in my earlier paper needs no substantial qualification.

The number of doctors active in Great Britain at September 1970 was about 70,700 (9). To this must be added the number active in Northern Ireland at the same date (a figure which I have not ascertained) to arrive at a total comparable with the figure of 'about 65,000' given in my earlier paper. Clearly the total number of doctors has increased by at least 10% in that period. The rate of increase and its distribution is more clearly reflected in annual figures for England and Wales for the six years 1967-73. In this period hospital medical staff in England and Wales (10) increased from 27,153 to 34,633, an increase over the period of 25%, while general practitioners in Great Britain increased over the same period from 24,005 to 25,561, an increase of only 6%. The average increase for the six years is over 17%.

The proportion of psychiatrists to the total of all specialities in the NHS in 1972 (the last figures available to me) remained at 10% as before, whether reckoned in individuals or in whole-time equivalents.

The total number of students entering medical schools in 1972 was 3438, as against the figure of 'about 2500' given in the earlier paper, so it would seem that the total number of medical students in training is increasing faster than the number of active doctors. I would therefore expect some increase in the proportion of medical time devoted to teaching. And since the time devoted to psychiatry has also increased, I should expect a more than proportionate increase in psychiatric teaching staff.

This is not clearly reflected in the figures available. The number of professorial chairs in psychiatry has indeed risen from twenty to thirty-four. All medical schools now have professorial chairs, except Cambridge and three of the London teaching hospitals (11). But the number of other whole-time academic posts has not risen correspondingly. The additional teaching load has been largely met by part-time appointments of psychiatrists who are also employed by the NHS. And even if these and the whole-time posts are added together, the total, for 1971 and 1972, amounted to only 6½% of the total medically qualified staff of universities, medical schools and institutes. The proportion of psychiatrists in these institutions who also held NHS appointments in these years was 80%, as against 63% for all specialities.

None the less the time given to the psychiatric element in general medical education has increased both in the clinical and in the pre-clinical years; and in the pre-clinical years it has broadened its content. These changes are reflected in a review published by Professor Crisp in 1973 (12) of the then state of the final and professional M.B. examination in psychiatry at the various medical schools of the country. This change in the volume and character of teaching in the field of psychiatry and more generally of the behavioural sciences is partly due, as Professor Crisp observes, to changes in the concept of medical education, to which the Todd Report contributed.

They doubtless owe something also to a major change in the status of psychiatry. The professional organization to which psychiatrists commonly belonged at the date of the earlier paper, The Royal Medico-Psychological Association, became in 1971 The Royal College of Psychiatrists. Psychiatry thus ceased to be one of many medical specialities and became a branch of the medical profession, comparable in its distinctness and autonomy with the five which had already attained the same distinction, medicine, surgery, gynaecology, pathology and general practice.

This change has both practical and symbolic significance. Practically it lays on the profession greater responsibility for determining its own standards of competence and excellence. Symbolically, it makes the profession more visible to medical students as one of the major fields which invite his interest. This symbolic effect must have some influence in meeting one of the needs identified in the paper—to make medical students more aware of psychiatry as a possible field of specilization and more able to evaluate its attractions before they have been carried past the point at which they could conveniently opt for it.

A welcome educational development is the report of a joint working party established by the Royal College of Psychiatrists and the Royal College of General Practitioners to consider the psychiatric education of general practitioners. This report, dated 17 December, 1973, but not yet published, deals with the postgraduate training of general practitioners. It concludes that the special relationship between psychiatry and general practice which should aid and support general practitioners in the exercise of their psychiatric skills is not reflected in the overall training of family doctors; that many of the clinical attachments offered in psychiatry are ill-suited for future general practitioners; and that some training schemes plainly ignore the importance of psychiatry. The report does however describe 'interesting and isolated experiments', and we may hope that its findings and recommendations will have an influence in this important field of psychiatric education.

There remains the key question whether psychiatric *research* is more active and better directed now than in 1966; and in particular whether it has improved what my earlier review showed to be its depressed position relative to research in other specialities. My information does not show whether it has improved its relative position, but leaves no doubt that it is more active and better directed.

I have been unable to arrive at figures comparable to those in the earlier paper to indicate the current volume of psychiatric research financed from decentralized research funds or from university funds. I have however obtained from the Medical Research Council and from the Department of Health and Social Security particulars which indicate the measure of both absolute, and to some extent, relative growth during the six years under review. Although the figures from the Department relate only to England and Wales they can scarcely fail to be a reliable indication of trends in the country as a whole. And since the MRC and the Department are by far the largest supporters of medical (including psychiatric) research, their information should be a fairly reliable index.

As regards the Medical Research Council, I am grateful to its secretary, Sir John Gray, for this account of changes since my previous paper.

About 1968 the Council gave specific instructions that priority should be given to work on mental health and the development of psychiatry as a discipline. From early 1968 there has been a special section of the office concerned with disorders, both behavioural and physical, of the nervous system and the officer in charge has special responsibility for promoting work in this area. There is a Psychiatric Committee giving advice on promotion of work in this field and by October 1974, the Council expects to have a special Neurobiology and Mental Health Board. Estimated expenditure on mental illness rose between 1968-69 and 1972-73 from £1,040,000 to £2,391,000, while the Council's grant in aid over the same period rose from £12,606,000 to £24,361,000, so expenditure on mental illness as a percentage of grant in aid rose from 8.3% to 9.8%.

The number of scientists paid for by the Council who work on various aspects of the nervous system rose from 17.3% in 1970-71 to 20.7% in 1973-74. Although two of the units listed in my earlier paper have been disbanded, their staff has been largely absorbed elsewhere, some into a new unit which is to work at the National Hospital, Queen Square, in relation to biochemical processes connected with subnormality. Two other new units have been created (13), and four new teams (14) concerned with psychiatric studies have been established within university departments by making relatively long-term grants rather than setting up MRC-employed units, a change in policy which has also developed during the period since the paper was written.

Finally, the Council's clinical research centre, referred to as a project in the earlier paper, has now been opened and a division of psychiatry was established in it from January, 1974. The building which will house this division (part of the third stage in the development of the Centre) has been completed and will soon be ready to admit patients. The division will have twelve beds, with access to a further seventy-five beds in the department of psychological medicine at Northwick Park Hospital, where it is situated. It will also have day-patient facilities and a full range of laboratories. The staff complement will number eighteen scientific and technical staff.

The research activities of the Department of Health and Social Security have expanded nearly twice as fast as those of the MRC. Departmental research rose from £610,000 to £2,987,000 and decentralized research from £703,500 to £1,200,000. Expenditure on research related to mental illness and mental handicap is estimated at about £280,000, a little less than 10% of the whole, a proportion similar to that in the MRC budget.

Increase in *expenditure* does not of course reflect corresponding rates of increase in *activity*. Rising costs, whether due to inflation or otherwise, account for a large part of the increase in the expenditure of both MRC and DHSS. And although the activities of the department at the date of their 1973 report (15) from which these figures are taken, have expanded faster than those of the MRC they remain small by comparison. They are none the less important in the greater degree of cooperation which the report shows to have developed between the DHSS and the MRC, both in finding and in designing research activities.

Three further changes should be noted, although I cannot evaluate them. First, both the number and the proportion of psychiatric hospital beds has dropped since 1966. This reflects the policy of the Service to transfer more psychiatric care to the community, a policy which accords ill with the relatively low increase of general practitioners. It may also reflect a reduced average duration of illness by some classes of the mentally ill and in at least some cases better liaison between hospital staff in out-patient clinics with general practitioners responsible for domiciliary care.

Second, there is evidence in some places at least, of increased inter-relation between NHS and university staff.

Finally this note makes no comment on any changes which may flow from the reorganization of the Health Service in April, 1974. All the information on which it is based was collected long before that date. It seems to me likely that those changes may be more momentous for the care of mental illness and retardation than for other fields of medicine, since these, more perhaps than any other, are related so closely and in so many ways to social structure, social function and social pathology, and hence to non-medical social services

Notes

(1) This figure is taken from the records of the British Medical Association. The BMA compiles records of non-members, as well as members, and classifies them by type of employment so far as its information permits; but of those in the United Kingdom who are not known to have retired or partly retired, about 10% are unclassified for lack of information. Thus, while its totals are believed to be substantially correct, the numbers in its several classifications can only be regarded as minima, unless they can be confirmed or corrected from some other source. These which I thus quote as minima in this paper are the figure of 5000 in this paragraph and its constitutents quoted on p. 243.

(2) I have counted as psychiatrists (i) all doctors who are so listed in the returns of the Ministry of Health and the Department of Home and Health for Scotland and in information supplied by the Northern Ireland Hospital Authority; (ii) all medically qualified occupants of posts in or attached to departments of psychiatry, the Institute of Psychiatry, and the nine MRC units with directly psychiatric remits; and (iii) medically qualified external staff on the MRC who are currently engaged on psychiatric work. This definition includes a few doctors who would not regard themselves as psychiatrists; and the number may be further inflated by the fact that some who are listed more than once by reason of honorary or part-time appointments may have been counted twice. I think, therefore, that it is likely to exaggerate the numbers of those who by any criterion would be regarded as psychiatrists. The exaggeration is significant in the count of MRC staff but not, I think, overall.

(3) These are the Social Psychiatry Research Unit; the Unit for Research on the Epidemiology of Psychiatric Illness; the Clinical Psychiatry Research Unit; the Psychiatric Genetics Research Unit; the Neuropsychiatric Research Unit; the Neuropharmacology Research

Unit; the Unit for Research on the Chemical Pathology of Mental Disorders; the Brain Metabolism Research Unit; and the Unit for the Study of Environmental Factors in Mental and Physical Illness.

(4) The number of medical teachers appearing in the BMA records should no doubt be supplemented by an uncertain number of the unclassified referred to in Note. 1. The larger this figure is, the stronger becomes the argument I have based on it.

(5) These are: London Hospital Medical School, Middlesex Hospital Medical School, St Bartholomew's Hospital Medical School, St George's Hospital Medical School (these four within the University of London); and the Universities of Aberdeen, Birminghan, Bristol, Edinburgh, Glasgow, Leeds, Liverpool, Manchester, Newcastle upon Tyne, St Andrew's, Sheffield, Wales, and Queen's University, Belfast.
I have described them all as Departments of Psychiatry, though their actual titles vary—three are entitled Departments of Mental Health.

(6) See *Education in Psychology and Psychiatry*, a report published by the Council of the Royal College of General Practitioners, September 1967, pp. 38, 39.

(7) *Ibid*, pp. 39-41.

(8) The ideal relationship is well described in Sir Harold Himsworth (ed.). *The Support of Medical Research* (1956) Blackwell Scientific Publications, pp. 10-12.

(9) I use the figure kindly supplied to me, with many others, by Dr Grey Turner, deputy secretary of the British Medical Association, because the corresponding figure used in the earlier paper came from the same source. The Department of Health and Social Security to which I am also much indebted gave me a somewhat smaller figure which appears in their published statistics; but whatever be the explanation of the discrepancy, the rate of growth is I think likely to be most faithfully indicated by drawing both figures from the same source.

(10) This figure excludes doctors holding 'para 94 appointments', of whom all but 1000 are general practitioners holding clinical assistant appointments in hospitals. The number of doctors holding such appointments rose from 4606 in 1967 to 5498 in 1973.

(11) St Thomas', University College and Westminster Hospital medical schools. Of the thirty-four chairs, three are at Edinburgh and five at the Institute of Psychiatry. Some of these last are 'personal', that is conferred on a particular individual and not necessarily continued when he retires.

(12) Crisp, A.H. (1973) Final and professional MB in psychiatry. *British Journal of Medical Education*, 7, 254-9.

(13) These are the Neurochemical Pharmacology Unit at Cambridge and the Clinical Pharmacology Unit at Oxford. The Unit formerly called the Unit for Research on the Chemical Pathology of Mental Disorders has been renamed the Unit for Metabolic Studies in Psychiatry.

(14) These are (i) Professor M.G. Gelder at Oxford for investigation of the psychological treatment of psychoneurosis, (ii) Dr R.P. Hullin at Leeds for biochemical and metabolic studies in psychiatry, (iii) Dr A. Kushlik at Winchester for epidemiological studies on and evaluation of services for the mentally subnormal and the elderly, and (iv) Dr I.M. Marks and Dr S. Rachman at the Institute of Psychiatry for therapeutic studies of resistant neuroses.

(15) Department of Health and Social Security Annual Report on Departmental Research and Development, 1973. London, HMSO.

14. Schizophrenics and their families: research on parental communication

Lyman C. Wynne

with the assistance of Margaret T. Singer, John J. Bartko and Margaret L. Toohey

In all comprehensive studies of the origin, development and perpetuation of schizophrenic disorders, the place of the family is an issue. This key proposition applies to both genetic and psychodynamic hypotheses. Although family studies from these seemingly diverse starting points have at times engendered considerable controversy, as well as dogmatism and misunderstanding, agreement is emerging both about what is now known and what is still unclear. This consensus, partial but promising, has provided a framework for fresh collaborative research now under way, for example, at the University of Rochester. Fortunately, a number of new research methods, biological, psychological, and diagnostic, can now be introduced into family studies of schizophrenia. These approaches are especially important because of their implications for revising the basic concepts of schizophrenic disorders and possibly of other forms of behavioural deviance as well.

Beginning in the mid 1950's, a number of investigators (e.g. 1, 2 3) initiated studies of family patterns from a psychosocial perspective, especially studying those current familial entanglements which appeared to sustain symptoms. These patterns of interaction and communication of the family as a social unit appeared to have an impact upon, and be linked with, individual symptoms, but were not a simple summation of the behaviour or symptoms of individual family members. Moreover, the family interaction patterns appeared to be extraordinarily stable over time. Families were observed to have self-equilibrating, 'system' properties; individual symptoms were viewed as integral ingredients in the processes of family disequilibrium and disorder and in the re-establishment of equilibrium.

Several basic conclusions about the relatives of schizophrenics emerged in these studies. First, it appears that ordinary psychiatric diagnosis grossly underestimates the frequency of psychological disturbance in the families of schizophrenics. Although initial interviews and conventional contacts often reveal nothing that would be recorded in ordinary hospital records, intensive family studies typically have found serious disturbance, clearly beyond the 'normal' range, in non-diagnosed family members.

Second, the quality of the psychiatric disturbances in the relatives of schizophrenics has been resistant to conventional diagnostic classification. Berze, in 1910, was apparently the first to report his impressions about these

A revised form of the Sir Geoffrey Vickers Lecture presented by Professor Wynne on 21 February 1968.

relatives on visiting days. He became convinced that 'any observer must notice' that abnormal characteristics are 'extraordinarily frequent' among the parents and siblings of 'praecox' patients, noting, among other things, that their emotional involvement with their psychotic offspring was abnormal (4). Usually, the term 'schizoid' has been used to describe the various eccentricities of these relatives. However, this label has been applied extremely loosely, so that sometimes *any* deviation in a relative of a diagnosed schizophrenic has been labelled schizoid. A variety of other terms which do not appear in standard nomenclatures, such as the borderline syndrome and schizophrenic character, have been applied to these family members.

Third, these clinical observations have raised questions about the boundaries and validity of the concept of schizophrenia, whether it should be narrowed (to exclude these 'borderline' relatives), be broadened (to include them), or, more fundamentally, be reformulated in different terms altogether.

Meanwhile, especially since the mid 1960s, genetic research on schizophrenia has been raising similar questions about the boundaries of the concept of schizophrenia. In this work, the terms 'schizoidia' (5) and the 'schizophrenia spectrum' (6) have recently been introduced to designate the atypical pictures found in the biological family members of schizophrenics.

These complex studies cannot be reviewed here in detail. Despite continuing uncertainty and unclarity about diagnostic criteria, the recent genetic research has confirmed the traditional assumption that *something* is in fact transmitted genetically in at least *some* persons diagnosed as schizophrenic. However, it is also true that the genetic factor seems to be weaker than was formerly claimed. For example, more recent, well controlled twin studies found concordance rates of 25% to 38% in monozygotic twins (7), in contrast to the traditionally quoted figure of 86% concordance (8). Both the twin research and recent adoption studies (6, 9) raise the important question of how to account for the substantial number of cases in which no evidence for a genetic contribution is discernible if the researchers rely on conventional diagnostic criteria for 'typical', 'nuclear' schizophrenia in relatives.

Although special versions of a monogenic Mendelian hypothesis for the aetiology of schizophrenia cannot be ruled out definitively, more and more genetic investigators, such as Gottesman and Shields (10), Kringlen (7) and Rosenthal (11), are turning to a polygenic theory which supposes that what is inherited is a multifactorial 'constitutional predisposition'.

This viewpoint is quite in accordance with the findings of the intensive psychological studies of schizophrenics and their families. At the present time the data are insufficient to decide on the question of genetic specificity for a type, or types, of schizophrenic disorder versus a concept of less specific underlying dimensions or processes. Either viewpoint is compatible both with polygenic theories and with psychosocial hypotheses. However, quantitative variations in degree of predisposition to schizophrenic disorders are not appropriately evaluated with usual diagnostic methods. These methods make all-or-none distinctions between diagnostic categories and have not provided for systematic measurement of underlying predispositions. Several newer approaches to diagnostic evaluation make standardized assessments of specific signs and symptoms and provide for alternative ways of deriving diagnostic assessments, both typologies and multidimensional profiles (12, 13).

In addition to further work on individual diagnostic procedures, a radically different kind of 'diagnostic' or classificatory evaluation needs to be considered. Here we refer to evaluations of families and other groups *as units,* with social system properties. Such assessments may be correlated with individual diagnoses, but only partially. Lidz *et al.* (2), Wynne (14), Alanen (15) and Reiss (16) have proposed typologies of family disorders. It would be unwise to assume that traditional, individual diagnostic approaches are the only meaningful way of looking at behavioural disorders. For the present, the important research point is that the criteria and methodology of assessment be carefully specified in every study so that provision can be made for seriously considering and comparing alternative concepts.

Another problem which has been understandably, but regrettably, neglected in research on the development of schizophrenia is the specification of environmental conditions in order to evaluate genetic factors, and vice versa. Even if a genetic factor is proved to be necessary, variations in environmental factors need to be studied in detail. MacMahon (17) has pointed out that even if the concordance of monozygotic twins were 100% and that of dizygotic twins were zero, environmental determinants can still be critical. For example, genetic vulnerability to favism is determined by a single, sex-linked recessive gene, but vulnerable individuals actually manifest the disease only with the variable environmental event of eating fava beans.

Similarly, if we hypothesize that genetic factors in schizophrenia are necessary but not sufficient to produce various clinical manifestations, the strength of the genetic factors may actually be *under*estimated if contributory environmental factors are relatively absent in a given sample of subjects. At the same time, if the significant environmental factors are not identified specifically, they too may be underestimated or erroneously discarded as unimportant, if biological relatives (such as twins or sibs of schizophrenics) are loosely assumed, without detailed study, to have been exposed to a 'schizophrenogenic' environment. Except in the case of monozygotic twins, they may not have in fact the same genetic vulnerability and, regardless of genetic similarities, they cannot be assumed to have had the same biological or psychological environment unless specific, relevant environmental factors are systematically assessed in all subjects. From this vantage point, then, genetic and environmental approaches are not antagonistic but complementary: both may be necessary and 'causative' for phenotypic manifestations. However, this possibility cannot be evaluated unless sophisticated measures of variables from *both* spheres are used with the same samples of subjects.

At the same time as genetic and biochemical studies have been moving forward, recent detailed studies of family communication, such as those conducted by Singer and Wynne (18, 19, 20, 21) and Wynne (22, 23), have tried to contribute to this long-range, collaborative task by delineating specific aspects of the 'environment', which may thereby become a less vague and global concept.

It is well recognized that psychological similarities between family members may derive either from genetic factors or from psychological identification processes. However, less attention has been given to the fact that social psychological role theory provides a basis for predicting *differences* between members of the same family. It is entirely naive to expect that being reared in the same family means that the psychological experience of the family members has necessarily been similar on dimensions relevant to schizophrenia, or to expect that persons adopted away or reared in different families will thereby necessarily differ from one another on these dimensions. Additional data, beyond the facts of 'reared together' or 'reared apart', are needed. For example, it is well known that even monozygotic twins reared together develop characteristic role complementarities in dominance-submission. On the other hand, persons *not* reared in the same family, but in the same social class, may in some respects share more of the same experience than siblings within a given family. For example, in many cultures first-born males from different families of the same social class undoubtedly have more experiences in common with one another than they do with their younger sisters. Without detailed study of all the relevant family members and their roles and transactions with one another, limited or faulty conclusions about the 'environment' are inevitable.

Another environmental influence needing careful evaluation, probably especially prevalent in socially and economically deprived groups, is a greater frequency of minimal brain damage in pregnancy and delivery due to poorer nutrition and inferior medical care. Just as the psychological environment varies for children of the same family, so also does the biological environment differ for children of the same mother during gestation and delivery. Particularly for twins, who often have unequal placental nutrition and a high frequency of pregnancy and birth complications, especially prematurity, it is possible to detect differences in activity and responsiveness at birth, even in monozygotic twins. Thus, any assumption that twins have shared the same environment, biologically or psychologically, is highly tenuous (24).

If one relies solely on clinical and symptomatic data, it is very unclear indeed what is being transmitted genetically and how and when the genetic influences interact with nongenetic factors. It is evident that a wide gap still exists between the presumed genetic endowment and the eventual symptomatic breakdown in adolescence or adulthood. What is needed is a redirected research strategy oriented to the specific study of *intermediate* variables which could fill this gap in our present understanding of the development of schizophrenia.

In Figure 1, a schema, by no means comprehensive, is outlined in which two of the major classes of intermediate variables are included. The first of these classes of variables, which we have called *response dispositions*, are aspects of 'temperament' that now can be measured with psychophysiological, neurophysiological, and perceptual methods (25, 26, 27, 28, 29, 30). As indicated in Figure 1, these response dispositions appear to be polygenically inherited to a substantial degree (31, 32). On theoretical grounds it seems probable that metabolic and biochemical processes mediate the genetic influences on the perceptual and psychophysiological response dispositions, but this has not yet been examined empirically. The degree to which minimal brain damage associated with pregnancy and birth complications contributes to these predispostions is currently disputed (33, 34).

We suggest that the genetic components in schizophrenia are not best

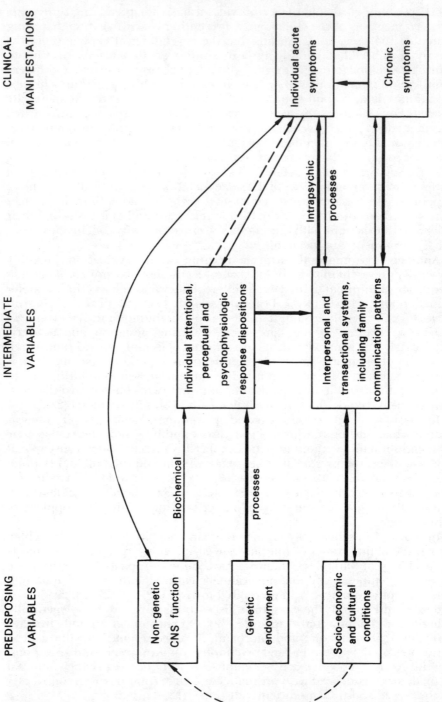

Figure 1 Simplified schema for studying the origin, development and perpetuation of the schizophrenias and similar disorders.

conceptualized as specific genotypes, but as non-specific, but genetically influenced response dispositions which are either extreme in degree or incongruent with one another. We further assume that if such response tendencies interact with certain non-genetic biological and psychosocial patterns, vulnerability to a diversity of forms of behavioural deviance is developed. We hypothesize that the vulnerability for developing the schizophrenic disorders *necessarily* involves both genetic and non-genetic factors. However, the same genetically influenced response dispositions, interacting with different environmental events, may alternatively lead to mere eccentricities or to 'inadequate personalities', or, on the other hand, to 'positive' deviance, as shown in certain forms of creativity and originality.

In accord with this formulation, the direct study of the measurable response dispositions, evaluated in their own right in patients, controls, and their relatives, is a more appropriate though complex approach to the genetic contribution to schizophrenia than is the traditional search for symptomatic and diagnostic concordance of relatives. The response dispositions can be measured in everyone so that *degrees* of concordance can be evaluated more systematically than is possible with traditional clinical studies of symptom patterns of diagnosis.

If the genetic contribution to schizophrenia is as non-specific as the term 'temperament' implies, a large portion of the general population may share in a biological vulnerability to schizophrenia without actually developing the clinical picture. The size of the vulnerable population will make a considerable difference in assessing the relative importance of the genetic contribution. For example, let us assume that 10% of the 'normal' population has highly deviant, attentional-response dispositions on a genetic basis. Let us further assume that all of those schizophrenics in the population with a genetically-contributed illness come from this 10%. However, only 1% or less of the population actually develops clinical schizophrenia. Perhaps, then, we face a two-stage research problem: (*a*) How do we differentiate the 10% who are vulnerable? (We have proposed the response-disposition hypothesis as a testable possibility.) (*b*) What has brought about the clinical illness in some and what possibly 'protected' most of these vulnerable 'normals'? How can we predict which will actually become symptomatic?

Thus, we hypothesize that experimentally measurable vulnerabilities, undiagnosed with traditional clinical methods, are indicators of a high 'heritability' of *underlying* predispositions which are usually *not* converted to symptomatic illness. This hypothesis is compatible with the evidence for a meaninfgul genetic contribution to the illness in some or all schizophrenics, but at the same time is consistent with the fact that a high proportion of relatives of schizophrenics are not diagnosably schizophrenic but do manifest a wide range of positively and negatively valued deviance. Clearly, this proposition is complex, but, in principle, empirically testable with methods now available. At the present stage of our understanding, it is premature to specify which of the various response dispositions are most highly relevant to schizophrenic illness. In current research, in which we are participating, a battery of measures producing a profile of response disposition scores is being obtained, instead of relying on a single test or dimension.

However, we suggest that research also turn to another level of investigation and another class of intermediate variables. Above all, we must study in more detail the interpersonal context in which the individual develops in order to understand why one outcome emerges rather than another.

Transactional processes and intrafamilial communication

In addition to individual response dispositions, transactional processes include, we believe, essential intermediate variables in the development of schizophrenic illness. The events, beyond the individual, which we call 'transactional' (35, 36), are related to phenomena given other labels such as interpersonal (37), interactional (38), interhuman and transexperiential (39).

The multiple variables in this area are interrelated conceptually. For convenience, they can be grouped into four classes: (*a*) intrafamilial communication patterns (1, 40); (*b*) family role structure (41, 42); (*c*) the intrafamilial *sub*culture of shared beliefs, myths, rules and values (3, 43, 44); and (*d*) extrafamilial factors, which may act *via* the family or separately and can be subdivided along lines such as peer-group, community network, social class, and the broader cultural context (35, 45, 46, 47).

In this report, we shall focus on only one aspect of the hypothesized transactional contributions to schizophrenic vulnerability, namely, intrafamilial communication patterns. Further, in this brief report we must restrict ourselves to only certain components of the communication patterns that we have studied. Methodologically, communication patterns are especially strategic because they are directly observable and can be specified operationally. Theoretically, communication patterns are a link between attentional, perceptual and cognitive response dispositions and a broader context of social learning and psychological development.

'Communication' patterns include, most importantly for schizophrenic processes, what we have called patterns of sharing attention and meaning (19, 48). We include here the individual's ability to focus attention selectively, flexibly, shifting with the transactional task and interpersonal context (49). Attentional styles and response dispositions ordinarily build into sustained, 'major sets' which make possible sequential thinking and purposive behaviour. However, major sets become segmentalized in schizophrenics (50).

Additionally, in order for 'normal' communication and the learning of language to occur, as well as for the learning of adaptive affective expression, foci of attention must be *shared* (48). Developmentally, the ways in which significant persons in the child's formative years communicate and share attention and meaning with the child are critical in the shaping of his own patterns of thinking, communicating, and experiencing (23, 40, 51).

From a slightly different perspective, communication patterns can be conceptualized as the overt manifestations of a family subculture of distinctive, often highly idiosyncratic, rules and role expectations. In addition, the value orientations of the broader culture and social class in modern Western society are typically transmitted through the nuclear family, especially in early life (35). Intimate peer relationships of children who later become schizophrenic are said to be impoverished and limited (52, 53). When this occurs, the impact of the intrafamilial life within the family psychological boundaries is correspondingly heightened (3).

Using this line of reasoning, we have proposed a quite radical hypothesis: Given a major, enduring relationship of parents and offspring, communication deviances of *parents* should be significantly related to the clinical psychiatric diagnosis and the symptomatic picture of their *offspring*. Further, we have hypothesized that the communication pattern of the parents, as a pair, and the family, when it has been an intact, enduring constellation or social unit, should be more decisively relevant to the offspring's psychiatric characteristics than either parent as an individual (40).

In our research, it should be noted that we have *not* been primarily concerned with familial contributions to the *immediate* 'stress' which could convert a 'predisposition' into a symptomatic breakdown. Rather, we have been interested in *patterns* of behaviour, *repeated* forms of communicating and relating which would contribute over years to the formation of character structure and personality, including the cognitive styles and response dispositions we have mentioned earlier. Thus, degrees of vulnerability-invulnerability to schizophrenic disorder are our primary concern (54, 55). Our objectives are to delineate a comprehensive picture of the predisposing factors, *both* 'constitutional' *and* experiential, as they are built up, maintained, and reinforced in the course of development.

Method

As part of our effort to assess these hypotheses, we shall present here a segment of the data obtained in a series of studies at the National Institute of Mental Health. These particular data were obtained with an unorthodox use of the Rorschach technique. We do not—and this is important—view Rorschach records in the usual way as an expression of intrapsychic projections. Rather, we regard them as samples of communication, as examples of how the subject relates to the examiner, organizes his attention in the testing task, and shares, or fails to share meanings with the examiner. We hypothesized that parents would bring to this situation some of the distinctive and enduring forms of communicating also found in their interpretive transactions with offspring, whose learning experience, both by identification and direct impact, would thereby be predictably influenced (19, 22, 23, 56).

The use of standardized, verbatim, individual Rorschach protocols is, of course, only one method of sampling communication. We have also applied the same principles with individual family members using the Thematic Apperception Test (21), the Object Sorting Test (57), and proverbs interpretation (58). Additionally, we have used these and other procedures with family members participating *together*, with and without a professional person present, as a means of examining certain characteristics of the family as a social unit or small social system (e.g., 16, 38, 59, 60, 61, 62, 63).

Methodological precautions

Certain methodological precautions are necessary in such research. First, it is essential that communication patterns be sampled in a comparable way from one subject to the next for any given body of data. Therefore, what the examiner says and does must be standardized as much as possible, including the provision of guidelines for his behaviour when the subject asks questions or diverts from the task. Also, the interviewer or tester should not be informed of the diagnosis or symptom picture of the subject because such information could covertly bias his attitudes and behaviour.

Second, communication samples must be verbatim, preferably tape recorded, and include comments of both subject and examiner. Otherwise, important, indeed essential, aspects of the communication may be omitted or selectively recorded, and independent checks on the comparability of the data will not be possible.

Third, the data must be analysed independently by raters or judges who have no information from or about the subjects other than the communication samples themselves, so that they can compare records from different kinds of subjects blindly. Thus, the communication samples from a parent should not include reference to the psychiatric symptoms of their off-spring.

Fourth, investigators who make the research diagnoses about the subjects should do so without knowledge of the tests or any clinical or research reports based upon them.

Fifth, interjudge reliability must be established and maintained at an adequately high level. This is a methodological criterion which is, unfortunately, too often neglected in psychiatric research.

Ideally, four separate staff members or groups of staff, should be available in research of this kind—for administration of the procedure to the subjects, for accurate transcription of protocols, for independent clinical diagnosis and evaluation, and for blind scoring or rating of the protocols. We have now achieved a considerable degree of success in applying these various criteria with several methods for studying communication.

Rorschach administration

In this study at the National Institute of Mental Health in Bethesda, Maryland, the Rorschach testing was done for research purposes and was not available to the diagnosticians or therapists of these subjects. When an adolescent or young adult family member was admitted to the clinical programme, the family members were asked to participate within a few weeks in a variety of research procedures. At the time the members of the families of the psychiatric patients were tested, the testing psychologists did not know the clinical history, symptoms, or diagnosis of the index family member. Usually one tester saw the index and another tested the other family members. The testing notes and tape recordings were then set aside for later transcription and research use. The twenty clinical psychologists who tested these families over a period of several years did so as part of their general clinical duties in accord with the needs of this project. In order to maintain a non-biased approach to the subjects, they did not participate in the planning of the project and were not familiar with the scoring categories, which were developed and published later on.

Thus, for all the families with disturbed members, the testers had no information that could have differentially influenced their behaviour toward the families of the schizophrenics compared with the families of the borderline or neurotic patients. When testing a subgroup of normal control families, the tester was not informed, but could infer that this family did not have a patient member because the appointments for testing entailed a slightly different procedure.

The testing psychologists, using a standard procedure to administer the ten Rorschach cards to each family member, made the following statement for the 'initial viewing':

'I have a series of cards here with inkblots on them. They look like different things to different people. I'll show them to you one at a time, and I'd like for you to tell me everything that each one looks like, everything that each one reminds you of. After you've finished with the first one, hand it back and we'll go on to the next one. Here's the first one.'

Thus, the primary task for the subject during the initial viewing was to focus attention selectively on particular aspects of the inkblots and to label his impressions so that they might be shared with the tester.

After the ten cards had been initially presented, the tester introduced the 'inquiry' as follows:

'I'd like to look through the inkblots with you once more. This time I'll remind you of the things the blots suggested to you the first time, and I'd like to ask you more about them.'

After restating each response in the subject's own words, the tester's standard requests were: 'Tell me more about it', or 'Tell me about the way you see it', or 'What about the inkblot suggested . . .?'

This use of a standardized but open-ended inquiry contrasts with some methods for administering the Rorschach in which the tester attempts to identify location and determinants (form, shading, color) as the objective of the inquiry. In our programme, the primary task in the inquiry portion of the Rorschach, unlike the initial viewing, was to facilitate a verbal transaction in which the subject might *reason about and elaborate on* his percepts. Thus, the tester was asked to limit his comments on the first cards to two, and later to one, of the standard, open-ended requests. There were, of course, occasional lapses from the standard procedures, but these appeared to be distributed randomly across the 20 testers and 483 subjects. Thus, both underproductive and overproductive subjects were presented with reasonably similar tester behaviour.

These details of administrative procedure are important, as we have found in reviewing protocols from other centres. Testers trained to obtain 'determinants' and 'location' in the inquiry as a primary goal, or testers using other approaches to Rorschach administration, will elicit protocols which either are not adequately standardized or do not permit the subject to reason and elaborate about his percepts or impressions. Such testers are prone to two extremes: (*a*) With subjects who give easily located responses, these testers too quickly move on during the initial viewing and later make an inadequate inquiry. Thus they do not wait to hear what might be deviant reasoning and communication about a response. (*b*) With subjects who are hesitant, vague, or impressionistic (particularly common with depressed persons), these same testers, in a non-standardized way, urge or even goad subjects to define or justify their percepts beyond what is characteristic for their perceptual and communicative 'style'; the tester thus induces communication which is atypical for these subjects.

Rorschach protocols obtained in these ways are not satisfactory for scoring with the manual we have developed (21), although such protocols may be quite adequate for more orthodox Rorschach scoring procedures which emphasize the location and inkblot characteristics. Regrettably, both types of pitfalls characterized the administration of the Rorschachs, especially in the inquiry portion, in an attempted replication of our work by Hirsch and Leff (64) with parents of schizophrenics and depressives.

Rorschach scoring

The tape recordings of the protocols were then transcribed in a standardized format and checked twice for accuracy by a research assistant who was unfamiliar with the clinical assessment of the subjects and the scoring categories.

In the study to be reported here, the sex and identifying code number for each subject were the only information on the transcripts given to the raters. Age and generation were not revealed; protocols were scored individually without knowledge of which records came from members of the same family.

The psychologists who scored the Rorschachs in this sample of families tested in Bethesda never saw the subjects themselves. Indeed, the primary rater (M.T.S.) lived 3000 miles away and had no direct or indirect information about these families.

The Rorschach scoring system derived from earlier research in which a battery of test protocols (Rorschach, TAT, Object Sorting, sentence completion, and proverbs interpretation) from 35 pairs of parents had been used for a series of blind predictions: first, the psychiatric diagnosis of the most disturbed offspring in each family; second, the severity of illness of the offspring, using a seven-point scale; and third, the form of thinking of the offspring. Also, offspring were matched blindly with the rest of the family from which they came (19, 65). All results were statistically significant (20).

We then delineated 41 categories of deviant communication which we believed appeared more frequently in the Rorschach records of parents of schizophrenics than in the records of other parents (21). We did not expect that this limited set of categories would tap all the clues that a skilled judge would find in a more comprehensive study of the kind previously conducted (19, 20). However, we wanted to go as far as possible in spelling out a portion of the criteria used in that study, especially certain aspects of communicating and reasoning. By so doing, other investigators might more easily use this method, replications might take place, a variety of other populations could be sampled, and the criteria themselves could evolve and be sharpened selectively.

We wish to emphasize that individual Rorschachs are only one of the procedures which we believe are important in studying the trans-actions within families. Furthermore, only a limited portion of the predictive features found in the Rorschach protocols are scored with the manual used in this report. We believe that our findings reported here and elsewhere suggest that this particular procedure can provide valuable data,

TABLE 1 Rorschach scoring categories

I. Closure problems

110 Uncorrected speech fragments
120 Unintelligible remarks
130 Unstable percepts
140 Gross indefiniteness and tentativeness
150 Responses in negative form
160 Subjunctive 'if' responses
170 'Question' responses
181 Contradictory information
182 Inconsistent and ambiguous references
183 Incompatible alternatives

Disqualifications

191 Derogatory, disparaging, critical remarks
192 Nihilistic remarks
193 Failures to verify own responses
194 Retractions and denials
195 Forgetting responses
196 Partial disqualifications

II. Disruptive behaviour

211 Interruptions of examiner's speeches
212 Extraneous questions and remarks
213 Odd, tangential, inappropriate remarks
220 Non-verbal, disruptive behaviour
230 Humour
240 Swearing
250 Hopping around among responses
260 Negativistic, temporary card rejection followed by a response
270 Concrete-set responses
280 References to 'they' and to the intent of others

III. Peculiar language and logic

A. Peculiar word usages, constructions and pronunciations

310 Ordinary words or phrases used oddly or out of context
311 Odd sentence construction
312 Quaint, private terms or phrases
313 Euphemisms
314 Slips of tongue
315 Mispronounced words
316 Foreign terms used for no particular reasons
317 Cryptic remarks
318 Clang associations, rhymed phrases and wordplay
319 Abstract, global terms

B. Reiteration

320 Repetition of words or phrases

C. Peculiar logic

330 Illogical combinations of percepts and categories
331 Nonsequitur reasoning
332 Assigning meaning illogically on basis of non-essential attributes of cards
333 Contaminations

IV. Word count: Initial Viewing, Inquiry, and Total.

but this pragmatic focus for this report should not lead to a neglect of other family features which we and others are scoring systematically in current research.

In the transactional principles guiding the selection of these scoring categories, we emphasized the importance of establishing and maintaining shared-task sets and foci of attention in a transaction—in this study, between subject and examiner (21). We were *not* attempting to evaluate 'thought disorder' in the parents *themselves*, but, rather, the *impact* that certain forms of communication hypothetically would have upon a listener, and especially upon a growing child. To be sure, some correlation of these communication disorder scores with 'thought disorder' measures would be expected, but traditional Rorschach indices of schizophrenia were not emphasized.

In Table 1, the headings are listed for the 41 categories in our present scoring system to be used with individual Rorschach protocols. (See 21 for details and examples of each category. A revised manual in current use regroups the items and contains additional examples and clarified scoring guidelines for improved reliability.)

The categories were tentatively grouped into three main classes:

(*a*) *Closure problems,* that is, problems in making a commitment to an idea or percept: (*i*) The percept offered by the speaker is not visualizable by the listener, or (*ii*) the speaker makes a premature and unwarranted assumption of shared meaning, or (*iii*) he secondarily disqualifies his own ideas as they are being expressed, or soon after.

(*b*) *Disruptive behaviour:* The speaker introduces material or behaviour which is extraneous to the task at hand.

(*c*) *Peculiar language and logic:* words, sentences and logic are scored if used in idiosyncratic ways which would ordinarily interfere with a listener's ability to give attention or ascribe meaning to what the speaker is saying.

In addition, we have made word counts for each subject. Payne, Caird and Laverty (66) have suggested that verbosity in a focused communication, such as proverb interpretation, is a measure of 'over-inclusive thinking'. They hypothesized that 'an over-inclusive individual should be unable to exclude from his answer associations to the proverb which are irrelevant to its explanation'. We obtained confirmatory evidence for this hypothesis in an analysis of the number of words used by a variety of patients and family members ($N=164$) in interpreting the 'rolling stone' proverb. Taking word counts from verbatim tape recorded responses, we found that the parents of schizophrenics were more verbose in this standardized task than were the parents of borderline, neurotic, and control parents (58). Therefore, in analysing communication deviances in Rorschach protocols, we have examined word count in some detail, both as a communication category in its own right and in combination with other categories.

Excerpt from a scored record: A short portion of a protocol from a father of a schizophrenic illustrates the use of the scoring categories. Note that the percept, 'bat', is an ordinary, popular response on this card, but it is the subject's style of expression which is of interest.

Card I

Initial viewing (following standard instructions from tester).
1. Well, you can read (310-odd word usage) it in a lot of different ways. It looks like a—bat or a—bug of some sort—
(one deviance score in this transaction).

Inquiry

1. Examiner: (Tell me more about the bat or bug of some sort, please.) Well, uh, was this the one I came out with the bat? (195-Forgetting response; 310-odd usage)
Well, all right, let me see—here's oh yeah, you what. (110-uncorrected speech fragment.) here's the un—this would be kind of the head and face looking at you, and the uh—wings like that—in here—with the body coming down this way and the feet in this area—sort of out of proportion.

Oh—I—I think I also started off in working (310) the bat to see if uh just as a—almost as a configuration over-all. As the whole thing as a—I get a kind of a bat to bat (318- wordplay) thing—there. (120- unintelligible remarks, applicable to the last major portion of this speech.)

(Six deviance scores in this transaction. As a scoring convention, in the data presented here we counted only one occurrence of any category in a given transaction. Thus, the second 310 score was not counted. However, in our current scoring procedure we now count all deviances.)

The Communication Deviance Index (D/T)

We have defined the basic unit to be scored as the 'transaction', which differs somewhat from the traditional Rorschach 'response'. We include everything communicated by the subject in describing a given percept and also other remarks interspersed before, during, and after the response itself. That is, all of the subject's communication is scored beginning immediately after the tester's comments with the presentation of each card, and continuing until the subject has begun to describe a different percept. Also included as a part of a 'transaction' are later disqualifying remarks by the subject about percepts described earlier on the same card. The communication in and around each response in the 'initial viewing' of each card is treated as one scorable transaction, and the later 'inquiry' about that percept is regarded as a separate scorable transaction. For the sample of families in this report, only the initial viewing and the inquiry for the first percept on each of the ten cards was scored. Thus, for the ten cards, a maximum of twenty transactions was scored (one response in the initial viewing of each card and the inquiry for that response).

One of the most useful measures for statistical manipulation is the total number of deviance scores divided by the number of 'transactions' (D/T). For example, if a parent had a total of ten deviance scores during twenty transactions, the D/T score would be 0.50. The highest D/T score for an individual in the present series was 6.18, 105 deviance scores in seventeen transactions. The total frequency of deviance scores is thus corrected for the number of responses the subject gives by taking the mean frequency for each transaction.

The D/T parental scores can be analysed from the standpoint of the parents either as individuals or as pairs (taking the mean, or midpoint, between the scores for the father and the mother in each pair). The analysis of parental pairs is of theoretical interest because we have hypothesized that in any intact family the problems posed by one of the parents may be either aggravated or counteracted by the other parent (20, 67). For example, the impact of guardedness or tentativeness of one parent is likely to be corrected by a spouse whose communication is clear and straightforward, but presumably would be aggravated if the spouse's communication is peculiar or tangential. This kind of qualitative 'fitting' together of parental pairs, although important, is difficult to take into account in simple numerical scoring from manuals of the kind we are reporting here. The method of computing the midpoint of the communication scores for each pair of parents is obviously an incomplete solution to this problem.

It should be noted that this way of looking at parents as pairs is different from that used when a genetic hypothesis of Mendelian dominance is used: *one* deviant parent in a pair would then be regarded as significant. From the standpoint of hypotheses of recessive genes, polygenes, or social psychological influences (in which the family as a unit is crucial), the scores of *both* parents are more important.

Scoring reliability

Testers and raters should be very familiar with the range of 'ordinary' and deviant behaviour shown by subjects in the Rorschach task, including the varieties of idiomatic language used by persons of a given social class, educational and cultural background. A period of training with the scoring system over a number of weeks is necessary to achieve reasonable reliability. Our current manual has been revised to provide additional guidelines to improve ease of learning the categories and to establish adequate reliability reasonably quickly. Even so, it should be recognized that periodic, detailed checks on reliability are necessary, both for total D/T scores and, more so, for qualitative, item-by-item comparisons. Raters differ in the degree to which they are willing or able to give sustained, consistent attention to this quite arduous task.

Six raters have now used this manual with reasonable inter-rater reliability after a period of training. An inter-rater reliability check was previously reported in which 82% agreement was obtained on 118 parental records (56).

Recently, in a test-retest reliability check, twenty records were rescored by Singer after a two-year interval. These records were selected by a research assistant from parental protocols in the present study. These records were a stratified sample in which the variables of sex of parent and of offspring, diagnosis of parent and offspring, and social class of family were varied systematically. Also, protocols from nine different testers were included. The intraclass correlation coefficient for the D/T scores was 0.96 (for specific categories the reliability was somewhat lower and varied from one category to another).

Sample characteristics

Encouraged by findings from scoring a sample of Rorschachs from 59 families tested elsewhere (68, 56, 22), we have collected and analysed data from a larger sample of 114 families studied at NIMH in Bethesda, Maryland. In these families, testing was carried out with 228 parents, 114 index offspring, and 141 siblings of the indexes, making a total of 483 individuals.

The 'index' family member was defined as the identified or presenting psychiatric patient in the offspring generation, or the oldest offspring if there were no identified patient (in normal control families).

Selection of patient-families

The index psychiatric patients in the present sample were hospitalized in the Clinical Center of the National Institutes of Health, Bethesda. Announcements had been previously circulated to local psychiatrists and psychiatric clinics and hospitals that the Clinical Center was available for referral of psychiatric patients who would not be charged a fee but would be asked to take part in certain research procedures. Among the patients thus admitted, the following criteria were applied for their selection in the present study: (a) The patient had to be seriously enough disturbed for a psychiatric team to believe that hospitalization was clinically justified. This criterion was severity of disturbance, *not* whether they were neurotic, delinquent, borderline, or schizophrenic. (b) The age of the identified patient was 15-45 years. (c) Patients with demonstrable brain lesions, including epilepsy, were excluded. Families were excluded if either parent showed evidence of organic changes associated with aging. (d) Both biological parents had to be available locally to take part in clinical evaluation interviews and psychological testing. The siblings of the index offspring were also asked to participate, and usually did so, but this was not a fixed requirement. (e) Families in which the patient or either parent were non-English speaking were excluded.

Many but not all of the families participated later in a clinical programme which stressed family psychotherapy, but this was not a requirement for inclusion in this study. The family members were subjects for a number of research procedures, among which the Rorschach was quite incidental.

Selection of normal control families

Seventeen of the twenty psychiatrically normal families were recruited by asking a local high school to provide a list of families with at least two same-sex adolescent offspring. These subjects were paid to participate; about 80% of those invited did so. The families of the normal control group were screened by a social worker who visited the home and interviewed each family member. The oldest offspring designated as the index was also given a standard diagnostic interview at the Clinical Center by a research psychiatrist. Families in which a parent or the index offspring had a brain disorder or in which any member had a recent symptomatic psychiatric disorder were excluded.

The other three families in the normal control group had an index offspring free of psychiatric symptoms but with a serious chronic medical illness requiring hospitalization—paraplegia from a spinal injury, mitral insufficiency, and Hashimoto's thyroiditis.

Diagnostic evaluations

All tested family members were individually diagnosed by a research psychiatrist. These evaluations were made by a single rater (L.C.W.) without seeing the Rorschach protocols or any reports about them, nor were the Rorschach protocols or evaluations available to the clinicians who treated and supplied information about the patients and the families. The research diagnostician drew upon information from multiple tape recorded interviews and extensive clinical contacts between each family member and a number of NIMH staff. A number of the index patients were interviewed with the WHO standardized interview schedules (12, 69). When these schedules had not been used in direct interviews, similar diagnostic criteria were applied in evaluating available clinical material. Follow-up information was also available on nearly all of the patient families, typically extending at least two years after discharge, and, in the case of some, for up to twelve or fifteen years.

Even though clinical evaluation is fraught with many difficulties for research purposes, these diagnostic assessments were based on unusually comprehensive data, with the diagnostic criteria held comparable from one patient to the next. A reliability check on the diagnostic ratings for fifteen of the patients revealed a product-moment correlation (r) of 0.96 between these research ratings and ratings on the same patients by a separate clinical research team that had examined this subsample of patients with special thoroughness.

Severity Rating Scale

In this report we shall primarily use a global mental health rating system which can be conveniently linked to the quantitative D/T scores. Other techniques for evaluating symptom clusters and diagnostic typologies and dimensions are of considerable interest. One system for classifying thought disorders of the patients and linking these distinctions to the qualitative study of parental communication has been previously reported (20, 68). The global scale used here is similar to the 'severity' rating scale we used previously (65), and it also has much in common with a global 'mental health' rating scale used by Kringlen (7). We refer the reader to Kringlen (7) for examples of how patients can be rated on such a scale.

Briefly, at levels 1 and 2, individuals are found who are within ordinary limits of psychiatric normality. At level 1 are persons about whom there have been no observations or reports of neurotic symptoms or personality deviations. At level 2 are persons who have slight eccentricities or have had temporary neurotic symptoms in times of unusual stress.

Level 3 includes persons with a history of definite symptomatic neurotic and personality disorders, including delinquency, but without evidence of psychotic features currently or in the past. In our sample, patients at level 3 were all quite markedly disturbed individuals. Most were hospitalized for a period of months or a year or two. Among the twenty-five index offspring diagnosed in this group, fifteen had severe neuroses, especially obsessional and depressive states, and ten had serious delinquency problems, particularly acting-out, such as promiscuity, group stealing, running away, group drug usage and assaultiveness.

Because these patients showed flagrantly deviant behaviour, their parents quite often were as much or more alarmed about these offspring rated at level 3 than were the parents of the patients who had a diagnostic rating at the 4 to 7 levels. The similarity in history of hospitalization and parental concern between these severe neurotics, the borderlines, and the schizophrenics is methodologically very important as Wynne and Singer (40) have pointed out: In *all* of these families, the index offspring was a seriously disturbed, usually hospitalized family member whose behaviour and patient status consistently and understandably was a significant feature of the family's life together. Thus, a control group for the families of the schizophrenics was built into this study by the presence of a serious psychiatric disorder and, usually, hospitalization in the neurotic and borderline index offspring. In contrast, the so-called normal control families did not have this experience of psychiatric hospitalization for a family member. If communication deviances in the parents could be induced by behavioural disorder or psychiatric hospitalization of an offspring, then one would hypothesize that the parents of the hospitalized neurotic offspring should have significantly higher scores than the parents of the normal controls. (As we shall report in the section on results, this hypothesis was not borne out.)

Level 4 includes what Grinker, Werble, and Drye (70) and others have called the 'borderline syndrome'. Persons at this level of severity have consistently given diagnosticians great difficulty. These patients sometimes have a history of transient psychotic episodes that are difficult to evaluate later on. Most of them have enduringly severe personality problems. Despite substantial impairment, the index patients and parents who were diagnosed borderline in this study have not become chronically psychotic during a long-term follow-up period.

Borderline persons have severe interpersonal difficulties, especially defects in their capacity for empathy. They often invite exploitation by others and are exploitative of others. Their work is less impaired than their interpersonal relationships, but work may suffer secondarily because of their unacceptable and unaccepting relationships with others. In the conventional nomenclature, which is unsatisfactory for this group, they are variously labelled as schizoid personalities, paranoid personalities, explosive personalities, and individuals with very ineffectual responses to emotional and social demands.

Some are called simple, latent or pseudoneurotic schizophrenics. The border-line syndrome needs to be considered in detail in studies of the families of schizophrenics because of the regularity with which relatives are given these or related labels.

Levels 5, 6 and 7 include persons who are, or have been, definitely psychotic for more than a brief episode. For the data analyses to be described here, we have subdivided these persons into what Vaillant (71, 72) has called the remitting versus the non-remitting schizophrenic psychoses. We have applied his criteria to the present sample of forty-four index persons who have been definitely psychotic. Fortunately, extended follow-up data have become available to check whether the prognostic indicators of remission actually have been borne out or not. We did not, however, include the family history of mental illness as a prognostic criterion, because we have examined family history as a separate variable.

Patients at our severity level 5 are often given labels of schizophreniform, schizo-affective, reactive or schizophrenia-like psychoses. They have in common a good premorbid history, an acute onset and, later, a definite remission. However, in this sample they all had, for weeks to months, a typically florid psychosis, including severe delusional and hallucinatory symptoms, sometimes with acute catatonic phases. They typically show what we have described as 'fragmentation' of the thinking processes (65). Typical manic-depressives and patients with neurologic or alcoholic syndromes were not included in this study.

The twenty patients at levels 6-7 have never shown a significant remission from a schizophrenic psychosis. Those at level 6 have done so only in a very limited, partial way. Patients at both levels would be called poor premorbid or 'process' schizophrenics, using the prognostic criteria of the Phillips Scale (73). With respect to form of thinking (65), thirteen were amorphous, six fragmented, and one constrictedly or coherently paranoid in their form of thinking. Because only families in which both parents were living and available were included, this sample was biased toward including younger schizophrenics than would be found in a general population of hospitalized schizophrenics. Consequently, chronic, organized paranoid schizophrenics were also under-represented. Most of the patients in this series at levels 6 and 7 were disintegrated, disorganized, incoherent individuals without systematized delusions. Several of them met the criteria that are usually implied when the term 'hebephrenic' is used.

We wish to emphasize that the diagnostic criteria applied in this study were much more stringent than is customary in the United States. The classifications were influenced by comparisons with diagnostic evaluations made with colleagues in the World Health Organization study of schizophrenia in which one of the authors (L.C.W.) has been participating (12, 69). A special feature of this study was that all of the parents and normal control index offspring were given mental health ratings on the same seven-point scale.

Demographic variables

The demographic features of the families have been partly demarcated by the

TABLE 2 Demographic variables for offspring

Severity of disorder of index offspring	No. of families	Sex of index offspring		Age of index	Years educ. of indexes	Sex of sibs	
		Males	Females			Males	Females
Normal 1-2	20	9	11	19.0 ± 0.7	12.5 ± 0.5	10	10
Neurotic 3	25	16	9	17.4 ± 0.4	11.0 ± 0.4	12	14
Borderline 4	25	17	8	18.2 ± 0.5	11.9 ± 0.4	10	17
Remitting schizophrenics 5	24	10	14	22.4 ± 1.3	13.1 ± 0.4	15	20
Non-remitting schizophrenics 6-7	20	10	10	23.0 ± 1.0	11.5 ± 0.5	12	21
Total	114	62	52	19.9 ± 4.6	12.0 ± 2.1	59	62

Means and standard error of the mean are given where applicable.

TABLE 3   Demographic variables for parents

Severity of disorder of index offspring		No. of families	Age of fathers	Age of mothers	Years educ. of fathers	Years educ. of mothers	Family social class
Normal	1-2	20	47.7 ± 1.9	45.0 ± 1.7	14.1 ± 0.8	12.7 ± 0.6	2.4 ± 0.2
Neurotic	3	25	48.0 ± 1.0	45.2 ± 0.8	15.5 ± 0.6	13.2 ± 0.3	2.1 ± 0.2
Borderline	4	25	50.2 ± 1.4	46.9 ± 1.1	16.1 ± 0.7	14.3 ± 0.5	1.8 ± 0.2
Remitting schizophrenics	5	24	50.4 ± 1.8	50.4 ± 1.6	14.1 ± 1.0	13.0 ± 0.6	2.2 ± 0.2
Non-remitting schizophrenics	6-7	20	56.2 ± 1.3	50.9 ± 1.1	12.2 ± 1.1	12.6 ± 0.6	3.1 ± 0.3
Total		114	51.0 ± 0.7	47.6 ± 0.6	14.5 ± 0.4	13.2 ± 0.2	2.3 ± 0.1

Mean and standard errors of the means are given where applicable.

criteria for selection of the sample, as described above. Further details are provided in Tables 2 and 3. It will be apparent that the mean age of the schizophrenics was somewhat greater than for the normal, neurotic, and borderline index offspring. Also, the fathers of the non-remitting schizophrenics were older than other parents. In years of education, the index offspring did not differ appreciably. However, the parents of the non-remitting schizophrenics tended to have less education and lower social class than the other parents. Social class was rated with the Hollingshead Two-factor Index of Social Position (74).

These demographic variations were examined in detail in the statistical analyses, reported below, to determine whether they might account for differences between groups in communication deviance scores.

Hypotheses

The central hypothesis assessed with the data in the present report is that the frequency of certain kinds of communication deviances by parents is significantly related to the severity of psychiatric disorder, especially schizophrenia, in their most disturbed offspring. Secondarily, we hypothesize that this measure of parental communication deviances is dimensionally different, and statistically separable, from clinically assessed psychiatric disorder in the parents themselves.

Further, although the index offspring, as primary patients, would of course be expected to be *clinically* more disturbed than their parents, we hypothesize that the parents will show more frequent communication deviances than the patients themselves. This hypothesis sould be confirmed if we were successful in our intention to construct the communication deviances manual so that communication features would be selected which, if repeated during the course of development, would be likely to have a schizophrenogenic *impact* upon a listener, especially a growing child. Because these parental communication features were not selected to be relevant to the diagnosis of schizophrenia in the parents, the schizophrenic offspring might well have fewer communication deviances than their non-schizophrenic parents. The concept of impact implies the expectation of differences between parents and offspring, not only similarities.

Additionally, we hypothesize that the siblings of the index offspring will have lower deviance scores than the index offspring and their parents, but that there will be a significant trend for more frequent deviances in sibs of schizophrenics than in sibs of non-schizophrenics. (Note: this hypothesis follows either from a genetic point of view or from a psychosocial formulation of the family as the small social system in which primary learning takes place.)

Finally, on the basis of other studies with families from a diversity of cultures and social groups (e.g. 35), we hypothesize that demographic variables, as well as such secondary phenomena as word count, will not account for the central hypothesized relationship between parental communication deviances and the severity of psychiatric disorder in the offspring.

Results

In the data analyses reported here, we shall focus upon the *total* frequency of communication deviances for the various subjects and not upon the frequency of the forty-one *component* categories which make up the scoring manual (21). In other publications, we shall report detailed findings with factor analyses, stepwise discriminant analyses, and other methods of distinguishing which of these deviance categories, plus word count, differentiate best the parents, index offspring, and their siblings, both on our seven-point severity scale and on a variety of qualitative clinical features. Also, in other reports we shall present a comparison with scorings made with other samples of families, including adoptive families, an investigation of tester effects upon scores, and an analysis of the relation of the present Rorschach communication data to scores on other tests with the same subjects.

The reader should understand throughout that the specific data presented here should not be considered as an ultimate test of the comprehensive theory and research strategy outlined earlier here and in previous papers by the authors (40, 65, 19, 22, 23, 35, 54). Rather, these findings are necessarily a component of a long-term series of investigations in which we have sampled diverse populations and studied families both with additional scoring procedures for the Rorschach records themselves, as well as with entirely different techniques for sampling communication. Further, these and related methods are now being utilized and evaluated more fully at the University of Rochester in a prospective, longitudinal study of families at genetic high risk for having a schizophrenic offspring.

Distribution of parental deviance scores

The distribution of communication deviance scores for parental pairs (taking the midpoint for each pair) is graphically depicted in Figure. 2.

The means and medians of parental scores and the spread of one standard deviation above and below each mean are shown for each of the five main diagnostic categories of the index offspring. Most noteworthy are the following points: (*a*) The parental deviance scores rise in a completely consistent, monotonically increasing fashion as the ratings of severity of illness of the index offspring increase. (*b*) The means and medians within each diagnostic group are quite similar, indicating that the distribution of intra-group parental scores is not highly skewed. (*c*) The scores for the two parental groups with schizophrenic offspring differ markedly from the scores for the two parental groups with normal and neurotic offspring. (*d*) The scores for the parents of borderline patients overlap both with those on the normal-neurotic side and on the schizophrenic side. It should be kept in mind that the parental Rorschach communication scores and the clinical diagnostic ratings of the offspring were obtained entirely independently.

Although the fathers tend to have slightly higher deviance scores than the mothers (mean D/T of 1.48 for fathers and 1.45 for mothers), this difference is not statistically significant. Except for a reversal for the mothers in which those with schizophrenic offspring at severity level 5 have somewhat higher deviance scores than those with offspring at levels 6 and 7, the means and medians for the scores of *both* fathers and mothers rise consistently as severity of illness of the index increases.

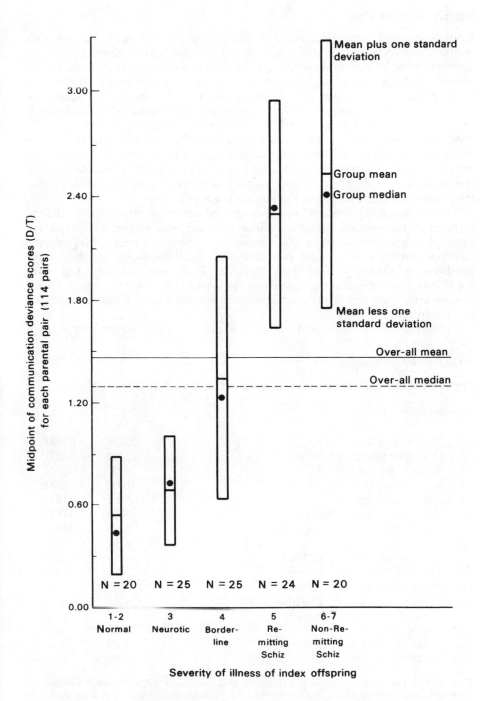

Figure 2 Parental communication deviances and severity of illness of index offspring.

Discriminant analysis

Geneticists and psychodynamicists alike (e.g. 2, 75) have agreed that concordance between relatives in severity of psychopathology should be expected, despite differences of views about the mode of transmission. In our present study, we have obtained ratings of severity of psychiatric disorder in both parents and offspring. These ratings differ from our scores of communication deviances which were not only obtained through independent procedures but also are based upon different conceptual premises. As we have noted, the deviance categories were selected because of the hypothesized transactional impact of these communicational features upon a listener, not because these features represented diagnostically relevant characteristics of the speaker. But do these two measures—severity of psychopathology and frequency of communication deviances—in fact differ?

To examine this question, we have applied several multivariate statistical techniques to our data, including a discriminant analysis (see Table 4) and a multiple regression analysis. All measures support our central hypothesis: parental deviance scores and parental psychiatric disorders are distinctive predictor variables, significantly different from one another, but both significantly discriminating severity of disorder in the index offspring. Of the two variables, the parental communication deviance score is somewhat more discriminating.

Table 4 shows the results of a discriminant analysis in which 16 predictor

TABLE 4   Discriminant analysis

Dependent variable: severity of disorder of index offspring

Independent variables	F	p
1. Deviance score, fathers	27.30	< 0.0005
2. Deviance score, mothers	25.22	< 0.0005
3. Severity of disorder, fathers	16.00	< 0.0005
4. Severity of disorder, mothers	10.69	< 0.0005
5. Age of indexes	8.84	< 0.0005
6. Deviance score, indexes	8.84	< 0.0005
7. Age of fathers	5.59	< 0.0005
8. Age of mothers	4.57	< 0.01
9. Occupational level, fathers	4.55	< 0.01
10. Years of education, indexes	3.75	< 0.01
11. Years of education, fathers	3.47	< 0.01
12. Years of education, mothers	1.83	n.s.
13. Total word count, indexes	1.59	n.s.
14. Sex of indexes	1.31	n.s.
15. Total word count, mothers	1.22	n.s.
16. Total word count, fathers	0.66	n.s.

This table is step 0 of a stepwise discriminant analysis. The F values for each variable are equivalent to an analysis of variance for that variable, indicating its power, considered separately from the other variables to discriminate among the index offspring at the seven levels of severity of disorder.

variables were compared as to their differentiation of the severity of disorder of the index offspring in this sample.

We have included in this analysis various demographic variables, noted in Tables 2 and 3, some of which do in fact discriminate among the groups of offspring, though less powerfully than the deviance scores and severity ratings of the parents.

In constructing the communication deviances manual, we had sought to identify features in Rorschach communication which would be especially frequent in the parents of schizophrenics, but not necessarily prominent in symptomatically ill schizophrenics themselves. Therefore, we hypothesized that the deviance scores of the *parents* would predict severity of illness of the index offspring even better than do the deviance scores of the *index offspring themselves*. Table 4 confirms that the communication deviance scores of the index offspring predict their own severity of disorder well but not so strongly as do the deviance scores of the parents.

Of special interest are the data on word count shown in Table 4. Hirsch and Leff (64) have attempted a replication of our study with forty pairs of parents, half with a schizophrenic offspring, and half with a neurotic offspring. We have noted above that their procedure for administration of the Rorschachs was not standardized in the manner that we have used. Nevertheless, despite limitations of their records, they found that the mean D/T scores for the parents of schizophrenics was 1.33 and for parents of neurotics was 0.88, a difference significant at the 0.05 level. However, noting in their data a high

TABLE 5 Communication deviance scores of parental pairs

Severity of index disorder	Parental pairs N	Unadjusted mean deviance score	Adjusted mean deviance score and standard error
1-2	20	0.54	0.63 ± 0.14
3	25	0.70	0.83 ± 0.10
4	25	1.35	1.38 ± 0.10
5	24	2.26	2.13 ± 0.11
6-7	20	2.50	2.37 ± 0.14

The parental pair deviance score is the midpoint between the deviance (D/T) scores of the father and the mother in each pair. These pair scores were compared across diagnostic groups, classified by the severity of disorder of the index offspring in each family. In an analysis of covariance, the effect of covariates on the parental pair deviance scores has been taken into account. The covariates were: (1) family social class, Hollingshead Index of Social Position, levels 1 to 5; (2) mean years of education for each parental pair; (3) mean severity of disorder for each parental pair on 7-point global mental health rating scale; (4) mean age of each parental pair; (5) mean total Rorschach word count of each pair. Analysis of covariance after adjusting with covariates: F $(4/104) = 25.51$.

TABLE 6   Communication deviance scores of fathers

Severity of index disorder	Fathers N	Unadjusted mean deviance score	Adjusted mean deviance score and standard error
1-2	20	0.49	0.68 ± 0.18
3	25	0.60	0.76 ± 0.14
4	25	1.47	1.41 ± 0.14
5	24	2.11	2.06 ± 0.15
6-7	20	2.85	2.59 ± 0.19

Adjusted means of deviance scores (D/T) were obtained by an analysis of covariance in which the effect of the covariates has been taken into account. Covariates were: (1) fathers' own severity of disorder (1-7 rating scale); (2) fathers' age; (3) fathers' years of education; (4) fathers' occupational level (Hollingshead code 1-7); (5) fathers' total Rorschach word count. Analysis of covariance after adjusting with covariates: F (4/104) = 18.34.

TABLE 7   Communication deviance scores of mothers

Severity of disorders of index offspring	Mothers N	Unadjusted mean deviance score	Adjusted mean deviance score and standard error
1-2	20	0.59	0.71 ± 0.16
3	25	0.82	0.89 ± 0.13
4	25	1.23	1.34 ± 0.13
5	24	2.42	2.16 ± 0.14
6-7	20	2.15	2.10 ± 0.15

Adjusted means of deviance scores (D/T) were obtained by an analysis of covariance in which the effect of the covariates has been taken into account. Covariates were: (1) mothers' own severity of disorder (1-7 rating scale); (2) mothers' age; (3) mothers' years of education; (4) mothers' total Rorschach word count. Analysis of covariance after adjusting with covariates: F (4/105) = 15.74.

correlation of word count and deviance scores, they suggested that number of deviances was primarily a reflection of word count. We have noted above that excessive verbosity can be regarded as a variety of communication deviance associated with overinclusive thinking.

In order to evaluate the question raised by Hirsch and Leff, we have examined the relationship between D/T scores and word count in both the present sample of subjects and in the sample of 59 pairs of parents previously studied (56). Using exactly the same statistical technique as that proposed by Hirsch and Leff, we have found that when the effect of word count is taken out, the difference in D/T scores between parental groups actually heightens, not diminishes as Hirsch and Leff expected. In Table 4, word count is shown to be a non-discriminating variable. Especially noteworthy is the contrast between the low discrimination with parental word count and the very high discrimination with parental D/T scores.

Analyses of co-variance

The statistical technique of analysis of co-variance is an especially powerful means of ascertaining whether a predictor variable, here the communication deviance scores, continues to discriminate when the effects of other variables are taken out.

Tables 5, 6, and 7 show that the parental deviance scores, for the parents as a pair and for the fathers and mothers separately, all continue to discriminate severity of disorder in index offspring even when the effects of major demographic variables and the parents' *own* severity of disorder, as well as their Rorschach word count, are taken into account. As we have hypothesized, the discriminations are most striking for the parents as pairs, but are very highly significant for fathers and mothers as well ($p < 0.001$).

In Tables 8 and 9, similar analyses are presented for the index offspring and their siblings. The parental differences in D/T scores are sustained, suggesting that family-wide phenomena are involved. All of the offspring have somewhat lower scores than their parents. This is striking because the mean

TABLE 8 Communication deviance scores of index offspring

Severity of index disorder	Index offspring N	Unadjusted mean deviance score	Adjusted mean deviance score and standard error
1-2	20	0.34	0.21 ± 0.17
3	25	0.64	0.67 ± 0.15
4	25	1.11	1.04 ± 0.15
5	24	1.52	1.51 ± 0.16
6-7	20	1.67	1.88 ± 0.18

As in Tables 4-6, an analysis of covariance was used to obtain the adjusted mean deviance scores for each diagnostic group. Covariates were: (1) sex of index offspring; (2) age; (3) years of education; (4) total Rorschach word count. Analysis of covariance after adjusting with covariates: $F (4/105) = 13.30$.

TABLE 9 Communication deviance scores of sibs of index offspring

Severity of disorders of index offspring	N of sibs	Unadjusted mean deviance score	Adjusted mean deviance score and standard error
1-2	20	0.29	0.32 ± 0.11
3	26	0.52	0.54 ± 0.10
4	27	0.62	0.73 ± 0.10
5	35	1.26	1.07 ± 0.09
6-7	33	1.25	1.32 ± 0.09

As in Tables 4-7, an analysis of covariance was used to obtain the adjusted mean deviance scores for sibs classified by the severity of disorder in the index offspring in the family. Covariates were: (1) sex of sib; (2) age of sib; (3) years of education of sib; (4) total Rorschach word count by the sib. Analysis of covariance after adjusting with covariates: $F (4/132) = 15.22$.

parental severity of disorder was lower than for the index offspring. While the mean severity of disorder for the 114 index offspring was 4.1, SD 1.72 (that is, about at the severity of the borderline syndrome), the mean severity of disorder for fathers was only about 2.6, SD 1.0 and for mothers, 2.7, SD 1.0 (that is, slightly less disturbed than neurotic).

Tables 5-9 show that the trends of the D/T scores are the same for all family members, including both the index offspring and their siblings. Once again, for the index offspring and sibs, taking out the effect of word count with the analysis of co-variance technique does *not* eliminate the distinctive, discriminating value of the deviance scores.

Concluding comments

We have proposed that research on schizophrenia be redirected to focus on variables intermediate between predisposing variables—such as genetic endowment—and eventual symptomatic schizophrenic breakdown. Two classes of intermediate variables, grouped under the headings of 'response dispositions' and 'transactional processes and communication', seem especially promising. In this paper, we have briefly reviewed our reasoning in selecting these variables for investigation. In more detail, we have described a specific method for studying family communication and reported some recent findings with this method. These results indicate that the method is useful in systematic research which links non-symptomatic parental behaviour with the severity of psychiatric illness in a late adolescent or young adult offspring.

We do not wish to imply that we are studying the only, or the best, intermediate variables which can or should be introduced into research with the families of schizophrenics. However, we have particularly emphasized intrafamilial communication and relationship patterns as a conceptually meaningful and researchable group of variables. Transactional processes build upon, and interact with, the genetically influenced response potentialities of the individual. Additionally, however, variables of the family and social organization, not predictable directly from individual characteristics, come into play as *patterns* of family communication and relatedness unfold over time.

The central hypothesis of this study has been strongly confirmed. We have shown that the frequency of communication deviances as scored in individual Rorschach records of parents and their offspring is significantly greater in families with an adolescent or young adult schizophrenic offspring; this relationship varies directly with severity of disorder in the offspring. We have also shown that severity of parental clinical disorder discriminates severity of disorder in the offspring, but these two measures—frequency of communication deviances and severity of psychiatric disorder—are not the same; each measure is strongly discriminatory in its own right.

Further, although the index offspring, as primary patients, are clinically more disturbed than their parents, we have shown that the parents have more frequent communication deviances of the kinds specified here than the patients themselves. However, both the index offspring and their siblings have communication deviance scores which are directly related to the severity of clinical disorder in the index offspring.

Finally, demographic variables and such secondary phenomena as word count do not account for the fact that frequency of communication deviances of any family member does discriminate severity of psychiatric disorder in the index offspring.

These various findings, part of a larger research programme, support the view that transactional processes need to be examined as intermediate variables in the development of schizophrenic disorders.

References

(1) Bateson, G., Jackson, D.D., Haley, J. and Weakland, J.H. (1956) Toward a theory of schizophrenia. *Behavl. Sci., 1,* 251-64.

(2) Lidz, T., Cornelison, A., Fleck, S. and Terry, D. (1957) The intrafamilial environment of the schizophrenic patient: II. Marital schism and marital skew. *Am. J. Psychiat., 114,* 241-8.

(3) Wynne, L.C., Ryckoff, I., Day, J. and Hirsch, S. (1958) Pseudo-mutuality in the family relations of schizophrenics. *Psychiatry, 21,* 205-20.

(4) Planansky, K. (1966) Conceptual boundaries of schizoidness: suggestions for epidemiological and genetic research. *J. nerv. ment. Dis., 142,* 318-31.

(5) Heston, L.L. (1970) The genetics of schizophrenia and schizoid disease. *Science, 167,* 249-56.

(6) Kety, S., Rosenthal, D., Wender, P. and Schulsinger, F. (1968) The types and prevalence of mental illness in the biological and adoptive families of adopted schizophrenics. *J. psychiat. Res., 6,* Suppl. 1., 345-62.

(7) Kringlen, E. (1967) *Heredity and Environment in the Functional Psychoses. An epidemiological-clinical twin study.* Oslo and London, Oslo University Press.

(8) Kallman, F.J. (1946) The genetic theory of schizophrenia: an analysis of 691 schizophrenic twin index families. *Am. J. Psychiat., 103,* 309-22.

(9) Heston, L.L. (1966) Psychiatric disorders in foster home reared children of schizophrenic mothers. *Br. J. Psychiat., 112,* 819-25.

(10) Gottesman, I. and Shields, J. (1967) A polygenic theory of schizophrenia. *Proc. natn. Acad. Sci. U.S.A., 58,* 199-205.

(11) Rosenthal, D. (1970) *Genetic Theory and Abnormal Behaviour*. New York, McGraw-Hill.
(12) WHO (1973) *Report of the International Pilot Study of Schizophrenia. Vol. 1.* Geneva, World Health Organization.
(13) Strauss, J.S. (1973) Diagnostic models and the nature of psychiatric disorder. *Archs gen. Psychiat., 29,* 445-9.
(14) Wynne, L.C. (1961) In *Exploring the base for family therapy*, pp. 95-115, Eds. Ackerman, Beatman and Sherman. New York, Family Service Assn. of America.
(15) Alanen, Y.O. (1966) The family in the pathogenesis of schizophrenic and neurotic disorders. *Acta psychiat. Scand., 42,* Suppl. 189.
(16) Reiss, D. (1971) Varieties of consensual experience: contrasts between families of normals, delinquents and schizophrenics. *J. nerv. ment. Dis., 152,* 73-95.
(17) MacMahon, B. (1968) Gene-environment interaction in human disease. *J. psychiat. Res., 6,* Suppl. 1, 393-402.
(18) Singer, M.T. and Wynne, L.C. (1963) Differentiating characteristics of parents of childhood schizophrenics, childhood neurotics and young adult schizophrenics. *Am. J. Psychiat., 120,* 234-43.
(19) Singer, M.T. and Wynne, L.C. (1965) Thought disorder and family relations of schizophrenics: III. Methodology using projective techniques. *Archs gen. Psychiat., 12,* 187-200.
(20) Singer, M.T. and Wynne, L.C. (1965) Thought disorder and family relations of schizophrenics. IV. Results and implications. *Archs gen. Psychiat., 12,* 201-12.
(21) Singer, M.T. and Wynne, L.C. (1966) Principles for scoring communication defects and deviances in parents of schizophrenics: Rorschach and TAT scoring manuals. *Psychiatry, 29,* 260-8.
(22) Wynne, L.C. (1967) Family transactions and schizophrenia: II. Conceptual considerations for a research strategy. In *The Origins of Schizophrenia.* Ed. J. Romano. International Congress Series 151, pp. 165-78. Amsterdam, Excerpta Medica.
(23) Wynne, L.C. (1968) Methodologic and conceptual issues in the study of schizophrenics and their families. *J. psychiat. Res., 6,* Suppl. 1, 185-99.
(24) Stabenau, J. and Pollin, W. (1967) Early characteristics of monozygotic twins discordant for schizophrenia. *Archs gen. Psychiat., 17,* 723-34.
(25) Gardner, R.W., Holzman, P.S., Klein, G.S., Linton, H. and Spence, D.P. (1959) Cognitive control: A study of individual consistencies in cognitive behaviour. *Psychological Issues, Monogr. 4,* New York, International Universities Press.
(26) Silverman, J. (1964) The problem of attention in research and theory in schizophrenia. *Psychol. Rev., 71,* 352-79.
(27) Silverman, J. (1967) Variations in cognitive control and psychophysiologic defense in the schizophrenias. *Psychosom. Med., 29,* 225-51.
(28) Silverman, J. (1968) A paradigm for the study of altered states of consciousness. *Br. J. Psychiat., 114,* 1201-18.
(29) Venables, P. (1964) Input dysfunction in schizophrenia. In *Progress in Experimental Personality Research,* Ed. B. Maher, pp. 1-47. New York, Academic Press.
(30) Witkin, H.A., Dyk, R.B., Faterson, H.F., Goodenough, D.R. and Karp, S.A. (1962) *Psychological Differentiation: Studies of Development.* New York, Wiley.
(31) Buchsbaum, M. and Wynne, L. (1974) Unpublished data.
(32) Scarr, S. (1969) Social introversion-extraversion as a heritable response. *Child Dev., 40,* 823-32.
(33) Mednick, S.A. (1970) Breakdown in individuals at high risk for schizophrenia: possible predispositional perinatal factors. *Ment. Hyg., 54,* 50-63.
(34) Sameroff, A. and Zax, M. (1973) Schizotaxia revisited. *Am. J. Orthopsychiat., 43,* 743-54.
(35) Wynne, L.C. (1969) The family as a strategic focus in cross-cultural psychiatric studies. In *Mental Health Research in Asia and the Pacific,* Eds. W. Caudill and T. Lin, pp. 463-77. Honolulu, East-West Center Press.
(36) Spiegel, J. (1971) *Transactions. The Interplay Between Individual, Family, and Society.* New York, Science House.
(37) Sullivan, H.S. (1931) Environmental factors in etiology and course under treatment of schizophrenia. *Medical Journal and Record, 133,* 19-22.
(38) Mishler, E.G. and Waxler, N.E. (1968) *Interaction in Families.* New York, Wiley.
(39) Laing, R.D. (1967) *The Politics of Experience.* New York, Pantheon.

(40) Wynne, L.C. and Singer, M.T. (1963) Thought disorder and family relations of schizophrenics: I. A research strategy. *Archs gen. Psychiat., 9*, 191-8.
(41) Lidz, T., Fleck, S., and Cornelison, A. (1965) *Schizophrenia and the Family*. New York, International Universities Press.
(42) Ryckoff, I., Day, J. and Wynne, L.C. (1959) Maintenance of stereotyped roles in the families of schizophrenics. *A.M.A. Archives of Psychiatry, 1*, 93-8.
(43) Ferreira, A.J. (1966) Family Myths. In *Family Structure, Dynamics, and Therapy*, pp. 85-90, Ed. I. Cohen. Washington, D.C.: American Psychiatric Association.
(44) Stierlin, H. (1973) Group fantasies and family myths—some theoretical and practical aspects. *Family Process, 12*, 111-25.
(45) Bell, N.W. and Vogel, E.F. (1962) *A Modern Introduction to the Family*. Glencoe, The Free Press.
(46) Bott, E. (1957) *Family and Social Network*. London, Tavistock.
(47) Kohn, M. (1969) *Class and Conformity: A Study in values*. Homewood, Illinois, Dorsey Press.
(48) Wynne, L.C. and Singer, M.T. (1966) Schizophrenic impairment in sharing foci of attention: A conceptual basis for viewing schizophrenics and their families in research and therapy. Presented as the Bertram H. Roberts' Memorial Lecture, Yale University, New Haven, Connecticut.
(49) Schachtel, E.G. (1954) The development of focal attention and the emergence of reality. *Psychiatry, 17*, 309-24.
(50) Shakow, D. (1962) Segmental set. *Archs gen. Psychiat., 6*, 1-17.
(51) Stierlin, H. (1969) *Conflict and Reconciliation: A Study in Human Relations and Schizophrenia*. New York, Doubleday.
(52) Sullivan, H.S. (1956) *Clinical Studies in Psychiatry*. New York, Norton.
(53) Fleming, P. and Ricks, D.F. (1970) Emotions of children before schizophrenia and before character disorder. In *Life History Research in Psychopathology*, pp. 240-64, Eds. M. Roff and D.F. Ricks, Minneapolis, University of Minnesota Press.
(54) Wynne, L.C. (1969) Family research on the pathogenesis of schizophrenia: Intermediate variables in the study of families at high risk. In *Problématique de la Psychose, Vol. 2*, Eds. Doucet and Laurin. Amsterdam, Excerpta Medica.
(55) Garmezy, N. and Streitman, S. (1974) Children at risk: the search for the antecedents of schizophrenia. Part I. Conceptual models and research methods. *Schizophrenia Bulletin, 8*, 14-90.
(56) Singer, M.T. (1967) Family transactions and schizophrenia: I. Recent research findings. In *The Origins of Schizophrenia*, Ed. J. Romano, International Congress Series No. 151, pp. 165-78. Amsterdam, Excerpta Medica.
(57) Wild, C., Singer, M.T., Rosman, B., Ricci, J. and Lidz, T. (1965) Measuring disordered styles of thinking. *Archs gen. Psychiat., 13*, 471-6.
(58) Singer, M.T., Wynne, L.C., Levi, L.D. and Sojit, C. (1968) Proverbs interpretation reconsidered: A transactional approach to schizophrenics and their families. Presented at Symposium on Language and Thought in Schizophrenia, Newport Beach, California (to be published).
(59) Loveland, N.T., Wynne, L.C. and Singer, M.T. (1963) The family Rorschach: a new method for studying family interaction. *Family Process, 2*, 187-215.
(60) Morris, G.O. and Wynne, L.C. (1965) Schizophrenic offspring and parental style of communication. *Psychiatry, 28*, 19-44.
(61) Reiss, D. (1967) Individual thinking and family interaction. I. Introduction to an experimental study of problem solving in families of normals, character disorders, and schizophrenics. *Archs gen. Psychiat., 16*, 80-93.
(62) Reiss, D. (1967) Individual thinking and family interaction. II. A study of pattern recognition and hypothesis testing in families of normals, character disorders, and schizophrenics. *J. psychiat. Res., 5*, 193-211.
(63) Waxler, N. and Mishler, E.G. (1970) Experimental studies of families. In *Advances in Experimental Social Psychology*, Ed. L. Berkowitz. New York, Academic Press.
(64) Hirsch, S.R. and Leff, J.P. (1971) Parental abnormalities of verbal communication in the transmission of schizophrenia. *Psychol. Med., 1*, 118-27.
(65) Wynne, L.C. and Singer, M.T. (1963) Thought disorder and family relations of schizophrenics: II. A classification of forms of thinking. *Archs gen. Psychiat., 9*, 199-206.

(66) Payne, R.W., Caird, W.K. and Laverty, S.G. (1964) Overinclusive thinking and delusions in schizophrenic patients. *J. abnorm. soc. Psychol., 68*, 562-6.

(67) Singer, M.T. (1968) The consensus Rorschach and family transaction. *Journal of Projective Techniques and Personality Assessment, 32*, 348-51.

(68) Fisher, S., Boyd, I., Walker, D. and Sheer, D. (1959) Parents of schizophrenics, neurotics, and normals. *Archs gen. Psychiat., 1*, 149-66.

(69) Lin, T. (1969) Reducing variability in international research. In *Social Psychiatry,* research publication, Association for Research in Nervous and Mental Disorders.

(70) Grinker, R., Werble, B. and Drye, R.C. (1968) *The Borderline Syndrome.* New York, Basic Books.

(71) Vaillant, G.E. (1964) An historical review of the remitting schizophrenias. *J. nerv. ment. Dis., 138*, 48-56.

(72) Vaillant, G.E. (1964) Prospective prediction of schizophrenic remission. *Archs gen. Psychiat., 11*, 509-18.

(73) Phillips, L. (1953) Case history data and prognosis in schizophrenia. *J. nerv. ment. Dis., 117*, 515-25.

(74) Hollingshead, A.B. and Redlich, F.C. (1958) *Social Class and Mental Illness.* New York, Wiley.

(75) Gottesman, I. (1968) Severity/concordance and diagnostic refinement in the Maudsley-Bethlem schizophrenic twin study. *J. psychiat. Res., 6*, Suppl. 1, 37-48.

Index